The Wolfe Pocket Medical Dictionary
Fourth Edition

GW00689744

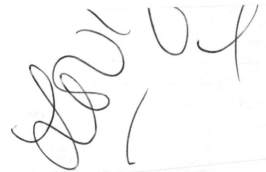

The Wolfe Pocket Medical Dictionary

Fourth Edition

formerly titled

The Faber Pocket Medical Dictionary

Revised by

Elizabeth Forsythe MRCS, LRCP, DPH

with David Bromham PhD, MRCOG

Wolfe Publishing Ltd

Published by
Wolfe Publishing, an imprint of
Times Mirror International Publishers Limited
Lynton House
7–12 Tavistock Square
London WC1H 9LB

Reprinted 1994 by Cox & Wyman Ltd, Reading, Berkshire

First published in 1966 by Faber and Faber Limited. Second
edition 1974, revised reprint 1977. Third edition 1979, reprinted
1985. Fourth edition 1989, reprinted 1990 (twice).

ISBN 0 7234 1836 5

For full details of all Wolfe titles please write to Times Mirror
International Publishers Limited, Lynton House, 7–12 Tavistock
Square, London WC1H 9LB, England.

A CIP Catalogue record for this book is available from the British Library.

Contents

Preface to the Fourth Edition

This dictionary is intended for paramedical workers, medical receptionists and secretaries, medical auxiliaries and the interested lay public. It is designed to provide a ready-to-hand, accurate, up-to-date and simple guide to medical terminology.

The first aim in this edition has been to revise the entries thoroughly and increase them to include many new words in current medical usage. The second aim has been to keep this dictionary a 'pocket' one both in size and price. To this end the number of appendices has been reduced.

My thanks are due to all those who have been so generous of their time and expertise in helping me and particularly to David Bromham, the assistant editor, to Philip Wood and to Roger Osborne, medical editor of Faber and Faber.

E.F.
1988

Dictionary of Medical Terms

A

AA   *Abbr.* Alcoholics Anonymous

a- or **an-**   Prefix indicating 'absence of' as in amenorrhoea, absence of menstruation, anoxia, absence of oxygen.

ab   Prefix meaning from, away from, *e.g.* abnormal, contrary to the normal type (Latin).

abdomen   The belly. The body cavity immediately below the thorax, bounded above by the diaphragm, below by the pelvis, behind by the lumbar vertebrae, and in front and at the sides by muscular walls. It contains many important organs, including the stomach, intestines, liver, kidneys, spleen, pancreas, bladder, uterus and ovaries. It is lined with a serous membrane called the peritoneum, which is reflected on to many of the organs in the abdomen.

abdominal   Pertaining to the abdomen.

abdominoperineal   Describes an operation with approach from both abdominal and perineal incisions.

abducent nerves   The sixth pair of cranial nerves, activating the external rectus muscle of the eyeball, which rotates the eyeball outwards.

abduct   To draw away from the midline.

abduction   The act of moving a limb away from the midline of the body.

abductor   A muscle which draws a limb from the median line of the body, *e.g.* deltoid.

aberration   Deviation from the normal. In optics, defect in focus of a lens. *Mental a.*: mental disturbance or peculiarity.

ablatio retinae   Detachment of the retina.

ablation   Removal or detachment of a part.

abort   To terminate a process before the full course is run.

abortifacient   A drug taken for the purpose of procuring abortion.

abortion   Discharge of the gestation sac from the pregnant uterus before the 28th week of pregnancy. Abortion may be *spontaneous* or *induced* and either may be complete or incomplete; spontaneous may be threatened (vaginal bleeding up to 28 weeks), or inevitable (products of conception passing through the vaginal canal). In *missed a.* the fetus is dead but not discharged immediately. In *habitual a.*, it recurs in successive pregnancies.

Also *therapeutic* or *legal a.*: termination of pregnancy when there are medical or social grounds to justify it; and *criminal* and *septic a.*

abortus The aborted fetus. *A. fever*: *see* BRUCELLOSIS.

abrasion A superficial injury to the skin or mucous membrane.

abreaction A state of mind brought about during the process of psychoanalysis. The patient lives again through past painful experiences which may unconsciously be causing the neurosis. *See also* NARCOANALYSIS.

abscess A collection of pus in a cavity, the result of infection. *Alveolar a.*: develops at the root of a tooth. *Pelvic a.*: arises in the pelvic peritoneum. *Stitch a.*: is formed around a stitch or suture.

abruption, abruptio placentae *See* ACCIDENTAL HAEMORRHAGE.

absolute values Actual figures, not the percentage figures, *e.g.* in blood counts,

the actual numbers of cells counted.

acantholysis Process of individual cell keratinization occurring in blistering diseases. *A. cell*: one that has undergone individual cell keratinization.

acanthosis Thickening of the epidermis. *A. nigricans*: pigmented warty outgrowths of epidermis.

acapnia *See* HYPOCAPNIA.

acardia Congenital absence of the heart.

Acarus The name of a group of animal parasites. *A. scabiei* is the parasite causing scabies.

acatalasia Genetic abnormality in which the enzyme catalase is absent from the red blood cells.

acataphasia Difficulty in expressing ideas in logical sequence.

accessory nerves The eleventh pair of cranial nerves. Developmentally a branch of the vagus.

accidental haemorrhage *Syn.* placental abruption: abruptio placentae. Bleeding from the pregnant uterus in the later months of pregnancy due to premature separation of normally situated placenta. It may be *concealed a.h.*, when the bleeding remains internal; or *revealed a.h.*, when the blood escapes by the vagina. *See* ANTEPARTUM HAEMORRHAGE.

accommodation The process of altering the focus of the eye by changing the curvature of the lens. When focusing on near objects, the lens becomes more convex by contraction of the ciliary muscles.

accouchement Childbirth.

accretion Accumulation of foreign matter.

acephalic Headless.

acetabulum The cuplike socket in the hip or innominate bone into which the head of the femur fits.

acetic acid The acid contained in vinegar.

acetoacetic acid *Syn.* diacetic acid. Produced at an intermediate stage of fatty acid oxidation. If metabolism is disturbed, as in diabetes mellitus, it is found in excess in the blood and the urine.

acetonaemia The presence of acetone in the blood.

acetone A colourless volatile solvent. This substance is formed in the body when metabolism is upset, as in starvation, excessive vomiting, diabetes mellitus. It is excreted in the urine and the breath.

acetonuria The presence of acetone in the urine.

acetylcholine A neurotransmitter causing parasympathetic effects, *e.g.* cardiac slowing, dilatation of surface blood vessels and contractions of the gut.

achalasia Failure to relax. Usually *a. of the cardia* when there is a disorder of motor function of the oesophagus and a failure of the cardiac orifice of the stomach to relax.

Achilles tendon The large tendon which attaches the calf muscles to the heel.

achlorhydria Absence of hydrochloric acid in the gastric juice; may occur in pernicious anaemia and cancer of the stomach.

acholia Absence of bile.

acholuria The absence of bile pigment from the urine.

acholuric jaundice *See* JAUNDICE.

achondroplasia A form of arrested development of the long bones, leading to dwarfism.

achromasia Absence of colour. Extreme pallor associated with severe illness.

achromatopsia Colour blindness.

achylia Absence of chyle. Usually *gastric a.* when an abnormally small amount of gastric juice is secreted.

acid A substance capable of combining with alkalis to form salts. Acids turn blue litmus paper red and when in liquid form have a sour taste *e.g.* vinegar and lemon juice both contain acids. (For individual acids *see under* special name.) *A. phosphate*

3

Phosphatases are enzymes which are able to split off phosphate groups from certain substances. The prefix 'acid' indicates that the enzyme is optimally active in acid solution; *cf.* alkaline phosphatase. *A. phosphatase* is present in lysosomes in all cells. The prostate gland is the source of most of the *a. phosphatase* in the serum.

acidaemia Abnormally acid blood, *i.e.* pH is below 7.3. Normal blood pH is 7.3–7.5.

acid–alcohol fast In bacteriology a term applied to bacteria which retain stain after application of acid and alcohol.

acid–base balance Balance between acidic and basic components which determines the pH of the body fluids.

acid-fast In bacteriology a term applied to certain bacteria which retain the red carbofuchsin stain after the application of an acid solution.

acidity The proportion of acid in a given substance. Thus gastric juice contains normally 0.2 per cent of hydrochloric acid.

acidosis A condition which tends to lower the pH of body fluids. Acidosis is generally classified as respiratory or metabolic.

aciduria An acid urine.

acinus (pl. acini) A minute grapelike structure whose cells secrete, as in the breast. *See also* ALVEOLUS.

acne Condition, occurring particularly in adolescents, on the face, neck, back and chest, resulting from a combination of hormonally induced hyperactivity of the sebaceous glands and bacterial infection and characterized by blackheads and pustules. *See* COMEDONES.

acneiform Acne-like.

acoustic Relating to sound or hearing.

acquired Contracted after birth, not congenital.

acquired immune deficiency syndrome *See* AIDS.

acrid Sharp, burning.

acriflavine Antiseptic yellow dye.

acrocephaly Congenitally malformed, cone-shaped head.

acrocyanosis Cyanosis of the extremities.

acrodynia Painful and red extremities.

acromegaly A disease marked by enlargement of the face, hands and feet, due to a pathological condition of the pituitary gland (giantism).

acromicria Abnormally small hands, face and feet.

acromion The outward extremity of the spine of the scapula. *See* SCAPULA.

acronyx An ingrowing nail.

acroparaesthesia Numbness and tingling sensation of the extremities.

acrophobia Fear of heights.

acrosclerosis Scleroderma affecting the hands.

acrosome Part of the head of sperm cells; involved in penetration of the ovum (*a. reaction*).

ACTH *Abbr.* adrenocorticotrophic hormone produced by the anterior lobe of the pituitary. It stimulates the release of steroid hormones from the adrenal cortex.

acting out Disturbed behaviour resulting from unresolved emotional conflicts.

actinic dermatoses Conditions caused by hypersensitivity of the skin to ultraviolet light.

actinism Chemical changes produced by radiant energy, *e.g.* light rays.

Actinomyces Group of filamentous bacteria.

actinomycosis Disease due to *Actinomyces* usually presenting as chronic discharging abscesses which may be localized, classically on the neck, or widespread in the body.

actinotherapy Treatment with infrared or ultraviolet radiation.

action potential Term applied to electrical changes which occur when a nerve conducts an impulse or when a muscle fibre contracts.

activator A physical or chemical agent which initiates some reaction in which the activator itself does not take part.

active assisted movements Active movements aided by the physiotherapist or by mechanical devices.

active movements Term used by physiotherapists to denote a movement done by the patient.

active principle The substance in a drug which gives it a therapeutic effect.

actomyosin Muscle protein complex composed of actin and myosin. The myosin component acts as an enzyme releasing energy by the breakdown to ATP. *See* ADENOSINE TRIPHOSPHATE.

acuity Sharpness and clearness.

acupuncture Skin puncture with fine metal needles. Used mainly by the Chinese for producing anaesthesia.

acute Of rapid onset; severe. *A. abdomen*: general term embracing surgical emergencies resulting from disease or damage of abdominal viscera, *e.g. a. appendicitis*.

acyanotic Without cyanosis, particularly in congenital heart conditions.

acystia Congenital absence of the bladder.

adactylia Absence of fingers or toes.

Adam's apple Laryngeal prominence due to thyroid cartilage.

Adams–Stokes syndrome *See* STOKES–ADAMS.

adaptation Adjustment by structural or functional change to new circumstances. (2) The process whereby the eye adjusts to sudden changes from light to dark and vice versa.

addiction State of physical and mental dependence on drugs including alcohol and tobacco, etc.

Addison's or Addisonian anaemia *See* PERNICIOUS ANAEMIA.

Addison's disease Syndrome, due to adreno-cortical insufficiency, characterized by wasting, hypotension, vomiting, malaise, weakness and hyperpigmentation of the skin and buccal mucosa.

adduct To draw towards the midline.

adductor A muscle which draws towards the midline of the body, *e.g. a. muscles of* the thigh draw the legs together.

adendritic Without dendrites.

adenectomy Excision of a gland.

adenine An amino purine base; one of two in both RNA and DNA.

adenitis Inflammation of a gland.

adenocarcinoma Malignant growth of glandular cells.

adenoid Lymphoid tissue, in the nasopharynx, which when swollen hinders breathing.

adenoidectomy Operation to remove adenoids.

adenoma Benign tumour of glandular cells.

adenomyoma Benign tumour composed of glandular and muscular elements.

adenomyosis Presence of endometrioiosis in the myometrium. *Syn.* internal endometriosis.

adenopathy A disease of a gland, especially a lymphatic gland.

adenosine An important member of the group of substances known as nucleosides, the phosphorylated derivatives of which are the key to energy reactions in the body. *A. diphosphate* (*ADP*): resulting from the removal of phosphate from ATP and is re-formed into ADP by respiratory metabolism, thus making the energy available for work in the cell. *A. monophosphate* (*AMP*): metabolically related to other adenosine phosphates. In its cyclic form (cAMP) exerts an important controlling influence on cellular physiology. *A. triphosphate* (*ATP*): a coenzyme of a large number of reactions. One of the phosphate groups is readily released by enzyme action resulting in the simultaneous liberation of utilizable energy.

adenotonsillectomy Operation to remove the tonsils and adenoids.

adenovirus A group of viruses affecting particularly the adenoids, pharynx and conjunctivae; usually associated with minor respiratory infections.

ADH *See* ANTIDIURETIC HORMONE.

adherent Fixed firmly to.

adhesion A sticking together of two surfaces or parts. Bands of fibrous tissue, usually the result of inflammation.

adiaphoresis Deficiency of perspiration.

Adie's syndrome Association of myotonic pupil with absent or diminished tendon reflexes.

adipose Fatty.

aditus An entrance, a portal. *A. ad antrum*: the narrow passage between the mastoid antrum and the tympanic cavity of the ear.

adjustment The change made by a person to adapt to circumstances.

adjuvant A secondary ingredient in a preparation aiding the action of the principal drug.

adnexa Appendages. Usually applied to the uterine appendages.

adolescence The period of

development during which full anatomical, physiological and emotional maturity is attained.

adoption To take voluntarily legal responsibility for a child who is not the natural offspring of the adopter.

ADP *See* ADENOSINE DIPHOSPHATE.

adrenal Pertaining to or produced by the adrenal glands. *A. cortex*: outer part of the adrenal gland which synthesizes and secretes the steroid hormones. Those of major importance are glucocorticoids, *e.g.* hydrocortisone, which tend to produce the conversion of tissue protein to glucose; mineralocorticoids, especially aldosterone, regulating sodium and potassium excretion and androgens. *A. glands*: a pair of endocrine glands, also called suprarenal glands, situated adjacent to the upper pole of each kidney. They consist of two regions, the cortex and the medulla. *A. insufficiency*: usually adrenocortical insufficiency. *See* ADDISON'S DISEASE. *A. medulla*: central part of adrenal gland which synthesizes and secretes adrenaline and noradrenaline. *A. nerves*: cholinergic, preganglionic sympathetic nerve fibres supplying the adrenal medulla. Stimulation causes the release of adrenaline into the circulation.

adrenalectomy The removal of one or both adrenal glands.

adrenaline Epinephrine. Hormone secreted by the adrenal medulla. Similar substance secreted at nerve endings of sympathetic nerves. Effects produced include increased heart rate, blood pressure and blood sugar, contraction of skin blood vessels, increase in muscle blood flow, dilatation of pupil, etc.

adrenergic Term applied to identify motor nerves by their transmitter substance, thus cholinergic, when the impulse is transmitted by acetycholine and adrenergic when the impulse is transmitted by adrenaline, noradrenaline or a drug with comparable action.

adrenocortical steroids *See* ADRENAL CORTEX.

adrenocorticotrophic hormone *See* ACTH.

adrenogenital syndrome Virilization occurring in women due to excessive secretion of androgens, usually as a result of hyperplasia or adenoma of the adrenal cortex. Rarely the syndrome is due to arrhenoblastoma or pituitary disorder.

adrenolytic Substance antagonizing the action of adrenaline.

adsorption The property possessed by certain porous substances, *e.g.* charcoal, of taking up other substances.

adulteration Addition to any substance of a component not normally present, making original substance, which may be a food or drug, of less value.

advancement Operation to move a tendinous insertion forwards. Can be used in curing a squint.

adventitia The connective tissue coat of any organ including a blood vessel.

Aëdes aegypti Species of mosquito transmitting yellow fever, etc.

AEG *Abbr.* air encephalogram or air encephalography.

aeration Charging with air or gas.

aerobes Term applied to bacteria requiring oxygen for respiration; *cf.* anaerobe.

aerobic respiration Respiration in the presence of free oxygen.

aerocele A diverticulum of larynx, trachea or bronchus.

aerodontalgia Toothache induced by reduction of atmospheric pressure.

aerogen Any gas producing bacterium, *e.g.* Clostridium welchii, the cause of gas gangrene.

aerophagy Excessive air swallowing.

aerosol Finely atomized solution ejected under pressure.

aesthesia Feeling.

aetiology The study of the causation of disease.

afebrile Without fever.

affect Term used in psychology for an emotion associated with ideas.

affective disorders Group of psychiatric illnesses primarily due to reaction to internal or external stress. They include anxiety states, depression, mania and hypomania.

afferent Leading to the centre, applied to the lymphatic vessels and to sensory nerves. *A. loop syndrome*: occasional complication of one type of partial gastrectomy.

affiliation The fixing of paternity of an illegitimate child on the putative father.

affinity Attraction. In chemistry the property of an element which prefers to combine with some other particular element.

afibrinogenaemia *Syn.* hypofibrinogenaemia: consumption coagulopathy. Clotting disorder of blood following absorption of clotting factors elsewhere. Triggered by thromboplastin release, *e.g.* from damaged myometrium after accidental haemorrhage or lung after amniotic fluid embolus.

aflatoxins Toxins present in spores of Aspergillus flavus, a contaminant of groundnut meal.

AFP *Abbr.* alphafetoprotein.

African tick fever Disease caused by a spirochaete, Spirochaeta duttoni, transmitted by ticks. Occasionally also applied to typhus transmitted by these insects.

afterbirth The placenta, cord and membranes as expelled after delivery of the infant.

aftercare Care of the convalescent, including rehabilitation.

after-image A retinal impression persisting although the stimulus of light has ceased.

afterpains Pains from uterine contractions following labour.

agammaglobulinaemia Absence or deficiency of gammaglobulin in plasma proteins, leading to inadequate response to infection. May be congenital or acquired.

agar-agar Polysaccharide obtained from seaweed, used in the culture of microorganisms.

agenesis Failure of an organ to develop embryologically.

agglutination The sticking together of cells, *e.g.* red blood cells, bacteria, due to an alteration of surface charge. Usually brought about by the effect of antibodies.

agglutinins Antibodies such as those found in the blood serum of persons suffering from typhoid or paratyphoid fever. They have the property of causing bacteria to clump together or 'agglutinate'. *See* WIDAL REACTION.

agglutinogen Factor promoting the mutual adhesion of cells.

aggregate To group together.

aggressin Substance believed to contribute to the virulence of pathogenic bacteria.

aggression A hostile attitude which may be a normal reaction to danger or a compensatory reaction to cover feelings of inferiority or frustration.

aglutition Inability to swallow.

agnathia Absence or underdevelopment of the jaw.

agnosia A disturbance in the recognition of sensory impression.

agonist In pharmacology, substance with positive action on system.

agoraphobia Literally a fear of the marketplace. In practice may mean a fear of open places.

agranulocytosis Absence or marked reduction in the blood of the polymorphonuclear cells. May be caused by drugs such as the sulphonamides or irradiation of the bone marrow.

agraphia Loss of the power to express words and ideas in writing.

ague *See* MALARIA.

AHG *Abbr.* antihaemophilic globulin. The blood-coagulating protein factor which is deficient in haemophiliacs. *See* BLOOD COAGULATION.

AID *Abbr.* artificial insemination by a donor.

AIDS *Abbr.* acquired immune deficiency syndrome. One of a spectrum of diseases due to infection of the T-lymphocytes of the immune system by the retrovirus HIV which is present in semen, blood and other body fluids. The clinical picture results from the activity of the virus itself and loss of the host's immunity resulting in opportunistic infections and certain tumours including Kaposi's sarcoma. *See also* ARC, HIV.

AIH *Abbr.* artificial insemination by a woman's legal husband.

air *See* ATMOSPHERE. *A. bed.* A mattress made of some distensible material such as rubber or plastic and filled with air. *Tidal a.*: the air breathed in and out in ordinary breathing. *A. embolism*: embolism caused by air entering the circulatory system. *A. encephalography*: radiography of brain after introduction of air into the subarachnoid space. *A. hunger*: respiratory distress caused by lack of oxygen.

akathisia Mental state

characterized by subjective feelings of unrest and outwardly by agitation and over-activity.

akinesis Loss or imperfection of movement.

ala A wing. *A. nasi.* The outer side of the external nostril.

Albers–Schönberg's disease Also known as osteopetrosis or marble-bone disease because of great increase in bone density seen radiographically. There are three types: fetal, juvenile and adult.

albinism Syndrome due to defective pigment production, resulting in deficiency of pigment in the skin, hair and eyes.

albino A person with albinism.

Albright's syndrome Polyostotic fibrous dysplasia of bone. Syndrome characterized by abnormal development of bone, hyperpigmentation of the skin and, in girls, precocious sexual development.

albumin Serum protein with relatively low molecular weight (MW = 70000) which is of great importance in controlling the water exchanges between the blood and the tissue fluids.

albuminuria Albumin in the urine; occurs in diseases of the kidneys.

alcohol Chemically the hydroxides of a great number of organic radicals are known as alcohols: the term usually refers to ethyl alcohol, the alcohol present in intoxicating drinks. *Absolute a.*: may contain up to 1 per cent by weight of water. Rectified spirit is 90 per cent alcohol.

Alcoholics Anonymous (AA) A self-help organization for those addicted to alcohol.

alcoholism Physical and psychological dependence on alcohol usually preceded by a varying period of excessive drinking.

aldolase Enzyme in muscle concerned in conversion of glycogen to lactic acid.

aldosterone One of the adrenocortical hormones which regulates metabolism of electrolytes.

aldosteronism Condition with excessive production of aldosterone causing muscular weakness and raised blood pressure.

Aldrich syndrome Sex-linked recessive condition occurring in male infants with eczema, thrombocytopenia, recurrent infections, usually fatal.

alexia Inability or difficulty in understanding the written or printed word, owing to a lesion of the brain. *See* DYSLEXIA.

algae Seaweeds, etc. A group of Thallophyta containing chlorophyll.

algesia Perception of pain.

algid Describing state of collapse with clammy skin and low blood pressure occurring in the course of severe fever. Often used in connection with malaria.

algogenic Pain-inducing.

alienation Term used in psychiatry meaning withdrawal of affection from a person or object.

alignment Bringing into line.

alimentary Pertaining to the absorption of nourishment. The *a. canal* is the whole digestive tract, extending from the mouth to the anus.

alimentation Nourishment.

aliquot A measured portion.

alkalaemia Abnormally alkaline blood with a pH above 7.5.

alkali A substance which combines with an acid to form a salt, and with a fat to form a soap. Turns red litmus paper to blue. Ammonia, soda and potash are examples of alkalis. *A. reserve*: this term is applied to the measurement of plasma bicarbonate concentration.

alkaline Containing alkali. Strictly, fluid with a pH greater than 7.0. *A. phosphatase*: enzyme(s), capable of splitting off phosphate groups from certain substrates, especially active in alkaline solution; *cf.* acid phosphatase.

alkalinity Proportion of alkali in a given substance.

alkalinuria An alkaline urine.

alkaloid An organic substance having some properties of an alkali, especially that of combining with an acid to form a salt. Morphine and quinine are alkaloids. Salts of these are morphine tartrate, morphine hydrochloride, quinine sulphate, etc.

alkalosis Circumstances tending to raise the pH of body fluids.

alkaptonuria Genetically determined defect of metabolism in which homogentisic acid is excreted in the urine which turns dark on standing.

alkylating agent Substance causing addition of an alkyl group into an organic compound.

all-or-none law Physiological law regarding irritable tissues, *e.g.* nerves, by which there are only two possible reactions to a stimulus, either no reaction or full response. There is no grading of response according to the strength of the stimulus.

allantois Saclike outgrowth from hindgut of embryo.

allele *See* ALLELOMORPH.

allelomorph Pair of genes which occupy the same relative position on homologous chromosomes and produce different effects on the same process in development.

allergen Substance which causes sensitization of tissues. Usually has a protein component.

allergy State of abnormal tissue sensitivity to chemical substance(s). The mechanism of sensitization is complex and involves prior contact of the allergic cells with the allergen. The release of histamine from mast cells plays a part in the reaction.

alloantibody Antibody which reacts with alloantigen.

alloantigen Antigen possessed by certain members of a species.

allocheiria Perception of touch referred to contralateral side of body.

allograft Graft in which both the donor and recipient are of the same species.

allopathy Treatment of disease by medicines that produce phenomena different from those of the disease treated, *cf.* homoeopathy.

alloplasty Surgical grafts to parts of body by foreign material.

alloy A mixture of two or more metals obtained by fusing them together.

alopecia Absence of hair, baldness.

alpha rays Nuclear radiation consisting of two protons and two neutrons. Will penetrate only a few millimetres into tissue.

alphachymotripsin A pancreatic enzyme. Used therapeutically as an anti-inflammatory.

alphafetoprotein (AFP) Major blood protein of the fetus. Present in liquor amnii or maternal serum in raised amounts with neural tube and intestinal anomalies. Also present in adults with primary liver and some ovarian cancer.

alphatocopherol Vitamin E.

alternating current Electrical current the polarity of which is phasically reversed.

alternative medicine Blanket term for non-conventional therapy, *e.g.* acupuncture, chiropractic, osteopathy, herbal medicine.

altitude sickness Malaise due to hypoxia resulting from decrease in partial pressure of oxygen in atmosphere at high altitudes.

aluminium hydroxide An antacid used to treat dyspepsia. Does not lead to alkalosis.

aluminium paste A compound containing aluminium powder used to protect skin around ileostomies.

alveolar block syndrome A thickening of the alveolar membrane impeding oxygen diffusion. Aetiology unknown.

alveolitis Inflammation of the pulmonary alveoli.

alveolus (pl. **alveoli**) (1) The socket of a tooth. (2) An air cell in the lung. (3) A secreting unit of the breast.

Alzheimer's disease Degeneration of the cerebral cortex. Loss of memory, aphasia and paralysis occur. Can be senile or presenile.

amalgam An alloy of mercury and other metals. *Dental a.* is of silver, tin and mercury. Used for filling teeth.

amastia Absence of breasts.

amaurosis Blindness from disease or defect of the nervous system of the eye.

amaurotic familial idiocy *Syn.* Tay–Sach's disease. An inherited inborn error of metabolism causing degeneration of the nervous system. Commonest in Ashkenazi Jews.

ambidextrous Equally skilful with each hand.

ambivalence Contrary emotions, such as love and hate, are experienced towards the same object or person.

amblyopia Indistinct vision; approaching blindness.

ambulance A vehicle for the conveyance of sick and wounded.

ambulant Able to walk.

ambulatory Relating to walking; moving about. *A. treatment of fractures* enables the patient to remain up and at work. The limb is im-

mobilized in plaster of Paris.

amelia Congenital absence of limbs.

amelioration Improvement; lessening of a patient's symptoms.

amenorrhoea Absence of menstruation. In *primary a.* menstruation has never been established. *Secondary a.* occurs after menstruation has commenced. There is amenorrhoea in pregnancy, and it may occur in certain endocrine disorders, anaemia, etc.

amentia Absence of intellect; idiocy.

ametria Congenital absence of the uterus.

ametropia Defective vision due to abnormal form or refractive power of the eye.

amino acid Organic compound containing both basic amino ($-NH_2$) and acidic carboxyl ($-COOH$) groups. Fundamental units in the structure of proteins. Of 20 different amino acids commonly found in proteins, eight cannot be synthesized in the body and must, as with vitamins, be obtained from food. These are known as essential amino acids.

aminoaciduria Presence of excessive amounts of amino acids in the urine.

amitosis Type of direct cell division without prior reduplication of chromosomes, said to take place in cartilage.

amnesia Loss of memory. *Anterograde a.*: inability to remember recent events. *Retrograde a.*: symptom of concussion. The patient cannot remember what happened immediately before the accident.

amniocentesis Aspiration of fluid from the amniotic cavity allowing tests for fetal normality and well-being.

amniography Radiographic demonstration of amniotic sac by injection of radio-opaque dye.

amnion The sac directly encircling the fetus in utero.

amniotic fluid *Syn.* liquor amnii. Fluid within the amnion which cushions the embryo from trauma and distortion.

amoeba A microscopic unicellular animal, one variety of which causes amoebic dysentery.

amoebiasis Infection by pathogenic amoebae. Complications include abscesses, cysts and amoeboma.

amoebicide Substance lethal to amoebae.

amoeboma Amoebic granuloma which may occur in the large intestine.

amorphous Formless.

AMP *See* ADENOSINE MONO-PHOSPHATE.

ampère Unit measure of electric current.

amphiarthrosis A slightly movable joint, *e.g.* the ar-ticulations of the spine.

amphoteric Substance with acidic and basic groupings capable of acting both as an acid or a base.

ampoule A sealed phial containing a drug or solution sterilized ready for use.

ampulla A flask-shaped dilation especially of a duct, *e.g. a. of Vater*, a dilation of the common bile duct just before it opens into the duodenum.

amputation The removal of a limb or organ. It is termed primary if performed immediately after the injury, secondary if performed later.

amylase Group of enzymes which split complex sugars, *e.g.* starch, glycogen, to disaccharides such as maltose. Present in saliva and pancreatic juice.

amyloidosis Lardaceous disease, characterized by deposition of globulin-like material in liver, spleen, kidneys, skin, etc. Classified as primary (cause unknown) and secondary when it follows long-standing infection.

amyotonia A form of muscular feebleness or paralysis, often congenital.

amyotrophic lateral sclerosis Syndrome comprising progressive muscular atrophy with upper motor neurone involvement. The clinical picture is variable according to the stage of the disease.

anabolism Synthesis, by living organisms, of complex molecules from simpler ones; *cf.* catabolism.

anacrotic Refers to ascending limb (Greek 'upstroke') of tracing of pulse wave.

anaemia Diminished oxygen-carrying capacity of the blood, due to a reduction in the numbers of red cells or in their content of haemoglobin, or both. The cause may be inadequate production of red cells or excessive loss of blood.

anaerobe Any microorganism that can live and multiply in the absence of free oxygen, *e.g.* tetanus.

anaerobic respiration Occurs when oxygen is in short supply and results in build-up of lactic and pyruvic acids.

anaesthesia Absence of sensation; loss of feeling. *Basal a.*: partial general anaesthesia obtained by a drug such as morphine given before an inhalation anaesthetic. *Dissociated a.*: loss of sensation to pain and temperature, sense of touch being retained. *Epidural a.*: induced by injection of anaesthetic agents into the epidural space surrounding the spinal cord. *General a.*: this gives loss of consciousness. *Glove a.*: loss of feeling in the area of the hand a glove covers, *Intravenous a.*: a general anaesthesia pro-duced by intravenous injection. *Local a.*: anaesthesia of a certain area only. *Nerve block a.*: local anaesthesia produced by injecting an anaesthetic near a sensory nerve. *Rectal a.*: general anaesthesia by administering an anaesthetic rectally. *Refrigeration a.*: anaesthesia produced by intense cold. *Spinal a.*: an anaesthetic injected into the subarachnoid space of the spinal cord producing anaesthesia in the lower part of the body.

anaesthetic An agent which produces insensibility. As an adjective it means insensible to touch.

anaesthetist The administrator of anaesthetics.

anal Of the anus.

analbuminaemia Absence of albumin from blood proteins.

analeptic A restorative. A drug which restores to consciousness, *e.g.* nikethamide.

analgesia Diminished sensibility to pain. A symptom in certain nervous diseases, *e.g.* syringomyelia.

analgesic Relieving pain; remedy for pain.

analogous Comparable in certain respects.

analysis In chemistry, the breaking down of a substance into its constituent parts. In psychiatric medicine, psychoanalysis.

anaphase A stage in cell division when the chromosomes move towards opposite poles of the cell. *See* MITOSIS.

anaphoresis Diminished activity of the sweat glands.

anaphylaxis A state of shock induced by an antigen–antibody reaction occurring in cells which causes the release of substances acting on the vascular system.

anaplasia The reversion of specialized tissue or cells to a less differentiated type.

anastomosis In anatomy the intercommunication of the terminal branches of two or more blood vessels. In surgery the establishment of some artificial connection, as, for instance, between two parts of the intestine.

anatomical position Standardized position of the body to which nomenclature of anatomical relations refers. Standing erect arms to side, palms facing forward.

anatomy The science of organic structure.

anconeus A small extensor muscle of the forearm.

ancylostomiasis *See* ANKYLOSTOMIASIS.

androgen A hormone producing male sex characteristics.

android pelvis Shaped like a male pelvis. In women associated with difficult labour.

androsterone A breakdown product of testosterone.

anencephaly Failure of development of the brain, resulting in perinatal death.

aneroid Without air.

aneuploid Having more or less than an integral multiple of the haploid number of chromosomes; *cf.* euploid.

aneurysm A permanent dilatation of an artery usually with rupture of the internal and middle coats. It may be (1) *fusiform a.* or (2) *sacculated a.* The thoracic aorta and the innominate artery are those usually affected, more rarely the abdominal aorta. *Arteriovenous a.*: a communication between an artery and a vein, usually the result of injury. *Dissecting a.*: results when blood is forced into the potential space between the layers of the arterial wall.

angiectasis Dilatation of blood vessels.

angiitis Inflammation of blood vessels.

angina Suffocating pain; most commonly *a. pectoris*, temporary pain from ischaemic heart muscle brought on by exercise. Also pain due to severe sore throat and respiratory tract, *e.g. Ludwig's a.* and *Vincent's a.*

angiocardiogram The x-ray film taken in angiocardiography.

angiocardiography To demonstrate the activity and function of the heart and great vessels by the injection of contrast medium.

angiogram X-ray film showing blood vessels.

angiography *See* ANGIO-CARDIOGRAPHY.

angioma A tumour composed of blood vessels, often called a naevus.

angioneurotic Having to do with the nervous control of the blood vessels. Thus *a. oedema* is a persistent or intermittent swelling of parts such as the eyelid or lip. It may be an allergic symptom.

angioplasty Plastic surgery of the blood vessels.

angiosarcoma A sarcoma composed of vascular tissue.

angiospasm The blood vessels contract in spasm.

angiotensin Polypeptide hormone which raises the blood pressure.

anhidrosis Deficiency of perspiration.

anhidrotics Drugs which reduce sweating.

anhydrous Without water.

aniline Phenylamine. Used in preparing dyestuffs.

anion An ion bearing a negative electrical charge.

aniseikonia Unequal magnification between two eyes or different meridia in the same eye.

anisochromatopsia Partial colour blindness.

anisocoria Inequality of the pupils.

anisocytosis Inequality of size of the red blood cells.

anisomelia Unequal limbs which should be a pair.

anisometropia Differing refraction between eyes.

ankle Joint between leg and foot; the weight is transmitted between tibia and talus. *A. clonus*, *see* CLONUS.

ankyloblepharon Adhesion of the edges of the eyelids.

ankyloglossia Inability to protrude the tongue fully and tendency for it to deviate to one side, usually the result of damage to the tongue muscles.

ankylosing spondylitis Disease of joints, of unknown aetiology, in which destruction of the joint space occurs and is followed by sclerosis and calcification. The sacro-iliac and spinal joints are predominantly affected. There is associated arterial disease.

ankylosis Immobility in a joint, following inflammation or prolonged immobilization. *False a.*: fixation or stiffness produced by conditions around the joint such as contraction of skin, *e.g.* after burns, or of tendons, by ossification of muscles, or by outgrowths of bone. *True a.*: fixation or stiffness produced by conditions in the joint such as injury or arthritis. *Fibrous a.*: fixation by fibrous tissue. *Bony a.*: the articular surfaces of the bones are fused together.

Ankylostoma duodenale A minute parasitic hookworm which may inhabit the duodenum in large numbers and cause profound anaemia.

ankylostomiasis Hookworm disease. Infection with Ankylostoma duodenale.

annular Ring-shaped. *A. ligament*: the ligament around the wrist or ankle.

anode Electrode with positive charge.

anodyne A pain-relieving drug.

anomalous Irregular. Out of the ordinary.

anomia Inability to name objects and recall names.

anonychia Absence of nails.

anoperineal Relating to anus and perineum.

Anopheles A genus of mosquito. They are carriers of the malarial parasite, their bite being the means of transmitting the disease to human beings.

anorchous Without testes. Sometimes applied incorrectly to undescended testes.

anorectal Pertaining to the anus and the rectum.

anorexia Lack of appetite, abhorrence of food. *A. nervosa*: a disease usually occurring in female adolescents. Dieting may start to lose real or imagined excess of weight

and the patient becomes progressively less able to eat any food. Amenorrhoea is common. Psychiatric treatment is usually indicated. *See also* BULIMIA.

anosmia Loss of sense of smell.

anovulation Cessation of ovulation.

anovulatory cycle Apparently normal menstrual cycle without ovulation.

anoxaemia Insufficient oxygen in the blood.

anoxia Absence of oxygen. Often implies insufficient oxygen available for normal respiratory metabolism, *i.e.* hypoxia.

antacid Any substance neutralizing an acid, *e.g.* sodium bicarbonate.

antagonist An organ such as a muscle that acts in opposition to another, or a drug neutralizing another drug.

antemortem Before death.

antenatal Before birth.

antepartum Before birth. *A. haemorrhage* may be inevitable when due to placenta praevia, accidental when it is due to partial separation of the placenta or incidental when it is due to diseases of the cervix.

anterior In front of. *A. chamber of eye*: the space, between the cornea in front and the iris and lens behind, which contains the aqueous humour. *A. commissure*: a bundle of nerve fibres crossing the midline in front of the third ventricle and serving to connect certain parts of the two cerebral hemispheres. *A. fontanelle*: see FONTANELLE. *A. root*: motor root. *Syn.* ventral root. Nerve root emerging from the spinal cord carrying motor fibres; *cf.* dorsal or posterior root.

anterograde Going forwards.

anteroinferior Lying in front and below.

anterointerior Lying to the front and internally.

anterolateral In front and to the side.

anteromedian Lying in front and near the midline.

anteroposterior From front to back.

anterosuperior In front and above.

anteversion The state of being inclined forward. It is the commonest position of the uterus.

anthelmintic A remedy for intestinal worms.

anthracosis Disease caused by inhaling coal dust or soot into the lungs. Seen in miners.

anthrax An acute, infectious disease produced by the anthrax bacillus. *Skin a.* and *pulmonary a.* are the two main forms.

anthropoid Man-like. *A. apes* include animals most closely

related to man. *A. pelvis*: the pelvis has a narrowed transverse inlet which is long anteroposteriorly.

anthropology The natural history of mankind.

antibiotic Opposed to life; drugs, derived from living cells, especially fungi, which prevent microorganisms from multiplying, *e.g.* penicillin.

antibody Protein substance, usually circulating in the blood, which neutralizes corresponding antigens. *Auto a.*: directed against a component normally present in the body. *Blocking a.*: inhibiting effect of another antibody. *Forssman a.*: specific for antigen unrelated to that providing immunizing stimulus. *Incomplete a.*: will not by itself form precipitate in vitro with corresponding antigen.

anticholinergic Substance antagonizing the action of acetylcholine.

anticholinesterase Generic term for substances which prevent the action of cholinesterases and specifically acetylcholinesterase which breaks down acetylcholine.

anticoagulant Substance which delays the clotting of blood.

anticodon Triplet of unpaired bases which are complementary to the triplet of the genetic code which specifies an amino acid.

anticonvulsant A drug used to prevent a convulsion.

antidepressant Drug used to treat depression.

antidiuretic hormone Posterior pituitary hormone regulating the amount of water reabsorbed from the uriniferous tubules into the renal substance.

antidote The corrective to a poison.

antigen Substance capable of stimulating the formation of antibodies. *Australia a.*: found in a proportion of people with viral hepatitis.

antigenic determinant Site on antigen molecule determining specificity of antibody evoked.

antiglobulin test Coomb's test, used to identify abnormal antibody in the blood.

antihaemophilic globulin (AHG) One of the factors essential for blood coagulation. Congenital deficiency causes haemophilia.

antihistamine Drug counteracting the effects of the liberation of histamine in the tissues.

antilymphocyte globulin (ALG) Immunoglobulin which binds to lymphocyte membrane antigens causing their inactivation and thereby reducing immune responses.

antilymphocyte serum Serum containing antilymphocyte globulins.

antimalarial Agent used for the prophylaxis or treatment of malaria.

antimetabolite Substitute for a metabolite which interferes with metabolism.

antimicrobial *See* ANTIBIOTIC.

antimigraine Agent used for the prophylaxis or treatment of migraine.

antimitotic Agent which inhibits cell division. Anticancer drug.

antimycotic Substance used to treat fungus diseases.

antinuclear factor (ANF) Antibody reacting with material in cell nuclei.

antiperistalsis Reverse peristalsis, *i.e.* from below upward. *See* PERISTALSIS.

antiphlogistic Relieving inflammation.

antipruritic Substance relieving itching.

antipyretic A drug which reduces the high temperatures of feverish conditions.

antirachitic factor *Syn.* vitamin D. Prevents rickets.

antiscorbutic *Syn.* vitamin C or ascorbic acid. Prevents scurvy.

antiseptic A substance opposing sepsis by arresting the growth and multiplication of microorganisms. Iodine, phenol, biniodide of mercury, chlorine, formalin, quaternary ammonium compounds, chloroxylenols, hypochlorites

are common antiseptics.
Many are poisonous.

antiserum Serum, usually
prepared from horses, containing a high titre of antibody to a specific organism or
toxin.

antisocial Disregard of the
normally accepted behaviour
in a particular society.

antispasmodic An agent relieving spasm.

antithrombin A substance in
the blood having the power of
retarding or preventing coagulation.

antithyroid drugs Substances
which restrict the secretion of
thyroid hormones by interference in the intermediary
metabolism of the gland.

antitoxin A specific antibody
produced in the blood in response to a toxin or poison.
The antibody is capable of
neutralizing that particular
toxin.

antitragus The prominence
of the lower portion of the
external ear.

antivenin An antidote to
animal or insect venom.

Anton's syndrome Cortical
blindness in which the patient
is unaware of inability to see.

antrostomy Incision of an
antrum.

antrum A cave; applied to
the maxillary sinus, called the
antrum of Highmore, and the
cavity in the mastoid bone
communicating with the

middle ear. *See* MAXILLARY
SINUS.

anuria Cessation of the production of urine; to be distinguished from retention of
urine, due to inability to
empty the bladder.

anus The rectal exit. *Imperforate a.*: a congenital malformation where a child is born
with no anal opening, or an
anus is present but does not
communicate with the bowel
above.

anxiety neurosis An illness in
which a patient's fears and an-
xieties are out of proportion to
reality.

aorta Large artery arising
from the left ventrical of the
heart and from which blood is
distributed to the whole body.

aortic Pertaining to the aorta.
A. incompetence: Blood from
the aorta regurgitates back
into the left ventricle, due to
inefficiency of the valve. *A.
stenosis*: narrowing of the aortic valve due to malformation
and/or disease. *A. valves*:
three semilunar valves guar-
ding the entrance from the left
ventricle to the aorta and
preventing the backward flow
of the blood.

aortitis Inflammation of the
aorta.

apathy Absence of emotion
or feeling.

apepsia Failure of digestion
due to deficiency of gastric
juice.

aperient A purgative medicine, *e.g.* cascara. *See* LAXATIVE.

aperistalsis Cessation of peristalsis.

apex Top, extreme point, summit. *A. of the heart*: narrow end of heart enclosing left ventricle. *A. beat*: the heart beat as felt at its most forcible point on the chest wall. This corresponds approximately with the position of the left ventricle.

Apgar score Rapid evaluation system for physical condition of newborn infants usually recorded at 1 minute and 5 minutes after birth.

APH *Abbr.* antepartum haemorrhage.

aphagia Inability to swallow.

aphakia Absence of lens.

aphasia Speechlessness; due to disease or injury to brain.

aphonia Loss of voice.

aphrodisiac An agent which increases sexual desire.

aphthae Small white ulcers in the mouth.

aphthous stomatitis Inflammation of the mucous membrane of the mouth due to herpes simplex virus; *cf. thrush*.

apicectomy Excision of the root-end of a tooth.

aplasia Non-development of an organ or tissue.

aplastic anaemia Anaemia resulting from destruction of bone marrow cells.

apnoea Suspended respiration.

apocrine glands Specialized sweat glands found in the axillae and genital regions.

aponeurosis A tendon-like fibrous tissue, which invests the muscles and transmits their movements to the structures upon which they act.

apophysis A bony protuberance or outgrowth.

apoplexy A stroke or cerebrovascular accident.

appendicectomy Removal of the vermiform appendix. Also called appendectomy.

appendices epiploicae Small bags of fat projecting from the peritoneal coat of the large intestine.

appendicitis Inflammation of the appendix.

appendix vermiformis A worm-like offshoot from the caecum, ending blindly, and 2–13 cm long.

apperception The conscious reception of a sensory impression.

applicator An instrument for applying local remedies, *e.g.* radium.

apposition The lying together or the fitting together of two structures.

apraxia Inability to carry out purposeful voluntary movements but without loss of muscle power.

APT *Abbr.* alum precipitated (diphtheria) toxoid.

aptitude A facility or a particular bent for certain work or actions.

aptyalism Absence of salivation.

apyrexia Absence of fever.

aqueduct Certain canals of the body, such as the *a. of Sylvius* which leads from the third to the fourth ventricle of the brain.

aqueous humour Fluid in the eye between the cornea and the iris and the lens.

arachnodactyly With spider digits. Developmental anomaly associated with Marfan's syndrome in which the digits are excessively long.

arachnoid Spider-like. *A. membrane* surrounds the brain and spinal cord. It is between the dura and pia mater.

arbor vitae Tree-like appearance seen in a section of the cerebellum and also applied to a similar appearance seen in the interior folds of the cervix of the uterus.

arborization Branching of processes of nerve cells.

arboviruses Arthropod-borne viruses. Viruses transmitted by the bites of insects including those causing yellow fever, sandfly fever and some viral haemorrhagic fevers.

arcus An arc or ring. *A. senilis*: an opaque circle round the edges of the cornea, occurring in the aged.

ARC *Abbr.* AIDS-related complex. Clinical state less severe than AIDS occurring in those carrying HIV.

areola The pigmented skin round the nipple of the breast.

areolar tissue Loose connective tissue.

ARF *Abbr.* (1) Acute renal failure. (2) Acute respiratory failure.

arginine An amino acid.

argininosuccinuria Inborn error of metabolism associated with mental retardation and sometimes abnormal hair. Inherited by a recessive gene.

Argyll–Robertson pupil Pupil of eye which is small, reacting to accommodation but not to light. Seen in diseases of the nervous system, *e.g.* tabes dorsalis.

argyria Discoloration of the skin and sclera due to the deposition of silver. Results from prolonged ingestion of preparations containing silver.

ARMS *Abbr.* Action for Research into Multiple Sclerosis.

Arnold–Chiari malformation Herniation of cerebellum and elongation of medulla oblongata, associated with spina bifida.

arrector pili Muscle fibres around the hair follicles which on contraction produce 'gooseflesh'.

arrhenoblastoma A neoplasm of the ovary associated with masculinization.

arrhythmia Disturbance of rhythm, usually the heart's rhythm. *Sinus a.*: increased pulse rate during inspiration; decreased during expiration; common in the young.

artefact A lesion produced by artificial means.

arterial Pertaining to an artery. Thus *a. tension* means the pressure of the blood circulating in a given artery.

arteriectomy Excision of an artery.

arteriography To demonstrate blood vessels following the injection of contrast medium opaque to x-rays.

arterioles Small arteries with contractile muscular walls which control the supply of blood to the capillaries.

arteriopathy Disease of the arteries.

arterioplasty Surgery to reform an artery, especially for aneurysm.

arteriorrhaphy Suture of an artery.

arteriosclerosis Degeneration of an artery with hardening of its walls, seen chiefly in old age. The condition is accompanied by high blood pressure.

arteriotomy Incision of an artery.

arteriovenous aneurysm *See* ANEURYSM.

arteritis Inflammation of the arteries.

artery A vessel carrying blood from the heart.

arthralgia Pain in the joints.

arthrectomy The removal by operation of the whole or part of a joint.

arthroclasia An operation for breaking up an ankylosed joint to produce free movement.

arthrodesis Fixation of a joint by means of a surgical operation.

arthrodynia Pain in the joints.

arthrography Radiography of joint after the injection of radio-opaque fluid to outline the joint space.

arthropathy Disease of the joints. Commonly used to imply secondary damage to joints as a result of other disease processes.

arthroplasty The making of an artificial joint.

arthroscope Endoscope for examining the cavities of joints.

arthroscopy Endoscopic examination of a joint.

arthrosis Disease of a joint.

arthrotomy Incision into a joint.

Arthus phenomenon Tissue necrosis after repeated antigen injections.

articular Relating to the joints; the articulation of a skeleton is the manner in

which the bones are joined
together.

articulation (1) A joint between two or more bones. (2)
The enunciation of words.

artificial feeding Feeding of
an infant with food other than
its mother's milk.

artificial insemination Artificial introduction of spermatozoa into the vagina.

artificial kidney Dialysing apparatus through which blood
from the patient is pumped so
that excretory products such
as urea may be extracted in
the event of the patient's own
kidneys not functioning.

artificial pneumothorax. *See*
PNEUMOTHORAX.

arytenoid The term applied
to two funnel-shaped car-
tilages of the larynx.

asbestos A mineral substance
which is incombustible and
which does not conduct heat.

asbestosis Disease of the lung
caused by inhalation of asbestos dust.

ascariasis Infestation of the
bowel by roundworms
(ascarides).

ascaricide Substance lethal to
intestinal worms.

Ascaris A genus of parasitic
roundworm. *A. lumbricoides*:
long roundworm.

ascending colon The first part
of the large intestine extending from the caecum to
the hepatic flexure in the right
side of the abdominal cavity.

Aschoff nodules The focal
lesions of acute rheumatic
fever consisting of peri-
vascular necrosis of collagen.
These nodules tend to occur
in the heart, muscles and connective tissue.

ascites Fluid collection in abdominal cavity.

aspirin A preparation containing salicylic acid with anti-
inflammatory, antipyretic and
analgesic activities.

assertiveness training Training by role-play to improve
self-confidence.

ascitic fluid Fluid of ascites
which can be aspirated.

ascorbic acid Vitamin C. It is
required for collagen formation in healing of wounds.
Deficiency causes scurvy.

asepsis The state of being
free from living pathogenic
microorganisms.

aseptic Free from bacteria. In
aseptic surgery all instruments, dressings, etc., are
sterilized before use.

asexual Having no sex.

Aspergillus A group of fungi,
some species of which are
pathogenic, causing asper-
gillosis, which may infect the
ear, eye or lungs.

aspermia Absence of live
spermatozoa in semen, *cf.*
azoospermia.

asphyxia Suffocation due to
reduced oxygen in inspired
air, obstruction in respiratory
tract, impaired alveolar

absorption or impaired oxygen carriage by blood. Associated cyanosis or pallor.

aspiration The operation of drawing off fluids from the body.

aspirator The apparatus used for aspiration.

assimilation The absorption and utilization of nourishment by the living tissues. *A. pelvis*: term indicating the incorporation of the fifth lumbar vertebra in the sacral body.

assisted ventilation Respiratory effort assisted by mechanical means. Usually with a ventilator via an endotracheal tube or tracheostomy.

association Co-ordination. 'Association of ideas', *i.e.* a phrase used to denote the secondary thoughts that arise on the receipt of any individual mental impression.

asteatosis Deficient action of sebaceous glands.

astereognosis Loss of power to recognize the shape of objects by touch.

asthenia Failure of strength; debility.

asthenopia Weakness of sight.

asthma Paroxysmal wheezing cough due to constriction of the bronchi of the lungs. May be due to various stimuli including inhalation of allergens, cold air, exercise and stress. Normally relieved by bronchodilators and, in severe cases, by inhaled or systemic steroids. *Cardiac a.*: wheezing associated with pulmonary oedema.

astigmatism Inequality in the curvature of the cornea or lens, with consequent blurring and distortion of the images thrown upon the retina.

astringent A substance applied to produce local contraction of blood vessels and inhibit secretion, *e.g.* tannin, adrenaline.

astrocytoma Tumour occurring in the central nervous system, composed of cells called astrocytes.

astroglia Star-shaped supporting cells of the central nervous system.

Astrup test Measurement of the pressures of oxygen and carbon dioxide in arterial blood to assess acidosis.

asymmetry Lack of symmetry.

asymptomatic Without symptoms of disease.

asynclitism Descent of the fetal head through the pelvis so that one parietal bone precedes the other.

atavism After an interval of several generations, recurrence in descendants of a character possessed by an ancestor.

ataxia, ataxy Literally, disorder; applied to any defective control of muscles and consequent irregularity of movements. *See also* LOCOMOTOR ATAXIA and FRIEDREICH'S ATAXIA.

atelectasis Imperfect expansion of the lungs of the newborn. Term also used for collapse of part of the lung from some other cause.

atherogenic Producing atheroma.

atheroma Degeneration of walls of arteries associated with deposition of cholesterol esters in the lesions.

atherosclerosis Narrowing of blood vessels resulting from atheromatous deposits.

athetosis A condition marked by continuous and purposeless movements, especially of the hands and fingers.

athlete's foot Infectious disease of the skin between and under the toes due to parasitic fungi.

atlas First cervical vertebra.

atmosphere The air surrounding the earth. The pressure, at sea level, measured by means of a barometer equivalent to approximately 15 psi or 1055 g/cm².

atomizer A spray for providing a shower of very minute droplets.

atony Wanting in muscular tone or vigour; weakness.

ATP *See* ADENOSINE TRIPHOSPHATE.

atresia Congenital absence of a natural passage, *e.g.* duodenal a., oesophageal a.

atria The two thin-walled chambers of the heart into which the veins drain.

atrial Pertaining to the atria. *A. fibrillation*: cardiac arrhythmia caused by the independent contraction of muscle bundles in the atrial walls. There is no coordinated atrial contraction and the ventricular contractions are stimulated irregularly. *A. flutter*: cardiac arrhythmia caused by rapid atrial contractions, 200 to 300 per minute, stimulated by an excitable focus in the atrial wall. The ventricles are unable to contract at this rate and respond only to every second or third atrial contraction. *See* HEART BLOCK. *A. septal defect*: defect in the development of the heart leaving a hole in the wall separating the right and left atrium.

atrioventricular bundle *Syn.* auriculoventricular bundle. Normally the contraction of the heart is initiated at the sinoatrial node. The impulse then passes through the atrial walls causing atrial contraction and reaching the atrioventricular (A-V) node which it stimulates. The A-V node is composed of specialized tissue continuous with the A-V bundle through which the impulse is conducted to the ventricles to initiate their contraction. Defects in the A-V bundle impairing conduction cause heart block.

atrophic Result of atropy. *A. rhinitis* is characterized by atrophy of the nasal mucosa; *a. vaginitis* is thinning of vaginal mucosa due to hormone lack.

atrophy Wasting of a part, from disuse or lack of nutrition.

atropine Active principle of belladonna. Parasympathetic antagonist.

ATS *Abbr.* antitetanus serum. Produces passive immunity because of tetanus antibodies.

ATT *Abbr.* antitetanus toxoid. Produces active immunity because of antigenically active but otherwise inactive toxins.

attenuation A weakening or dilution.

atypical Not typical.

audiogram Chart showing the responsiveness of the ear to sounds of differing pitch.

audiologist A specialist in the diagnosis and treatment of hearing problems.

audiometer Instrument used for audiometry.

audiometry Measurement of hearing ability. The results are usually plotted as an audiogram.

auditory Pertaining to the sense of hearing.

Auer bodies Blue-staining granules seen in myeloblasts in leukaemia.

Auerbach's plexus The collection of nerve fibres (terminations of vagus and sympathetic nerves) and ganglia situated in the intestinal walls. Its function is to regulate peristalsis.

aura A sensation, which is usually auditory or visual, arising indigenously in the patient; it may precede an epileptic fit.

aural Pertaining to the ear.

auricle (1) The external ear. (2) Small ear-like appendage on atrium of heart.

auricular Pertaining to the ear or to the auricles of the heart.

auriculotemporal syndrome Results from injury to the fibres of the auriculotemporal nerve. When the patient eats, the cheek becomes red, hot and sweats.

auriculoventricular bundle *See* ATRIOVENTRICULAR BUNDLE.

auriscope An instrument for examining the drum of the ear. An otoscope.

auscultation Listening to sounds of the body for the purposes of diagnosis. Usually using a stethoscope.

Australia antigen Antigen associated with hepatitis B. Blood positive for this antigen can transmit infection.

autism A condition, usually of childhood, involving a

failure to develop normal
relationships.

autistic Usually describing a
child who withdraws from
contact with people and fails
to use speech as a means of
communication.

auto A prefix (Greek) meaning self, or itself.

autoagglutination Red cell
clumping because of auto-
antibodies, *e.g.* in acquired
haemolytic anaemia.

autoantibody Antibody produced by the body against one
of its own components.

autoantigen Antigen against
which autoantibodies are
produced.

autocatalytic Catalysing production of self.

autoclave An apparatus for
sterilizing by steam.

autodigestion Process of self-
digestion.

autoeroticism Masturbation.

autogenous Self-produced.

autograft Graft taken from
the patient's own body. *See*
GRAFT.

autographism Same as
dermographism.

autohypnosis Self-induced
hypnotism.

autoimmune disease Disease
characterized by and resulting
from the production of antibodies against components of
one's own body.

autoimmunity State of sensitization to products of one's
own organs, *e.g.* as in Hashi-

moto's disease.

autoimmunization Sensitization to a component or components of one's body
resulting in the production of
autoantibodies.

autoinfection Self-infection.

autointoxication Poisoning by
toxins generated within the
body.

autolysis Process of self-
digestion.

automatism A condition in
which actions are performed
without consciousness or
regulated purpose; sometimes
follows a major or minor epileptic fit.

autonomic nervous system
Motor supply to smooth
muscle and glands. Divided
into sympathetic and parasympathetic systems and
characterized by synapsing in
ganglia after fibres leave the
central nervous system.
Generally speaking the
effector fibres (postganglionic
fibres) of the sympathetic system are adrenergic and the
parasympathetic are cholinergic, not directly under conscious control but there is
considerable cortical repre-
sentation.

autoplasty *See* AUTOGRAFT.

autopsy A postmortem examination.

autoradiography Photo-
graphy showing localization
of radioactive substance in a
tissue section.

autosomes All chromosomes excluding the sex chromosomes.

autosuggestion Self-suggestion: used in the treatment of functional nervous disorders.

autotransfusion The return to the patient's circulation of blood shed by haemorrhage usually into the abdominal cavity.

avascular Bloodless.

aversion therapy Treatment by conditioning based on association of a disagreeable stimulus with an abnormal desire.

avian Bird-like. Usually refers to zoonoses carried by birds, *e.g.* a. tubercle.

avirulent Not virulent.

avitaminosis Lack of vitamins. Usually the particular vitamin deficiency is specified, *e.g.* a. A.

avulsion A tearing apart.

axilla The armpit.

axillary artery The artery of the armpit, connecting the subclavian and brachial arteries.

axis (1) The second cervical vertebra on which the atlas rotates. (2) Line passing through the centre of a body. *A. of pelvis*: a curved line which is everywhere at right angles to the planes of the pelvic cavity. *A. traction*: force so applied to the fetus by forceps that its effect is al-ways exerted along the axis of the pelvis.

axon The long process of a nerve cell conducting impulses away from the cell body; *cf.* dendrites.

axonotmesis Damage causing discontinuity of axons but the supporting tissue remains intact.

azoospermia Absence of viable sperms in the semen causing male sterility.

azotaemia Excess urea in the blood.

azoturia An increase of urea in the urine.

azygos Single, *i.e.* not paired as in azygos vein.

B

Babinski's reflex Extensor plantar response, *i.e.* the toes go up when the sole of the foot is stroked. This is normal in infants and abnormal after about two years.

bacillary dysentery Infection of the gut with Shigella bacilli; *cf.* amoeba.

Bacille Calmette-Guérin *See* BCG.

bacilluria Presence of bacilli in the urine.

bacillus *See* BACTERIA.

bacteraemia Bacteria in the blood.

bacteria Microscopic unicellular living organisms; some cause disease and are called pathogenic. The principal forms are: (1) cocci, those which are rounded in shape. When these are disposed in pairs they are called diplococci. These occur in pneumonia, some forms of meningitis, and gonorrhoea. When in chains they are called streptococci, when in clusters staphylococci. (2) Bacilli are rod-shaped bacteria which include the Gram-positive organisms causing anthrax, tetanus and diphtheria; Gram-negative causing dysentery, typhoid and plague and the acid-fast organisms of tuberculosis and leprosy. (3) Spirochaetes are corkscrew-like germs, or spiral rods with several twists, occurring in relapsing fever and syphilis. The majority of bacteria are immobile, but some have power of movement. Bacteria have the power of multiplying by splitting across their centre; this is known as binary fission; others form spores, which are small, round, glistening bodies able to withstand great extremes of heat and cold.

bacterial Pertaining to bacteria.

bactericidal Capable of killing bacteria; *cf.* bacteriostatic.

bacteriology The study of bacteria.

bacteriolytic Capable of breaking down the cell membranes of bacteria.

bacteriophage A virus which destroys bacteria.

bacteriostatic Preventing the growth of bacteria; *cf.* bactericidal.

bacteriuria The presence of bacteria in the urine.

bagassosis Disease of lungs caused by the inhalation of sugar cane dust.

Bainbridge reflex Inhibition of vagal impulses caused by raised right atrial pressure.

Baker's cysts Cysts originating from synovial pouches connected with joints.

BAL *Abbr.* British antilewisite (dimercaprol), an antidote for heavy metal poisoning.

balanitis Inflammation of the glans penis.

baldness *See* ALOPECIA.

Balkan beam Frame erected over bed to enable limb to be suspended.

ballooning The distension of a cavity by air, or by its natural contents.

ballottement The sensation of a return tap against the fingers when the hand is suddenly pressed on the pregnant uterus and temporarily displaces the contained fetus as it floats in the liquor amnii. Ballottement may be elicited externally, or per vaginam.

bandages Materials used for binding wounds, fractures, etc.

Bandl's ring Retraction ring in the uterus.

Bankart's operation Operation to repair the glenoid cavity after repeated dislocation of the shoulder joint.

Banti's syndrome Characterized by anaemia with recurrent bleeding from the alimentary tract, leucopenia and splenomegaly, due to portal hypertension.

Bárány's chair test A test for labyrinthine function in aviators assessed by rotating chair.

Barbados leg Elephantiasis.

barber's rash *See* SYCOSIS BARBAE.

barium enema Radiological investigation of the rectum and large bowel following the introduction of barium-containing contrast medium via the anal canal.

barium meal Radiological investigation of the oesophagus, stomach and small bowel following the ingestion of barium-containing contrast medium. The progress of contrast medium through the bowel is demonstrated by means of serial radiographs.

barium swallow *See* BARIUM MEAL.

Barlow's sign Test for congenital dislocation of the hip. *See also* HIP, CONGENITAL DISLOCATION OF.

baroreceptors Aortic nerve-endings of afferent branches of vagus and glossopharyngeal nerves. Receptors of pressure stimuli in reflex control of blood pressure.

Barr body Sex-chromatin body. Small dark-staining mass underneath nuclear membrane in majority of female cells. Represents an inactive X chromosome.

barrier nursing The nursing of a patient with an infectious disease in a general ward, or a ward with patients having a variety of infectious diseases. Adequate precautions are taken so that cross-infection does not occur.

Bartholin's glands Two small glands, one each side of the vulva. An abscess may develop there or the duct may distend into a cyst.

bartholinitis Inflammation of Bartholin's glands.

basal ganglia Four deeply placed masses of grey matter within the cerebral hemisphere, known as caudate, lentiform and amygdaloid nuclei, and the claustrum. Little is known of their function but disease involving the basal ganglia gives rise to athetosis and Parkinsonism.

basal metabolism The rate of combustion of foodstuffs to produce energy when the body is at rest.

basal metabolic rate (BMR)
Also known as resting metabolic rate or RMR, the rate of consumption of oxygen by the patient after an overnight fast and at least an hour's complete rest. This figure is expressed as a percentage of the normal average. Normal range ± 15 per cent.

basal narcosis Deep sleep induced by drugs.

base (1) The bottom. (2) The chief substance of a mixture. (3) In chemistry, an alkali, the substance which combines with an acid to form its salt.

basement membrane Substance probably secreted by the basal cells of an epithelium, which forms a fine membrane separating the epithelium from the underlying structures.

basic (1) Basal. (2) Alkaline. *B. life support*: Assisted ventilation and cardiovascular support.

basilar vertebral insufficiency
See VERTEBROBASILAR INSUF-FICIENCY.

basilic The name of a vein on the inner side of the arm.

basophil Cell whose cytoplasm stains with basic dyes, *e.g.* basophil granulocytes of the blood, basophil cells of the anterior pituitary. *B. adenoma*: tumour of the basophil cells of the pituitary *See* CUSHING'S DISEASE.

basophilic Readily stained with basic dyes in which the cation is the active part.

battered baby syndrome
Physical and/or emotional trauma to any infant or child intentionally inflicted by an adult attending the child. Also known as child abuse, non-accidental injury.

Bazin's disease Purple, tender nodules which may ulcerate. Characteristically on the lower legs of young women with tuberculosis.

BBA *Abbr.* baby born before arrival of mother at delivery suite.

BCG Bacille Calmette-Guérin. A vaccine used for inoculation against tuberculosis.

bearing down Popular term for the expulsive contractions during the second stage of labour when the cervix uteri is fully dilated.

beat Applied to the beating of the heart and pulsation of the blood.

bed bug Insect, the Cimex lectularius, living in furniture

bedsores Ulcerated lesions occurring on pressure areas, *e.g.* buttocks, heels, ankles, elbows, in chronically debilitated patients. More commonly called pressure sores.

behaviour Conduct; or response to certain stimuli. *B. disorder*: abnormal pattern of behaviour in child or adult. May be of physical origin but usually considered a psychological problem.

behaviourism Psychological analysis of behaviour patterns.

Behçet's syndrome Association of ulcers in the mouth and genitalia with often serious eye involvement.

Bell's palsy Peripheral paralysis or palsy of facial nerve.

belladonna Deadly nightshade, the source of atropine.

belle indifférence Abnormal lack of emotional response to distressing circumstances. The cause of this absence of integration is not known.

Bence–Jones protein A protein found in the urine in myelomatosis.

bends *See* CAISSON DISEASE.

Benedict's solution Used in testing urine for sugar.

benign Non-malignant. *B. myalgic encephalomyelitis (BME)*: also known as Royal Free disease or ME, postviral fatigue syndrome or postviral syndrome. It is of unknown aetiology but is said to follow a viral infection; characterized by myalgia, easy fatiguability lasting several months or longer after the original infection. Some doubt about its validity as a single disease.

Bennett's fracture Fracture of the base of the first metacarpal due to a blow on the point of the thumb.

beriberi Polyneuritis some-

times associated with oedema due to deficiency of thiamine, vitamin B_1.

berylliosis Pneumoconiosis from inhalation of beryllium oxide particles.

beryllium window Apparatus designed to allow minimum penetration of the beam in X-ray therapy.

bestiality Intercourse with animals.

beta blockers A group of drugs acting as antagonists at the beta-adrenergic receptor of the sympathetic nervous system. They cause a decrease in heart rate and cardiac output and are commonly used to lower arterial blood pressure in essential hypertension.

beta cells Insulin-producing cells of the islets of Langerhans in the pancreas. Two types of cells are found which were originally distinguished as alpha (α) and beta (β) by the differential solubilities of their cytoplasmic granules.

beta rays *Syn.* beta particles. Electrons emitted by radioactive substances. They will penetrate up to about 1 cm in tissue.

Betz cells Large motor nerve cells present in the cerebral cortex.

bezoars Masses of foreign material present in the gastrointestinal tract of ruminant animals and occasionally man.

bi Prefix meaning two or twice.

biceps The two-headed muscles in front of the humerus and behind the femur. The latter is known as biceps femoris.

bicornuate Having two horns. *B. uterus*: a congenital abnormality due to incomplete development. The uterus may be double or a single organ possessing two horns. Pregnancy may take place in one half and be normal. Very rarely twins may develop, one in each horn.

bicuspid (1) Having two points or cusps. (2) The two teeth immediately behind the canines in each jaw are bicuspids. (3) *B.* or mitral *valve*: the valve between the left atrium and the left ventricle of the heart. Rarely the aortic valve is bicuspid.

bifid Cleft.

bifocal With a double focus. *B. spectacles* can be used for near and distant vision.

bifurcate Forked.

bigeminal pulse Applied to the pulse when a double impulse is produced by 'coupled' heart beats. An extra heart beat occurs just after the normal beat.

bilateral Two-sided. Pertaining to both sides.

bile The secretion of the liver; greenish, bitter, viscid and alkaline. Specific gravity 1010 to 1040. It consists of water, inorganic salts, bile salts, bile pigments. About 570–850 ml secreted daily. *B. duct*: duct transporting the bile from the liver to the duodenum. *B. pigments*: breakdown products of haemoglobin. When red blood cells are broken down their content of haemoglobin is split into two fractions: an iron-containing part which is retained by the body, an iron-free part, porphyrin, from which bilirubin is derived. Bilirubin is converted to a water-soluble glucuronide (conjugated) by the liver and this conjugated bilirubin passes in the bile into the duodenum where it is converted to stercobilinogen which gives the faeces their normal colour. Some of this is reabsorbed and small quantities occur in the urine, urobilinogen.

bilharzia *Syn.* schistosoma. A parasitic worm infesting the portal vein and lymph spaces. The worm's eggs are the main cause of the symptoms in those affected; they are spiny, and therefore cause bleeding wherever they lodge. They are found in enormous numbers in the bladder and rectum.

biliary cirrhosis Liver disease which is considered to affect first the cells adjacent to the bile canaliculi. Two forms are recognized: *primary b.c.* of unknown cause, and *obstructive b.c.*

bilious Connected with bile. Term often used to denote nausea.

bilirubin *See* BILE PIGMENTS.

biliverdin Bile pigment related to bilirubin.

Billroth I gastrectomy Excision of ulcer-bearing lesser curvature of stomach, pyloric antrum and pylorus, followed by gastroduodenostomy.

Billroth II gastrectomy Excision of ulcer-bearing area of stomach or duodenum followed by gastrojejunostomy.

biluria Presence of bile in the urine. Choluria.

bimanual With two hands. By the use of both hands.

binary fission Division of a cell into two equal parts.

binaural Pertaining to both ears.

binge and purge syndrome *See* BULIMIA.

binocular Relating to both eyes.

binovular Produced by two ova. Binovular twins develop from two separate ova fertilized at the same time.

bioassay Quantitative estimation of biologically active substances, *e.g.* hormones, by comparing with a standard preparation, their action on living organisms.

biochemistry The chemistry

of life-processes.

biofeedback Regulation of a body system by a product of the system. In a negative feedback accumulation of the product inhibits further production. In a positive feedback accumulation of the product stimulates further production. Can be used with the help of auditory or visual aids to help a person control a normally unconscious regulation of body function such as heart rate or blood pressure.

biogenesis The birth of living matter from living matter.

biology The science of life and living organisms.

biometry Application of mathematics to biological problems.

biophysics Application of physics to biology.

biopsy Removal of living tissue from the body for pathological examination.

bios The Greek word for life; hence the derivation of such words as 'biology', 'biogenesis'.

biosynthesis Synthesis by living things.

biotin Part of vitamin B complex. Formerly called vitamin H.

Biot's respiration Completely irregular respiration seen in meningitis.

bipolar version *See* VERSION.

birth Being born. *B. injury*: injury to the newborn

sustained at birth. These may be relatively slight, *e.g.* bruising of the scalp, or may be severe, *e.g.* fracture of the skull or long bones, various nerve injuries causing paralysis. *B. mark*: congenital skin defect. Usually denotes abnormal development of dermal blood vessels which give rise to florid areas of skin. *B. paralysis*: birth injury. *B., premature*: an infant is said to have been born prematurely if its birth weight is 2.5 kg or less. The premature baby tends to be drowsy, to suck feebly, and does not cry.

bisexual Person having sexual attraction towards both sexes, *cf.* heterosexual, homosexual.

bistoury A surgical knife.

bitemporal hemianopia Loss of vision in the outer part of the visual field of each eye.

Bitot's spots Conjunctival lesions found in vitamin A deficiency.

blackhead *See* COMEDONES.

black stools Sign of bleeding from the intestine. May also occur in patients taking large quantities of iron tablets.

blackwater fever Acute haemolysis occurring in malaria and leading to excretion of altered haemoglobin in the urine.

bladder A hollow organ for the reception of fluid. *Urinary b.*, receives the urine from the kidneys. *See* GALL BLADDER.

Blalock's operation The subclavian artery is anastomosed to the pulmonary artery. Performed in cases of congenital pulmonary stenosis. *See* FALLOT'S TETRALOGY.

bland Mild, non-irritating.

blast cell Primitive cell which can usually divide to yield more mature forms.

blast injury Injury sustained as a result of blast wave from explosion.

Blastomyces A genus of pathogenic fungi.

blastomycosis A skin disease caused by the invasion of a yeast-like organism.

blastula Early stage in development of fertilized ovum.

bleb *See* BLISTER.

bleeder *See* HAEMOPHILIA.

bleeding time The duration of bleeding following puncture of the skin.

blennophthalmia Mucoid discharge from the eye.

blennorrhoea Mucous discharge from urethra.

blepharitis Inflammation of the eyelids.

blepharoptosis *See* PTOSIS.

blepharospasm *See* BLINKING.

blind loop syndrome Disconnection of a loop of small intestine from alimentary tract mainstream which causes decrease in fat absorption from intestine.

blind spot Point where the optic nerve enters the retina.

blindness Lack of sight. *Colour b.*: an inability to distinguish certain colours. *Cortical b.*: blindness due to a lesion of the visual centre in the brain. *Night b.* or nyctalopia: vision subnormal at night, thought to be due to a deficiency of vitamin A in the diet. *Snow b.*: dimness of vision with pain and lacrimation due to the glare of sunlight upon the snow. *Word b.*: inability to recognize familiar written words owing to a lesion of the brain.

blinking Normal spasmodic closure of eyelids. Increased frequency commonly due to a foreign body in the eye.

blister Usually refers to collection of fluid in or under the epidermis. Blisters greater than 5 mm in diameter are termed bullae; those smaller are termed vesicles.

blood Fluid circulating through blood vessels which serves as a transport system for oxygen, food materials, waste products, etc. It may be divided into cellular and non-cellular components. The cellular component consists of the red blood cells (RBCs or erythrocytes) and a smaller number of white cells (leucocytes). The non-cellular component (plasma) is a complex solution containing many proteins. One of these, fibrinogen, is important in the blood-clotting mechanism and can be removed by allowing the plasma to clot. This leaves the serum which contains albumin and globulins.

blood bank Store containing blood of various groups and also blood products. In the UK blood is donated and treated to remove possible pathogens before being released for transfusion.

blood–brain barrier Term used to denote the fact that a number of substances which are found in the blood do not appear in the cerebrospinal fluid. Apart from academic interest, it is important as some antibiotic drugs are unable to cross the blood–brain barrier.

blood casts Small shreds of coagulated blood present in the urine in renal injury.

blood cells Usually divided into red blood cells (RBCs or erythrocytes) and white blood cells (WBCs or leucocytes). The RBCs are biconcave in shape and measure about 7 μm in diameter. They have no nuclei and contain haemoglobin. The WBCs are divided into three groups: (1) Cells which contain granules in the cytoplasm; these are classed as basophil, neutrophil or eosinophil (acidophil) granulocytes according to the staining of the granules. (2) Lymphocytes, which have an even nucleus and relatively little clear cytoplasm. (3) Monocytes, relatively large cells with kidney-shaped nuclei. The function of the RBCs is to transport oxygen. The function of the various WBCs is in the defence of the body against infection by phagocytosis and the production of antibodies.

blood coagulation Also clotting of blood. The mechanism for stopping haemorrhage after injury to blood vessels. The two processes involved are the aggregation of platelets to form a plug which seals the leaking vessel, and the so-called clotting cascade which results in the conversion of fibrinogen to fibrin which forms the basis for the repair of the damaged vessel. Absence of clotting factors results in bleeding disorders such as haemophilia, Christmas disease, afibrinogen aemia.

blood count By the use of special dilution techniques and a counting chamber the number of cells in a sample of blood may be estimated by microscopic examination. The figure is expressed as the number of cells per mm³. The normal range is approximately 5 million RBCs and 5000–10 000 WBCs. In a *differential b.c.*, the number of different types of WBC, *see above*, are expressed as a percentage of the total WBC count.

blood destruction The normal processes of destruction of old blood cells occur in the spleen. Abnormal destruction of RBCs may take place in the blood vessels and this is known as haemolysis. *See* HAEMOLYTIC.

blood dyscrasias Any abnormal features of the blood cells.

blood formation Except in infants and in certain disease states the blood cells are manufactured in the bone marrow. Some lymphocytes are produced by lymphoid tissue (lymph glands).

blood grouping For a blood transfusion it is essential that the blood of the donor be compatible with that of the patient. Blood grouping is decided according to the presence or absence of certain agglutinogens in the corpuscles, two in number, A and B. The international nomenclature of the different groups is as follows: AB, A, B, O. In group AB are those who may receive blood from any other group and are called universal recipients. Group A may receive blood from groups A and O. Group

B may receive blood from groups B and O. Group O may receive only from group O. From the above it will be seen that group O can give blood to all other groups, and therefore is a universal donor. Before transfusion a direct match is always made between the red cells of the donor and the serum of the recipient. Any clumping together or agglutination of the corpuscles which can be seen even with the naked eye means incompatibility. The rhesus (Rh) factor: in human beings of most races 85 per cent possess this agglutinogen in their red cells, and are termed 'Rh positive'. The remaining 15 per cent, 'Rh negative', are liable to form an antibody (agglutinin) against the agglutinogen, if it is introduced into their circulation. It may occur in an Rh negative woman if she becomes pregnant with a fetus whose blood cells are Rh positive or if an Rh negative person is transfused with Rh positive blood. Other blood groups include M, N, P, Lewis, Duffy, Kell, Lutheran, etc.

blood-letting Bleeding, phlebotomy, venesection. The withdrawal of blood for therapeutic purposes from a vein.

blood plasma *See* PLASMA.

blood platelets These are small fragmentary bodies produced by the breakdown of special cells, megakaryocytes, in the bone marrow. *See* BLOOD COAGULATION.

blood pressure The pressure exerted by the blood in the vessels in which it is contained. It is taken in the brachial artery and estimated in terms of the number of millimetres pressure of mercury (mm Hg) required, on the upper arms, just to obliterate the pulse at the wrist. This figure is the *systolic b.p.* The average systolic pressure in a young adult is 100–120. The *diastolic b.p.* is the pressure in the artery during the resting phase of the cardiac cycle, *i.e.* the lowest pressure. The average diastolic pressure is 70 to 90 in a young adult. It rises with age. High blood pressure is present in arteriosclerosis, and some kinds of kidney and heart disease.

blood sedimentation rate Also called erythrocyte sedimentation rate (ESR). It is a measure of the rate at which red cells clump together. Clumping of RBCs, and therefore a raised sedimentation rate, is increased by the presence of certain proteins in the blood. The test is a nonspecific index of disease.

blood serum *See* SERUM.

blood sugar The amount of sugar normally in the blood is about 0.08 to 0.12 per cent or 4.6 to 7.0 mmol/l of blood. This figure rises slightly after a meal but not to more than about 10 mmol/l and returns to a normal level within 2 hours. Above this figure, sugar leaks through into the urine. The amount in the blood can be raised artifically by a meal of glucose; and the blood sugar is raised in diabetes mellitus.

blood transfusion The transference of blood from a healthy individual to one suffering from a grave degree of anaemia due to either haemorrhage or disease. The donor's blood must belong to the same or to a compatible group. *See* BLOOD GROUPING. Clotting is prevented by the addition of 3.8 per cent sodium citrate solution. The blood is taken from a suitable vein of the arm; the quantity is usually 0.5 litres (1 pint). This is allowed to flow from the needle in the arm along a piece of short tubing into a vacuum bottle containing citrate solution; all needles and tubing have previously been run through with citrate solution. The blood is injected into the patient (1) the closed method, through a thick hollow needle into the vein, (2) the vein of the patient is cut down upon, isolated and lifted; an incision is made into it, a small cannula slipped into the opening and tied there. The blood is then slowly run in from a giving set through a drip cannula. After the cannula in the arm is withdrawn, the vein is tied above and below and the skin incision closed.

blood urea Normally between 2.5 to 6.6 mmol/l of blood, rising to a higher figure with increasing age. An abnormal amount of urea present usually shows deficient kidney function.

blood volume The calculated amount of blood in the whole body, about 4.5 litres in the normal adult.

blue baby Cyanosed infant due to circulatory defects which prevent adequate oxygenation of the blood, or which mix venous and arterial blood.

blue-dome cyst A bluish-coloured benign cyst which appears in the female breast at age 40–50, associated with fibrous overgrowth of surrounding stroma.

blue line Present on gums in lead poisoning.

blue sclera A feature of osteogenesis imperfecta.

BME *Abbr.* benign myalgic encephalomyelitis.

BMR *Abbr.* basal metabolic rate. *See* BASAL METABOLISM.

BMT   *Abbr.* bone marrow transplant.

BNA   *Abbr.* Basle Nomina Anatomica. Naming of anatomical terms agreed in Switzerland in 1895.

BNF   *Abbr.* British National Formulary.

Bodecker index   The ratio between the number of tooth surfaces (five to a tooth) which are carious and the total number of surfaces of the teeth which could be affected.

body image   The image one has of one's own body. Characteristically distorted in the eating disorders such as anorexia and bulimia in which subjects see themselves as overweight.

body language   Non-verbal, often subconscious communication by facial expressions and body movement.

body rocking   One of a variety of rhythmic movements seen in infancy and childhood. Occurs most commonly in children deprived of an adequate feeling of security.

Boeck's disease   *See* SAR-COIDOSIS.

boil   Furuncle. A staphylococcal infection of the skin, causing inflammation round a hair follicle.

bolus   A large round mass such as that of food before it is swallowed.

bonding   The development of the relationship between a mother and her newborn baby in the immediate postnatal period.

bone   Hard material forming the skeleton. It is made up of organized connective tissue in which calcium salts are deposited. *B. graft*: a portion of bone is transplanted to remedy a defect. *B. marrow*: fatty substance contained within the marrow cavity of bones. In the flat bones, and with children in the long bones as well, the fat is replaced by active blood-forming tissue, which is responsible for production of the granular leucocytes, the red cells and platelets. *B. m. puncture*: method by which specimen of blood-forming marrow tissue is obtained. The bone is punctured and a specimen of marrow cells withdrawn through a needle.

borborygmus (pl. **borborygmi**) Rumbling of intestinal flatus.

Bordetella pertussis   Organism causing whooping cough.

Bornholm disease   Epidemic diaphragmatic pleurodynia.

boss   A projection.

botulism   Follows ingestion of food contaminated by the toxin of Clostridium botulinus. Usually fatal.

bougie   Instrument used to dilate passages.

bougienage Dilation of a structure by bougie.

bowel The intestine. The gut. It consists of the small and large intestine. The small intestine is about 6.1 m long and divided into duodenum, 30 cm long; jejunum, about 2.4 m long; ileum, about 3.65 m long. The large intestine is about 152 cm long and consists of (1) the caecum with the vermiform appendix; (2) ascending colon, running up the right side; (3) transverse colon, running from right to left; (4) descending colon, running down left side; (5) sigmoid or pelvic colon, passing to (6) rectum which opens externally via (7) the anal canal.

Bowen's disease A premalignant condition affecting exposed skin. May progress to squamous carcinoma if untreated.

Bowleg Genu varum.

Bowman's capsules Malpighian capsules which surround glomeruli in the kidney. *See* MALPIGHIAN CORPUSCLE.

BP *Abbr.* blood pressure.

brachial Pertaining to the arm. *B. artery*: the main artery of the arm, a continuation of the axillery artery. *B. plexus*: the plexus of nerves supplying the arm, forearm and hand. *B. neuralgia*: *Syn.* brachial neuritis. Pain in the arm due to pressure on the

roots of the brachial plexus. Comparable with sciatica in the leg.

brachium The arm.

brachycephaly Descriptive of shape of head in which the anteroposterior diameter is relatively short. Principally of anthropological interest but may be of some importance in obstetrics.

bradycardia Slow heart beat.

bradykinin Peptide formed by enzymatic degradation of protein.

brain The main integrating mass of nervous tissue situated in the skull. It may be divided into cerebral hemispheres, cerebellum and brain stem.

branchial Pertaining to the gills. Thus *b. cysts* are sometimes found in certain regions of the neck as vestiges of the gill stage of fetal development.

Braun's splint Type of lower limb splint with extension frame.

breast (1) The milk-secreting gland. (2) The anterior surface of the thorax. *See also* MAMMAE.

breath Air taken into and expelled from the lungs. *B. of life*: kiss of life. Mouth-to-mouth respiration used as a resuscitatory measure. *B. sounds*: the sounds heard by auscultation of the chest during respiration. *B.-holding*: a behaviour disorder of infants and children.

breathing exercises Physiotherapy to improve ventilation of the lungs.

breech The buttocks. *B. presentation*: presentation of buttocks of fetus.

bregma *See* FONTANELLE.

Brenner tumour Fibromatous ovarian tumour with epithelial cells generally benign.

Bright's disease Kidney disease, now classified as type II nephritis characterized by albumin in the urine and oedema.

brittle bones *See* OSTEOGENESIS IMPERFECTA.

broad ligaments The folds of peritoneum with the contained ligaments, blood vessels, fallopian tubes, etc., which pass outwards on each side of the uterus.

Broca's area On left side of brain exercising control of movement of lips, tongue and vocal cords, and therefore the motor speech area. *See* APHASIA.

Brodie's abscess Chronic abscess of bone. The tibia is most commonly affected.

bromidrosis Offensive sweating, most common in the feet.

bromism Poisoning by bromides.

bronchi (sing. **bronchus**) Tubes into which the trachea divides.

bronchial Pertaining to the bronchi. *B. breathing*: abnormal breath sounds heard on auscultation over consolidated lung as in lobar pneumonia. *B. carcinoma*: cancer arising from the lining of a bronchus. *B. tubes*: *see* BRONCHI.

bronchiectasis Pathological dilatation of bronchi.

bronchiole A small bronchus.

bronchiolitis Inflammation of the bronchioles.

bronchitis Acute bronchitis may follow an upper respiratory tract infection. Chronic bronchitis is often associated with the pathological changes of emphysema and is most commonly due to cigarette smoking.

bronchogenic Originating from a bronchus.

bronchography Instillation of radio-opaque dye in the bronchi, so that they are apparent on x-ray.

broncholith A bronchial calculus.

bronchophony Voice resonance heard over bronchi.

bronchopneumonia Pneumonia, beginning in the bronchioles, affecting scattered lobules of the lung and also the finest or capillary bronchioles.

bronchoscope An instrument for seeing into the main bronchi.

bronchoscopy Examination of the bronchi with a bronchoscope.

bronchospasm Spasm of the muscles in the bronchial walls, usually associated wtih copious secretion of mucus into the bronchi, results of respiratory difficulty. *See* ASTHMA.

brow presentation Presentation of brow in fetus.

Brown's splints Metal splints for correction of talipes equinovarus.

Brownian movement Oscillatory movement seen under the microscope in fine particles suspended in a liquid.

Brown–Séquard syndrome Complex neurological syndrome resulting from damage to one-half of the spinal cord.

Brucella abortus Organism causing brucellosis. It causes abortion in cows and is present in the milk of infected cows. Similar organisms are present in infected goat's milk.

brucellosis Undulant fever. Infection with an organism of the Brucella group.

Brudzinski's sign Passive flexion of the thigh causes spontaneous flexion of the opposite thigh. Sign of meningeal irritation.

bruise A contusion. The skin is not broken but is discoloured due to bleeding in the underlying tissues.

bruit The French for 'sound', used with regard to the sounds heard in auscultation.

Brunner's glands Glands of the duodenum.

Bryant's gallows traction A device for holding the hips flexed and in abduction and used for the treatment of congenital dislocation of the hip.

bubo Inflammatory swelling of lymph glands, particularly of groin.

bubonic plague Oriental plague, which in some forms is characterized by the development of buboes.

buccal Pertaining to the mouth.

buccinator The muscle of the cheek; one of the muscles of mastication.

Budd–Chiari syndrome Syndrome consisting of vomiting, jaundice and enlargement of the liver and ascites due to thrombosis of the hepatic vein.

Buerger's disease Thromboangiitis obliterans. Rare disease of blood vessels resulting in reduction of blood supply to extremities.

buffer A substance stabilizing changes in the pH of a solution.

bulb A rounded expansion of an organ.

bulbar palsy Paralysis due to disease of the medulla oblongata.

bulimia A disorder characterized by alternate excessive eating and purging or vomiting. One of the so-called eating disorders. *See also* ANOREXIA NERVOSA.

bullae Large blisters, *cf.* vesicle.

bundle branch block Term applied to ECG evidence of delay in conduction in either the left or right branch of the atrioventricular bundle.

bundle of His *See* ATRIOVENT-RICULAR BUNDLE.

bunion Inflammation of a bursa situated over the meta-tarsophalangeal joint of the great toe.

burette Graduated tube with a tap which allows measured volumes of a reagent to be dispensed.

Burkitt's lymphoma A malignant lymphoma occurring most commonly in the jaw, orbits and retroperitoneum. The geographical distribution parallels with malaria. It may be due to infection with the Epstein–Barr virus.

burns Burns may be produced by various physical and chemical agents. They may be local or widespread and are classified according to the depth of tissue destruction. (1) First degree burns involve only the epidermis. (2) Second degree burns involve dermis and epidermis. (3) Third degree burns extend into deep structures, *cf.* scald.

Burns–Marshall technique Method of delivering a breech presentation.

burr hole Circular hole cut in cranium to allow access to the brain.

bursa A small sac interposed between movable parts.

bursitis Inflammation of a bursa.

buttock Breech. Nates.

byssinosis A type of pneumoconiosis caused by in-halation of cotton dust.

C

cachet Capsule in which powders of disagreeable taste are enclosed.

cachexia A chronic state of malnutrition and debility produced by absorption of toxins.

cadaver A corpse.

caecostomy Operation to provide an opening into the caecum through the abdominal wall.

caecum The blind intestine, a cul-de-sac at the commencement of the large intestine. *See* BOWEL and APPENDIX VERMIFORMIS.

caesarean section Delivery of the fetus through an incision in the abdominal and uterine walls.

café au lait pigmentation Areas of skin pigmentation characteristic of neurofibromatosis.

caffeine The alkaloid of coffee and tea; a cerebral stimulant and diuretic.

caisson disease Also known as 'the bends'. The effect on those working under a greater atmospheric pressure than normal, *e.g.* in deep mines or under water. Return to normal pressure should be effected gradually or nitrogen bubbles form in the blood and tissues.

calcaneal spur A bony outgrowth from the calcaneum leading to persistent local tenderness on the sole of the foot.

calcaneus The os calcis or heel bone.

calcareous Containing calcium phosphate.

calciferol Vitamin D. Its function is to regulate calcium metabolism.

calcification Deposition of insoluble calcium salts, *e.g.* calcium phosphate, in tissue. This is normal in bone but may occur in other sites.

calcitonin Hormone which regulates blood calcium levels.

calculus A stone. The term generally refers to a concretion in the urinary tract.

Caldwell-Luc operation Operation to drain the maxillary antrum.

calibrate To graduate an instrument for measuring according to a given standard.

calipers or **callipers** (1) Surgical instruments for measuring the chest, the pelvis, etc.

(2) *Icetong c.*: a two-pointed instrument used for fixing a bone by actual penetration of some of it, as in the treatment of fractures. (3) *Walking c.*: an instrument fixed at the lower end to a boot. At the upper end is a padded ring which fits round the groin and under the ischial tuberosity. This takes the weight off an injured leg when walking.

callosity Thickened horny layer of epidermis formed on palmar and plantar surfaces which are subject to much friction.

callus (1) Material which first joins broken bone. It consists predominantly of connective tissue and cartilage, which later calcifies. (2) Callosity.

calor Heat.

calorie Scientific term for the standard unit of heat. One kilocalorie (kcal, Cal) is the amount of heat required to raise 1 litre of water by 1°C. The amount of heat produced in the body by the combustion of food can be estimated. A diet should yield an adequate number of calories per day. One calorie is the amount of heat necessary to raise 1 g H_2O by 1°C. The unit is now the joule. 1 kcal = 4.2 kJ.

calorific Producing heat.

calorimeter An apparatus for determining the amount of heat yielded by combustion of a substance.

calvarium The upper half of the skull. The cranial vault.

calyx A cup-shaped organ or cavity such as those of the recesses of the pelvis of the kidney.

canal of Nuck A narrow passage along which the round ligament passes to the region of the pubes; it is sometimes the seat of inguinal hernia and occasionally of cysts.

canaliculus A small canal.

cancelli The uncalcified spaces of bone.

cancer A malignant growth usually classified according to its tissue and organ of origin. *See* CARCINOMA, SARCOMA.

cancerophobia Excessive fear of cancer.

cancroid Cancer-like.

cancrum oris Ulceration of the mouth. Has nothing to do with cancer.

candida A genus of fungi, commonly infecting the mouth, vulva and vagina as oral or vaginal thrush. Systemic candidiasis may occur in immunosuppressed patients, *e.g.* those with AIDS.

canicola fever Disease produced by Leptospira canicola. Characterized by malaise, fever, muscle pains, and occasionally jaundice.

canine teeth The four eye teeth, next to the incisors. *See* TEETH.

canker Ulceration.

cannabis Hemp, hashish.

cannula Surgical name for a tube used to withdraw fluid from a cavity. *See* TROCAR.

canthus The angle of the eyelids, outer or inner.

capelline bandage Bandage for the head.

capillaries The network of microscopic vessels which communicate with the arterioles and the venules. The walls are formed of a single layer of endothelium.

capillary fragility test Fragility of capillary vessels is measured by applying suction to a small area of skin and recording the negative pressure required to produce haemorrhage. *See also* HESS'S TEST.

capillary naevus Also known as a congenital abnormal dilatation of capillary blood vessels.

capitate (1) Like a head. (2) One of the carpal bones.

capsular ligament A ligament surrounding a movable joint.

capsule Connective tissue sheath investing an organ.

capsulitis Term usually used to describe pain in the shoulder joint causing limitation of movement.

capsulotomy An incision of the capsule of the lens of the eye.

caput succedaneum Swelling on infant's scalp, due to pressure during labour.

carbohydrate Compound of the general formula C_x $(H_2O)_y$ such as sugar and starch. Carbohydrates are of central importance in cell metabolism.

carbon dioxide (CO_2) A gas which is a product of combustion. It is formed in the system by the metabolic process of the body, and excreted through the lungs. It is a respiratory stimulant and is administered diluted with oxygen when respiration is depressed. At extremely low temperatures this gas forms a liquid, and lower still a substance resembling snow. The latter is often used for destroying naevi and similar superficial growths on the skin.

carbon monoxide poisoning Poisoning by inhalation of carbon monoxide, CO, *e.g.* from coal gas or motor vehicle exhaust. Symptoms begin as giddiness and singing of ears, then lividity of face and body; later, owing to combination of the gas with the blood, the patient may have a rosy tinge; loss of muscular power; violent action of heart and lungs; fixed dilated pupils, convulsions, coma or asphyxia. Treatment: fresh air, oxygen and artificial respiration if necessary.

carboxyhaemoglobin A compound of carbon monoxide and haemoglobin formed in coal-gas poisoning.

carbuncle Severe staphylococcal inflammation of an area of skin and subcutaneous tissue. There is necrosis and liquefaction of the subcutaneous tissue and several points of discharge.

carcinogenic Term applied to substances producing or predisposing to cancer.

carcinoid syndrome Collection of symptoms associated with carcinoid tumour. These include flushing, diarrhoea and bronchospasm.

carcinoid tumour A tumour of the argentaffin cells of the gut, usually appendix or occasionally ovary. Secretes serotonin (5-hydroxytryptamine) causing carcinoid syndrome.

carcinoma Cancer of epithelial tissue.

carcinoma-in-situ Early stage of carcinoma in which the growing cells have not invaded surrounding tissues.

carcinomatosis The spread of carcinomatous metastases.

cardia (1) The heart. (2) The aperture between the oesophagus and the stomach.

cardiac Relating to the heart. *C. arrest*: stopping of the heart. *C. catheterization*: investigation carried out to diagnose certain heart conditions. A catheter is introduced through a vein in the arm into the chambers of the heart from which pressure recordings can be obtained. *C. cycle*: the recurrent train of events which produce a heart beat. *C. failure*: when the contraction of the heart is insufficient to expel a volume of blood equal to that which fills it there is a damming back of blood on the venous side of the circulation with the consequent production of the clinical signs of congestive cardiac failure (CCF). *C. massage*: direct cardiac massage consists of squeezing the heart rhythmically to stimulate the normal heart beat in an attempt to restart the circulation, having first gained access to the heart through an incision in the chest. More recently external cardiac massage has been widely used to restart the heart. This consists of pressing on the chest with patient lying flat on his back so that the heart is rhythmically compressed between the front and back of the thoracic cage. *C. tamponade*: the action of the heart is impeded by the accumulation of fluid in the pericardium.

cardinal ligaments Fan-shaped fibromuscular expansions passing from the cervix and vault of the vagina to the pelvic wall which forms part of the support of the uterus and vagina.

cardiograph Also known as electrocardiograph (ECG or EKG). Instrument which records the electrical potentials which reflect the conduction of impulses and other electrical events in the heart.

cardiology Study of the heart and circulatory diseases.

cardiomyopathy Disease of heart muscle not caused by specific infection.

cardiomyotomy Operation to relieve muscular spasm at the lower end of the oesophagus.

cardiospasm Achalasia of cardia.

cardiovascular Pertaining to the heart and circulatory system.

carditis Inflammation of the heart muscle.

caries Decay of teeth.

carina Literally a 'keel'. Term sometimes applied to ridges.

carminative A remedy for flatulence, *e.g.* oil of peppermint.

carneous Flesh-like. *C. mole*: term sometimes used to describe retained products of conception.

carotene A yellow pigment occurring in some plants. It is a precursor of vitamin A.

carotid Name given to the two great arteries of the neck, and to structures connected with them. *C. body*: specialized tissue found at the bifurcation of the carotid artery (into internal and external carotids) which is sensitive to chemical changes in the blood. *C. sinus*: region of the carotid artery just below its bifurcation which is sensitive to pressure and acts as one of the blood pressure regulating mechanisms. *C. sinus syncope*: may occur in individuals who have hypersensitive carotid sinuses; loss of consciousness may follow pressure on the sinus by an abrupt movement of the neck, etc.

carpal tunnel syndrome Numbness and tingling in the fingers and hand as a result of compression of the median nerve at the wrist.

carpometacarpal Relating to a carpus and metacarpus.

carpopedal spasm Cramp in hands and feet which occurs typically in conditions in which there is a deficiency of ionized calcium in the blood.

carpus The wrist.

carrier An individual who transmits disease without showing symptoms of it. (1) Genetic defects may be masked by other genes in a carrier. (2) Microorganisms may be harboured in the body, *e.g.* typhoid bacilli. In families with inherited diseases an unaffected female may carry the defect in her genes and if sex-linked her sons may inherit the disease

and her daughters become carriers.

cartilage Gristle; a transparent substance of the body, very elastic and softer than bone.

caruncle Small pedunculated granulomatous mass. *Lacrimal c.*: the small red globe at the inner corner of the eye. *Urethral c.*: pea-sized vascular growth in the urethra which may give rise to urinary symptoms in elderly women.

caseation Conversion into cheesy material, as in breaking down of tuberculous glands.

casein An albuminous component of milk.

Casoni test Intradermal test used for the diagnosis of hydatid disease.

castration Removal of the testes, *cf.* sterilization.

casts Pieces of material taking shape of cavity from which they have been expelled, *e.g.* blood or epithelial debris found in the urine in kidney disease, membranous casts from large bowel in mucous colitis.

cat scratch fever Fever transmitted by the scratch of apparently healthy cats. The causative organism has not been isolated.

catabolism Biochemical reactions taking place in living tissues (metabolism) are divided into those involved in building up or synthesis of material (anabolism) and those involved in breaking down or lysis of material (catabolism).

catalepsy A period of trance, during which the limbs remain in any position in which they are placed.

catalyst A substance which takes part in a reaction, not itself being changed. Enzymes are catalysts.

cataphoresis Introduction of positively charged ions.

cataplexy A rigid muscular condition produced by fear or shock.

cataract May be congenital or acquired. Congenital cataracts occur in rubella syndrome. Acquired cataracts may be associated with age and with certain disorders such as diabetes.

catarrh Inflammation of the mucous membrane, generally applied to the nose and throat, and also to internal organs, *e.g.* the bile ducts.

catatonia State of generalized muscular inhibition in schizophrenia.

catgut Material prepared from sheep's intestine and used for absorbable ligatures.

catharsis Emotional relief brought about by the conscious realization of suppressed desire.

cathartic Literally can be a drastic purge. Can also be

used in sense of release of pent-up emotions.

catheter Instrument used for the passage of fluids, usually from the bladder where there is urethral obstruction. *Nasal c.* (Ryle's tube): used for the administration of fluid feeds. The tube passes through the nose down the throat into the stomach. *Eustachian c.*: a special tube used to inflate the pharyngotympanic (Eustachian) tube.

cathode The negative pole of an electric battery.

cation exchange resin *See* ION EXCHANGE RESIN.

cauda equina The bundle of sacral and lumbar nerves at the base of the spine.

caudal analgesia Regional anaesthesia of the rectum and perineum produced by injecting local anaesthetics into the sacral canal through the sacral hiatus.

caul Fetal membranes about the face and head of some infants at birth.

causalgia Pain referred to the distribution of a cutaneous nerve which persists long after an inquiry to that nerve. Causalgia often follows herpes zoster (shingles). The cause is not known.

caustic Substance, usually a strong alkali or acid, which destroys cells and causes chemical 'burns'.

cautery Application of

heated metal to living tissue in order to destroy it or to arrest haemorrhage.

cavernous naevus Abnormal development of blood vessels which are greatly enlarged and dilated.

cavernous sinus A blood sinus on the body of the sphenoid bone. Related to optic nerve. *C.s. thrombosis*: thrombosis within the cavernous sinus. A rare complication of head and neck sepsis and can cause blindness.

cavitation Process whereby cavities are formed.

cavity of pelvis The space between the pelvic inlet and outlet.

cell Discrete mass of protoplasm bounded by a membrane which forms the basic reproducible structural unit of living organisms. There are about 10^{12} cells in a human. Generally speaking cells contain a nucleus which harbours the genetic material – the DNA blueprints – which provide the instructions for the synthesis of materials by the cytoplasmic component. The advent of electron microscopy has revealed the cytoplasm to be exceedingly complex. The nuclear material (which contains one or more nucleoli, the function of which is unclear) is discontinuously bounded by a double membrane which projects and branches into the cytoplasm forming a complex network of interconnecting canals. In places this network opens exteriorly to the cell, becoming continuous with the cell wall. The canalicular system in the cell is called the endoplasmic reticulum (ER) and it is thought that it is made by the Golgi apparatus. In some places the endoplasmic reticulum is closely associated with ribosomes, tiny granular structures which are the sites of protein synthesis. The cytoplasmic material between the canals of the endoplasmic reticulum contains mitochondria which are the centres housing the respiratory enzymes, and lysosomes which are specialized organelles containing catabolic enzymes.

cellulitis Inflammation of cellular tissue. *Pelvic c.*: *see* PARAMETRITIS.

cellulose The woody, fibrous part of plants. It has no food value but forms bulk in the colon and so stimulates peristalsis. In the form of wood wool, cellulose is used as an absorbent dressing.

Celsius In SI units the equivalent of the centigrade scale which is now obsolete.

censorship Freudian term for the barrier preventing repressed memories, ideas and impulses from easily coming into consciousness.

centigrade *See* CELSIUS.

centimetre (cm) Metric unit of length, one hundredth of a metre. Approximately 2.5 cm equal 1 inch.

central nervous system (CNS) General term incorporating the brain and spinal cord, as opposed to the peripheral nervous system which includes the nerves and sensory receptors outside the brain and spinal cord.

centrifugal nerve fibres Usually called efferent nerves; those which conduct impulses leaving the central system.

centrifuge An instrument for separating liquids of different specific gravity by rotation.

centriole Small granule situated just outside the nuclear membrane and found in many resting cells. Just before mitosis this granule divides and at mitosis the two resulting centrioles move apart and form the poles of the spindle.

centripetal nerve fibres Usually called afferent nerves; those which conduct impulses entering the central nervous system.

centromere Spindle-attachment. The region of the chromosome which attaches it to the spindle which is composed of long protein molecules passing between chromosomes and the centriole when the cell is dividing.

centrosome Region of differentiated cytoplasm in which the centriole is situated.

cephalhaematoma A subperiosteal haemorrhage on the head of an infant, usually due to pressure during a long labour. It is gradually absorbed.

cephalic Of the head. *C. presentation* is infant in utero with head over the pelvis. *C. version*: the production artificially of a cephalic presentation, from a breech presentation or transverse lie. *See* VERSION.

cephalocele Hernia of the brain.

cephalometry Estimation of the size of the head of a fetus, usually by radiographic means.

cephalotribe An instrument consisting of two blades and a screw, used to crush the fetal head when intact delivery is impossible.

cerebellum Outgrowth from the hindbrain overlaying the medulla oblongata. Concerned with the coordination of movement.

cerebral Of the brain. *C. cortex*: outer rim of grey matter of the brain. *C. embolism*: embolism of vessels supplying the cerebral cortex and its major connections. *C. haemorrhage*: rupture of an artery of the brain, due to either high blood pressure or disease of artery. Escape of blood causes destruction of brain tissue, and paralysis occurs of that side of the body which is opposite to the injured side of the brain. If the haemorrhage has occurred on the left side of the brain, then speech is affected in right-handed subjects. *C. palsy*: a condition in which the control of the motor system is affected due to a lesion in the brain resulting from a birth injury or pre-natal defect. The popular term is 'spastic'. *C. thrombosis*: thrombus formation in vessels supplying the cerebral cortex or its major connections.

cerebration Thinking: activity of the brain related to conscious thought processes.

cerebrospinal fluid (CSF) The clear watery fluid which lies in the subarachnoid space, surrounding the brain and spinal chord. It also fills the cavities or ventricle of the brain.

cerebrovascular accident General term referring to cerebral embolism, thrombosis or haemorrhage.

cerebrum The larger part of the brain occupying the cranium. *See* BRAIN.

cerumen Secretion of the ceruminous glands situated in the external auditory meatus. The secretion is a wax-like substance closely related to sebum, the oily secretion of the sebaceous glands.

cervical From Latin = neck. Hence the neck or the cervix uteri. (1) Pertaining to the neck. *C. rib*: an outgrowth from the seventh cervical vertebra passing out and down to join the rib below. It may press on nerve trunks to the arm causing pins and needles in hands and fingers. *C. spondylosis*: degenerative changes in the intervertebral discs of the cervical spine with associated secondary osteoarthritic changes in the intervertebral joints of the neck. (2) Pertaining to the cervix or neck of the uterus. *C. dystocia*: failure of relaxation of the external os of the cervix. A rare cause of mechanical obstruction to the delivery of a child. *C. intraepithelial neoplasia (CIN)*: premalignant changes within the cervical epithelium. CIN III includes severe dysplasia and carcinoma-in-situ. Must be confirmed histologically and may respond to local therapy, *e.g.* laser. *C. smear*: sample of mucosa taken from the cervix uteri, smeared on to a glass slide and examined microscopically for the appearance of the cells it contains.

cervicectomy Excision of the cervix uteri.

cervicitis Inflammation of the cervix of the uterus.

cervix uteri The neck of the uterus. The lowest third of the uterus, about 2.5 cm in length. It is traversed by a canal which opens into the vagina.

Cestoda Class of platyhelminths: tapeworms.

CF *Abbr.* cystic fibrosis.

CFT *Abbr.* complement fixation test.

chalazion Meibomian cyst. A small retention cyst in the eyelid, due to blocking of a meibomian follicle.

chancre Syphilitic ulcer of the first stage; occurs at the site of infection. Contagious.

chancroid A venereal ulcer due to infection by Haemophilus ducreyi.

Charcot–Marie–Tooth disease *See* PERONEAL MUSCULAR ATROPHY.

Charcot's joint Painless destructive changes in a joint due to loss of sensation.

Charcot's triad Nystagmus, intention tremor and scanning speech; manifestations of advanced multiple sclerosis.

cheilitis Inflammation of the lip.

cheiloplasty Plastic operation on the lips.

cheilosis Condition affecting the lips and angles of the mouth which can be caused by riboflavin deficiency.

cheiropompholyx An eczematous eruption on the hands characterized by the appearance of tense vesicles.

chelating agent Substance which forms a complex with metals, thus rendering them chemically inactive.

chemoreceptor Nerve ending capable of detecting and differentiating substances according to their chemical structure by contact with the molecules of the substances, *e.g.* taste, smell.

chemosis Oedema of the conjunctiva.

chemotaxis Tendency for cells to move through a chemical gradient.

chemotherapy Treatment of disease by administration of drugs. Hence: *antibacterial c.*: use of antibiotics; *antiviral c.*: use of antiviral drugs; *anticancer c.*: use of anti-cancer drugs, etc.

chemotropism *Syn.* chemotaxis.

Cheyne-Stokes breathing Irregular respiration, at first shallow, then increasing in depth till a maximum is reached, when it decreases again until imperceptible and a pause ensues, during which breathing is absent. Usually a bad sign, and due to a poor supply of oxygen to that part of the brain containing the respiratory centre.

chiasm A crossing.

chiasma opticum *See* OPTIC CHIASMA.

chickenpox A virus disease.

57

Varicella. Rash appears on the chest on the first day; the disease runs its course in a fortnight. Incubation period, 10–16 days. Quarantine period for contacts, 20 days.

chilblain Pernio. Inflammation of the skin due to cellular damage as a result of local deficiency in the circulation.

chimera Organism whose tissues are composed of cells of two or more genetically different sorts.

chiropodist One qualified in the treatment of the feet and hands.

chiropractic Manipulation of the spine to relieve pain from compressed nerve roots.

chiropractor A person skilled in chiropractic and its application to the relief of pain and other symptoms.

chirurgical Surgical.

chloasma Usually *c. gravidarum*. A patchy hyperpigmentation of face associated with pregnancy.

chloroform Anaesthetic agent. In disrepute since it may cause sudden cardiac arrest and liver damage.

chloroma A green-coloured sarcoma especially affecting the bones of the skull.

choana An opening like a funnel such as one of the posterior nasal openings.

cholaemia Bile in the blood.

cholagogue Preparation reputed to increase flow of bile.

cholangiogram X-ray showing the biliary system.

cholangitis Inflammation of the biliary system.

cholecystectomy Removal of the gall bladder.

cholecystenterostomy Operation for forming an artificial communication between the gall bladder and the intestine.

cholecystitis Inflammation of the gall bladder.

cholecystography Radiographic examination of the gall bladder and bile duct by the introduction of a radioopaque substance which is usually ingested some time before the procedure is undertaken.

cholecystolithiasis Removal of a stone from the gall bladder.

cholecystostomy Operation for making the gall bladder open to the exterior.

choledocholithotomy Incision of the common bile duct for the removal of gallstone.

choledochotomy Incision of the common bile duct.

cholelithiasis Formation of gallstones.

cholera Epidemic tropical disease due to infection by the cholera vibrio.

cholesteatoma Small tumour containing fat-like material. May occur in the middle ear as a complication of chronic otitis media.

cholesterol A sterol widespread in animal tissues, first isolated from bile. One of the substances which on precipitation gives rise to gallstones.

choline An organic base which is a constituent of some important substances, *e.g.* phospholipids, acetylcholine.

cholinergic Nerves which release acetylcholine as a transmitter substance.

cholinesterase Specific or acetylcholinesterase: an enzyme found at motor endplates and other sites, which breaks down and inactivates acetylcholine. Non-specific or pseudocholinesterases are found in the blood.

choluria Bile in the urine.

chondralgia Pain in cartilage.

chondritis Inflammation of cartilage.

chondroma Benign tumour of cartilage cells.

chondromalacia Roughening and softening of cartilage, typically occurring in the cartilage lining the patella.

chondrosarcoma Malignant tumour of cartilage.

chordae tendineae Thin musculotendinous bands extending between the walls of the ventricles of the heart and the tricuspid and mitral valves.

chordee Painful erection of penis, common in gonorrhoea.

chorditis Inflammation of the vocal cords.

chordotomy Division of an anterolateral column of the spinal cord.

chorea *Huntington's c.*: dominantly inherited disease with an incidence of about 6 per 100000 of the population. The disorder does not manifest itself till the age of about 40 and begins with choreiform movements with progressive dementia. *Sydenham's c.* (also known as St Vitus' dance): it is a disease of children associated with rheumatic fever which is characterized by involuntary movements.

chorion Layer enclosing embryonic structures and forming the placenta. *C. epithelioma*: malignant tumour arising from chorion.

chorionic villi Vascular processes developing on the external surfaces of the chorion.

choroid The posterior five-sixths of the middle coat of the eye, containing blood vessels and pigment. It lies between the retina and the sclerotic. *C. plexus*: specialized vascular epithelium which produces the cerebrospinal fluid. One choroid plexus is situated in each of the four ventricles of the brain.

choroiditis Inflammation of the choroid.

choroidocyclitis Inflammation of the choroid and ciliary body.

Christmas disease *See* HAE-
MOPHILIAS.

chromatography Separation
of components of a mixture
by their physical properties.

chromatosis Abnormal pigmentation.

chromophobe adenoma
Tumour of chromophobe
(unstained) cells of anterior
pituitary. Prolactin-secreting.
See PROLACTIN.

chromosomes When a cell
divides, the genetic material
present in the nucleus becomes segregated into thread-
shaped bodies which are visible under the microscope.
These are known as chromosomes and consist of connected strands of DNA
molecules known as genes. In
man there are 46 chromo-
somes per cell: 22 pairs of
autosomes and two *sex c.*;
females have two X chromosomes, males one X and one
Y. The Y chromosome is
shorter than the X
chromosome.

chronic A disease or symp
toms persisting over a period
of time; *cf.* acute.

Chvostek's sign A spasm of
the facial muscles produced
by tapping the facial nerve.
This sign is present in tetany.

chyle Lymph draining from
the villi of the small intestine.

chylomicron Tiny emulsified
droplets of neutral fat which
are absorbed into the lym-

phatics of the small intestine.

cicatricial Pertaining to a
scar, or cicatrix.

cicatrix The scar of a healed
wound or ulcer.

cilia Fine protoplasmic
threads projecting from the
surface of a cell which beat in
a constant direction moving
material surrounding it.

ciliary body Consists of the
ciliary muscle and processes,
forming part of the middle
coat of the eye.

ciliated epithelium Epithelial
cells with cilia forming the lining of certain tubes, *e.g.* respiratory passages.

Cimex lectularius The common bed-bug.

CIN *Abbr.* cervical intraepithelial neoplasia.

cinchonism Intolerance to
quinine, indicated by buzzing
in the ears, nausea, vomiting.

circa About.

circadian Relating to 24-hour
cycle of physiological events.

circinate Ring-shaped.

circle of Willis Circular intercommunication of arteries
supplying the brain.

circulation *See* HEART. *Systemic or general c.*: arterial
blood received into the left
atrium passes through the
mitral valve to the left ventricle. It then passes into the
aorta and through its smaller
branches to the capillaries,
into small veins, then larger,
until on reaching the superior

and inferior venae cavae it passes into the right atrium. *Pulmonary c.*: the venous blood which is received into the right atrium passes through the tricuspid valve into the right ventricle. From there into the pulmonary artery, which divides into two branches, one going to each lung. The artery divides in the lung into capillaries, and here the blood by means of the haemoglobin in the red cells takes up oxygen from the inspired air. Oxygenated blood returns to the heart by the four pulmonary veins, two from each lung, entering the left atrium. *Portal c.*: veins from the pancreas, spleen, stomach, intestines, unite behind the pancreas and form the portal tube or vein. This takes blood, rich in the products of digestion, to the liver where it divides into smaller vessels and capillaries. Blood leaves the liver by the hepatic veins which enter the inferior vena cava.

circumcision Surgical removal of the foreskin or prepuce. May be performed because of local disease, *e.g.* preputial warts, or to relieve constriction (phimosis, paraphimosis), as well as for religious reasons. *Female c.*: involves removal of the clitoris and part of introitus with labial folds.

circumflex nerve This arises from the brachial plexus to supply the deltoid and teres minor muscles.

circumoral Around the mouth. *C. pallor*: especially seen in scarlet fever, when the white area around the mouth is in great contrast to the colour of the rest of the face.

circumvallate Surrounded by a wall.

cirrhosis Usually referring to the liver: generic term applied to chronic diffuse liver damage of multiple aetiology. Characterized by destruction of the normal liver architecture and fibrosis.

cirsoid Resembling a varix.

cisterna magna A subarachnoid space at the back of the hindbrain between cerebellum and medulla oblongata.

cisternal puncture A puncture made with a hollow needle at the nape of the neck into a space called the cisterna magna which contains cerebrospinal fluid. Used when the fluid cannot be obtained by lumbar puncture.

citric acid cycle Krebs cycle or tricarboxylic acid cycle (TCA): cycle of enzyme initiated reactions whereby pyruvic acid is broken down yielding water, carbon dioxide and energy. It is the final oxidative step in the breakdown of carbohydrates

61

and occurs in the mito-
chondria.

CJD *Abbr.* Creutzfeld–Jakob
disease.

clamps Instruments used to
compress vessels or to secure
a grip on a structure.

claudication Limping. *Intermittent c.*: limping with severe
pain on walking which disappears with rest; due to insufficient blood supply.

claustrophobia Fear of
confined spaces.

clavicle Collar bone.

clavus A corn.

claw foot The foot is shaped
like a claw and has a very pro-
nounced arch.

claw hand Claw-shaped hand
due to flexor spasm followed
by contracture of the muscles
flexing the fingers. Often
caused by ulnar nerve
damage.

cleft palate Failure of fusion
of the lip and palate during
development. The cleft is
variable in extent. The
deformity can be remedied by
plastic surgery.

cleidocranial dysostosis Rare
hereditary condition in which
there is a failure of development of membranous bone;
consequently there may be
partial or total absence of the
clavicles and imperfect ossification of the skull in the region of the fontanelle. The
striking feature is the ability
to approximate the shoulders

in front of the chest.

cleidotomy Cutting the collar
bone.

climacteric Gradual reduction in and eventually end of
cyclical ovarian activity. Associated loss of ovarian follicles reduce fertility.
Climacteric is the hormonal
cause of the menopause but
usually precedes it by two
years.

clinic An institution to treat
patients.

clinical Relating to disease.

Clinitest Proprietary tablets
containing reagent for testing
urine for sugar.

clitoris A small organ of
erectile tissue, found in the
female in front of the urethra.

clone Descendants by division of a single cell and therefore of the same genetic
constitution.

clonic Spasmodic contractions, short and irregular.
They occur in the second
stage of an epileptic convulsion and in certain other fits.

clonus Reflex irregular contractions of muscles.

Clostridium Large spore-
bearing anaerobic bacilli. The
genus includes *C. botulinum*,
C. tetani and the gas gangrene
group.

clubbing The appearance of
fingers and sometimes toes
when the normal angle at the
base of the nail is lost. It results from hyperplasia of con-

nective tissue. Clubbing is associated with long-standing respiratory or cardiovascular disease.

club foot *See* TALIPES.

clumping Packing together of cells, usually red blood cells, due to loss of membrane charge resulting from reaction with antibody.

Clutton's joints Swelling of the knee joints found in congenital syphilis.

CMV *Abbr.* cytomegalovirus.

CNS *See* CENTRAL NERVOUS SYSTEM.

coagulase test Test used for identification of pathogenic staphylococci which depends on the demonstration of the enzyme coagulase which breaks down fibrinogen and clots plasma.

coagulation Thickening of a fluid into curds or clots. Almost always applied to blood. The *c. of blood* is a complex cascade of interactions resulting in the formation of fibrin from fibrinogen.

coarctation The compression of the walls of a vessel. When this occurs in the aorta it is narrowed where it is joined by the ductus arteriosus.

cobalt Trace element. Its absence from the diet of young animals may lead to anaemia. *C. bomb*: source of irradiation in deep x-ray therapy.

COC *Abbr.* combined oral contraceptive.

cocaine A powerful local anaesthetic, much used by oculists. It enlarges the pupil of the eye. Included in the Misuse of Drugs Act because it is a drug of addiction.

coccus (pl. **cocci**) Any spheroidal-shaped microorganism. *See* BACTERIA.

coccydynia Pain in the coccygeal region.

coccyx The tail-like termination of the spine.

cochlea The spiral cavity of the internal ear, containing the nerve endings of the eighth cranial or auditory nerve.

cock-up splints For hand and wrist. Usually made of metal or polythene.

codeine One of the alkaloids of opium. It allays cough, and is used in diarrhoea for its constipating effect.

codominance Of genetically transmitted conditions in which two traits are expressed in heterozygote.

codon Triplet of consecutive bases in unit of messenger RNA.

coeliac Related to the abdominal cavity. *C. disease*: a condition caused by the sensitivity of the intestine to gluten. It is usually diagnosed in infancy. Marked by failure to thrive, diarrhoea and marked wasting of the buttocks and thighs. A malabsorption syndrome.

coelioscopy Type of laparoscopy.

coenzyme Compound which plays an essential role in a reaction or reactions catalysed by an enzyme, usually acting as a carrier of an intermediate product of the reaction.

coffee ground vomit Appearance of vomit when it contains partly digested blood.

cognition Awareness. Part of a mental process. There is cognition when there is perception or memory of a material thing or idea.

coil. INTRAUTERINE DEVICE.

coitus Heterosexual intravaginal intercourse. *C. interruptus*, also called withdrawal: removal of the penis from the vagina before ejaculation. An ineffective method of contraception.

colectomy The operation of removing the colon.

colic Severe abdominal pain due to muscular spasm of a hollow viscus. Frequently caused by obstruction.

coliform Bacteria resembling coli.

colitis Inflammation of the colon. *Acute ulcerative c.*: due to an infection, *e.g.* dysentery. *Chronic ulcerative c.*: cause unknown. *Mucous c.*: thought to be of nervous origin and associated with constipation.

collagen Fibrous protein forming a major part of the intercellular connective tissue. *C. diseases*: a group of diseases in which one of the principal pathological features is the presence of fibrinoid necrosis usually in relation to blood vessels. To what extent the collagen is affected has not been determined but it seems that basically there is a deposition of abnormal material, possibly globulins, in the connective tissue rather than an alteration in the material normally present. Diseases such as systemic lupus erythematosus, scleroderma and periarteritis nodosa are examples of 'collagen' diseases.

collapse Severe sudden prostration. Symptoms: *see* SHOCK.

collar bone Clavicle.

collarstud abscess Abscess having two cavities joined by a narrow channel.

collateral Accompanying or accessory.

Colles' fracture Transverse fracture of the radius just above the wrist with displacement of the hand backwards and outwards.

collodion Pyroxylin dissolved in alcohol and ether; used in surgery to form a false skin. When painted over an incipient pressure sore it forms a protection over the skin. Highly inflammable.

colloid Physicochemical state

of certain non-electrolytes in solution. Colloids are unable to pass through semipermeable membranes and thus exert an osmotic pressure (colloid osmotic pressure).

coloboma A fissure or gap in the eyeball or in one of its component parts, *e.g.* coloboma iridis.

colon The part of the large intestine between the caecum and the rectum. *See* BOWEL.

colony A group of cells. Usually refers to circular collections of bacteria growing on culture medium.

colostomy Operation to make an artificial opening so that the colon opens on to the anterior abdominal wall.

colostrum A milky fluid flowing from the breasts the first 2 or 3 days after confinement, before the true milk comes.

colotomy An incision into the colon.

colour blindness Inability to distinguish certain colours, known sometimes as Daltonism.

colpitis Inflammation of the vagina.

colpocele A tumour or hernia in the vagina.

colpohysterectomy Removal of the uterus through the vagina. Usually called vaginal hysterectomy.

colpoperineorrhaphy Opera-

tion for repairing a torn vagina and perineum.

colporrhaphy Operation for repairing a torn vagina or for preventing prolapse of the vaginal walls. *Anterior c.*: repairing the anterior vaginal wall and preventing recurrence of a cystocele. *Posterior c.*: repairing the posterior vaginal wall and preventing the recurrence of a rectocele.

colposcope Instrument for performing colposcopy.

colposcopy Examination of the cervix. Usually performed in a hospital outpatient department when a cervical smear has shown cervical intraepithelial neoplasia (CIN). Surgical procedures such as biopsy or laser treatment may be done at the same time thus avoiding hospital admission and general anaesthetic.

colpotomy Incision of the vagina.

coma Insensibility, stupor, sleep.

comatose In a state of coma.

combined oral contraceptive The 'pill' containing both oestrogen and progestogen.

comedones Accumulations of sebaceous secretion in the hair follicles, commonly called blackheads. *See* ACNE.

commensal Refers to members of different species living in close association but without influencing each other, *cf.* symbiosis.

comminuted fracture Fracture in which the bone is broken into more than two pieces.

commissure Bundle of nerve fibres connecting the right and left sides of the brain and spinal cord.

communicable disease Disease caused by microorganisms which can be transmitted directly or indirectly between hosts.

compatibility Able to be mixed together without ill result: thus *compatible blood* is used for transfusion since it can be mixed with that of the recipient. *Compatible drugs* are those which can be mixed without producing undesirable chemical interactions.

compensation (1) A psychological way of making up for real or imagined deficiencies in personality. (2) *C. neurosis*: term used in psychiatry of patient who remains ill or disabled after an accident when monetary compensation is involved. There may be malingering or an unconscious mechanism. (3) *Cardiac c.*: is a way the body has to balance what would otherwise be an inadequate function.

compensatory hypertrophy Increase in size of residual organ or part of tissue in response to the removal of part, *e.g.* if one kidney is removed then the other enlarges.

complement A protein present in the blood which forms an essential component of certain antibody–antigen reactions. *C. fixation test*: the disappearance of complement from the serum is used to detect antigen–antibody reactions. This complement 'fixation' forms the basis of certain serological tests such as the Wassermann reaction.

complex A group of ideas with an emotional background. Partially or entirely repressed in the unconscious mind, it may be the underlying cause of a neurotic illness.

complicated fracture Fracture combined with injury to other important structures.

complication In illness, a disorder arising from the circumstances produced by the primary disease.

compos mentis Of sound mind.

compound Consisting of more than one element. *C. fracture*: fracture communicating with the surface.

comprehension The understanding of ideas and the relationship between them.

compress (1) A tightly folded pad of lint, gauze or other material used to secure local pressure. (2) A sterile dressing applied over an area which has been prepared for a surgical operation.

compression The state of being compressed. *Cerebral c.*: increased intracranial pressure from a tumour, etc.

computerized tomography *Abbr.* CT scanning. The technique of examining body sections in the axial plane using very sophisticated equipment.

concavity A depression or indentation.

concentric With a common centre.

conception (1) The impregnation of the ovum. (2) An idea.

concha auris Deepest hollow of pinna of the outer ear.

concordance Of twins, when both have same physical trait.

concretion A calculus. An abnormal deposit in the body such as stone in the gall bladder.

concussion Interruption of function of the brain as the result of compression wave set up by a blow to the head. The wave of compression transmitted through the cerebrospinal fluid and the brain substance obliterates momentarily the blood capillaries supplying the brain. Recovery may take many hours.

condensation Transformation of gas into liquid.

condenser Apparatus to cool and thus cause condensation of gas.

conditioned reflex A reflex which is modified by experience in such a way that the original afferent (sensory) stimulus is replaced by a different 'learned' stimulus, *e.g.* Pavlov's dog salivated at the sound of a bell, associating this with the introduction of food into its mouth.

condom Rubber sheath for the penis preventing conception.

conduction Passage of a physical disturbance through matter. Biologically, the passage of a nerve impulse.

conductor An instrument used to direct surgical knives, called also a director. In electricity, a substance which allows the passage of electric currents.

condyle A round projection at the ends of some bones, e.g. humerus.

condyloma Wartlike growth about the anus or pudendum.

cone biopsy Excision under anaesthetic, of a cone of tissue from the cervix uteri if it cannot be completely identified and treated under colposcopy. Used to confirm and treat CIN.

confabulation The narration of fictitious occurrences.

confection Medication with sweet covering.

confinement Childbirth.

conflict Psychological term to denote antagonism between conflicting desires.

confusion Inability to think clearly.

congenital Existing at birth. *C. heart disease*: heart disease present from birth. Due to developmental abnormalities of the cardiovascular system.

congestion Hyperaemia. Accumulation of blood in a part of the body, as in the lungs or brain. *C. of the lungs*: pneumonia.

conization Part of the cervix is removed by excision or diathermy.

conjugate or **conjugate diameter** An important diameter of the pelvis, measured from the most prominent part of the upper half of the sacrum to the nearest point on the back of the symphysis pubis. This is the *true* c., which should measure not less than 10cm, and is sometimes as large as 12cm. If less than 10cm, the pelvis is deformed. The *diagonal c.* is measured from the lower edge of the symphysis to the sacrum, and can be determined clinically, whereas the true conjugate cannot. The diagonal conjugate is about 1–2cm longer than the true conjugate. The *external c.* is measured from the spine of the last lumbar vertebra to the front of the symphysis pubis (this can only be done with calipers), and is normally about 20cm.

conjunctiva The mucous membrane which covers the sclerotic and lines the eyelids.

conjunctivitis Inflammation of the conjunctiva.

connective tissue Supporting or packing material consisting of a fibrous gel made up of collagen and elastin fibres in a mucopolysaccharide ground substance, bathed in extracellular fluid with scattered cells, blood vessels, lymphatics and nerve fibres traversing it.

Conn's syndrome Also called primary aldosteronism. Rare disease characterized by periodic attacks of severed muscular weakness, tetany, paraesthesiae, hypertension and impaired renal function. The cause is usually an adenoma of the adrenal cortex with overproduction of aldosterone, which results in reduced levels of potassium and raised sodium in the blood.

consanguinity Blood relationship.

conservative Aiming at preservation or repair, e.g. conservative treatment of a tooth.

consolidation Becoming solid, as with a lung in pneumonia.

constipation Undue delay in the passage of the residue of a meal.

constitutional Affecting the whole body, not local.

constrict Contract or draw together.

consumption Popular term for tuberculosis.

contact One who has been exposed to an infectious disease. *C. lens*: plastic or glass lens worn directly on the cornea.

contagious Communicable disease which is transmitted by contact, *i.e.* not communicable through atmosphere.

contraception Preventing conception.

contraceptives, oral Drugs, usually a combination of synthetic oestrogens and progestogens, which inhibit ovulation and thus depress fertility. They prevent blastocyst implantation and make cervical mucus unfavourable to sperm migration.

contraction Shortening. A drawing together.

contracture Permanent contraction of structure due to the formation of fibrous tissue which is inelastic. *Dupuytren's c.*: localized thickening of palmar fascia which involves the overlying skin of the psalm. There is a strong tendency for this to contract, drawing the affected fingers into rigid flexion.

contragestation Preventing or aborting pregnancy by using antiprogestogen drugs to antagonize the luteal output of progesterone.

contraindication Reason for considering a particular treatment to be unsuitable.

contralateral On the opposite side.

contrecoup Injury due to the transmission of the force of a blow. Contrecoup injuries often affect the brain which is damaged by striking the skull at a point diametrically opposite the site of the blow.

controlled drugs Drugs whose distribution and use is subject to the restrictions of the Misuse of Drugs Act 1971.

contusion A bruise.

convalescence Period of regaining full health after an illness.

convection The heat of liquids and gases transmitted by a circulation of heated particles.

convergence A coming together.

conversion *C. symptom*: term used in psychiatry for a symptom representing an emotional conflict but presenting as a physical illness.

convex With outline curved like exterior of circle.

convolutions The folds and twists of the brain or the intestines. *See* BOWEL and BRAIN.

convulsions Violent spasms of alternate muscular contraction and relaxation, due to disturbance of cerebral function. A fit.

Cooley's anaemia Also called

thalassaemia major. It is a dominantly inherited haemolytic anaemia found in Mediterranean peoples, and due to a metabolic fault leading to the continued production of fetal haemoglobin.

Coomb's test Test for the presence of globulin on the surface of red cells such as may occur in certain haemolytic anaemias in which antired cell antibody is produced. *Direct C.t.*: cells on which the antibody has combined with the antigen and thus coated the surface with globulin, are suspended in a medium containing anti-human globulin which reacts with the coating globulin causing agglutination of the coated red cells. *Indirect C.t.*: normal (compatible) red cells are incubated with the serum thought to contain antibody and subsequently tested for adsorbed antibody.

copulation Sexual intercourse.

cor pulmonale Heart disease resulting from affection of the lung.

coracoid A process of bone on the scapula which resembles a crow's beak. *See* SCAPULA.

cord Any string-like body such as the spinal cord or umbilical cord.

corn Local hyperkeratosis due to pressure on the skin.

Frequently occurs on the foot, *cf.* callus.

cornea Transparent epidermis and connective tissue which forms the front surface of the eye.

corneal graft Healthy cornea is given by grafting to replace a diseased cornea.

corneal reflex Important superficial reflex whereby a light touch on the cornea provokes a blink in both eylids.

corona dentis Crown of a tooth.

coronal suture The suture which joins the parietal and frontal bones of the skull.

coronary vessels Arteries and veins carrying the blood supply of the heart muscle. Arterial blockage results in myocardial infarction.

coroner Crown officer in England and Wales, usually legally and/or medically qualified who holds the responsibility of determining cause of death where violence may have occurred. Any deaths within 24 hours of hospital admission or after anaesthesia of surgery must be notified to the coroner. And death without recent medical attendance also demands notification, postmortem and coroner's inquest. In Scotland many of the roles of coroner are carried out by the Procurator Fiscal, and the equivalent of the coroner's inquest is

the Fatal Accident Inquiry
conducted by the sheriff.

coronoid Like a crow's beak
as with certain bony pro-
cesses.

corpora quadrigemina Four
rounded bodies consisting
chiefly of grey matter in the
midbrain.

corpulence, corpulency Undue
fatness. Obesity.

corpus A body. A large mass
of tissue. *C. callosum*: the
band of nervous tissue which
connects the two hemispheres
of the cerebrum. *C. luteum*: a
temporary organ secreting the
hormone progesterone which
favours the establishment and
continuity of a pregnancy. It
is formed, under the influence
of luteinizing hormone of the
pituitary, by growth of the
wall of a Graafian follicle
after ovulation. If ovulation
does not result in fertilization,
the corpus luteum de-
generates, but if fertilization
occurs, the corpus luteum
persists. *C. striatum: see*
BASAL GANGLIA.

corpuscle Usually refers to a
cell, especially red blood cell.

corrective A drug which
modifies the action of another
drug.

corrosive Eating into, con-
suming.

cortex The outer layer of an
organ.

Corti's organ The collection
of nerve endings of the auditory nerve in the cochlea.

corticosteroids Generic term
used to refer to steroid hormones from the adrenal cortex such as cortisol and
cortisone and also similar
metabolic actions.

corticotrophin Hormone
from the anterior pituitary
gland stimulating the adrenal
cortex.

**cortisol, hydrocortisone and
adrenal corticosteroid** Excess production results in
Cushing's syndrome and deficiency in Addison's disease.
Natural cortisol used in treat
topical eczema and asthma.

cortisone An adrenal corticosteroid. It is converted to
cortisol before become active
and therefore has similar
actions.

Corynebacterium diphtheriae
The bacillus causing diphtheria.

coryza The common cold.

cosmetic Action taken to improve the appearance. *C. surgery*: plastic surgery to alter
facial or other body ap-
pearance.

costal Relating to the ribs.

costochondritis Inflammation
of the costal cartilage. The
cause is unknown.

costoclavicular syndrome
Also called thoracic outlet
compression syndrome.
Characterized by pain in the
arm, wasting of the muscles
of the hand, paraesthesiae,

sensory loss and sometimes transient obliteration of the blood supply to the hand. It is due to compression of vessels and nerves between the clavicle and the top rib.

cot death *Syn.* sudden infant death syndrome (SIDS). Occurs most commonly in the first year of life during the night in an apparently healthy baby.

cotyledon Portion of the placenta.

counselling An interactive conversation between patient and counsellor (who may be doctor or other health care worker, volunteer or specified trained counsellor). The purpose is to increase the patient's knowledge of the problem facing them and to uncover any doubts and fears about their problems and help them come to a realistic decision which is right for them.

counterirritation The application of an irritant stimulus to the skin in order to divert attention from sensory information coming from another site, *e.g.* application of hot water bottle to relieve abnormal pain.

Courvoisier's law An adage to the effect that in jaundice the palpation of an enlarged tender gall bladder favours the diagnosis of obstructive jaundice, since a gall bladder which is the seat of chronic inflammation is usually incapable of distension.

Cowper's glands Two small glandular structures associated with the male urethra. Their function is unknown.

coxa The hip joint. *C. vulga*: deformity of the hip joint in which the angle made by the neck and shaft of the femur is greater than normal. *C. vara*: in this case the angle is less than normal.

coxalgia Pain in the hip joint.

coxsackie virus Group of viruses which may cause epidemic myalgia, Bornholm disease, and benign lymphocytic meningitis, and possibly other relatively mild diseases.

crab louse The phthirus pubis which infests the pubic region.

cradle cap Seborrheic dermatitis usually affecting the scalp of newborn babies.

cramp Sudden painful tonic contraction of the muscles.

cranial nerves Peripheral nerves emerging from the brain, as distinct from those emerging from the spinal cord. There are twelve pairs of cranial nerves: (1) *Olfactory c.n.*: the sensory nerves of the nose; (2) *optic c.n.*: the sensory nerves from the eyes; (3) *oculomotor c.n.*: motor nerves supplying the eye muscles; (4) *trochlear c.n.*: supplying eye muscles;

(5) *trigeminal c.n.*: sensory from parts of face and tongue and motor to jaw muscles; (6) *abducens c.n.*: supplying eye muscles; (7) *facial c.n.*: sensory from face and motor to muscles of expression; (8) *auditory c.n.*: sensory nerves from the ear and vestibular apparatus; (9) *glosso-pharyngeal c.n.*: concerned with sensory and motor aspects of swallowings; (10) *vagus c.n.*: parasympathetic nerve, with motor and sensory fibres distributed to oesophagus, stomach, heart and lungs; (11), *accessory c.n.*: nerve to trapezius and sternomastoid muscles; (12) *hypoglossal c.n.*: motor nerve to muscles below the pharynx.

cranioclast An instrument for breaking up the fetal skull when it is impossible to deliver the fetus intact.

craniometry Measurement of skulls.

craniopharyngioma *Syn.* Rathke pouch tumour. Cystic tumour arising from remnants of a developmental pouch in the pituitary region of the skull.

craniostenosis Abnormally early fusion of bones of the vault of the skull with the effect that further growth of the skull in the direction at right angles to the line of the obliterated suture is prevented.

Compensatory growth elsewhere in the skull produces a distorted head.

craniosynostosis Premature fusion of the cranial sutures giving rise to distortion of shape of head and face.

craniotabes Thinning of the bones of the vault of the skull; occurs in rickets.

craniotomy Operation in which openings are made in the skull.

craniotribe *See* CEPHALO-TRIBE.

cranium The skull.

creatine A constituent of muscle. Creatine phosphate acts as an energy storage substance.

creatinine A substance formed from creatine and excreted in the urine.

Credé's method Expelling the placenta by means of compression of the fundus of the uterus.

crepitation, crepitus (1) The grating of ends of a fractured bone. (2) Type of 'clicking' sound heard on auscultation of the chest when the alveoli contain fluid.

cretinism Congenital deficient thyroid secretion, causing impaired mentality, small stature, coarseness of skin and hair and deposition of fat on the body. Treated early with thyroid extract, great improvement may result.

Creutzfeld–Jakob disease Fatal presenile cerebral degeneration.

cribriform Perforated like a sieve.

cricoid cartilage A ring-shaped cartilage below the thyroid.

'cri du chat' syndrome Congenital abnormalities causing mental retardation and characteristic mewing sound.

criminal abortion *See* ABORTION.

crisis The deciding point of a disease, from which the patient either begins to recover or sinks rapidly; often marked by a long sleep, profuse perspiration, or other phenomena.

Crohn's disease Chronic form of enteritis affecting the terminal part of the ileum.

crossed laterality Combination of either right-handedness with left-eyedness or of left-handedness with right-eyedness.

crossinfection Hazard in hospitals where, owing to proximity of patients to each other, infection is easily transferred. Particularly dangerous in surgical and obstetric wards where wound infection is a problem despite stringent efforts to minimize the spread of bacteria.

cross-resistance Microorganisms which are resistant to one antibiotic tend to have resistance to other antibiotics of the same type.

croup Dyspnoea and stridor due to obstruction of the larynx. It may be due to inflammation, or spasm of the muscles.

crucial Critical or decisive.

cruciate Cross-shaped.

crural Relating to the thigh.

crus Latin for leg. A limb-like structure.

crush syndrome As the result of extensive crushing of muscles, toxic substances pass into the circulation which cause the medullary circulation of the kidney to be opened up so that blood is diverted from the glomeruli in the renal cortex. This results in oliguria.

crutch paralysis Caused by pressure on the axillary nerves and vessels by a crutch.

cryaesthesia Sensitivity to cold.

cryoanalgesia Application of cold to block pain perception.

cryosurgery Method of surgical removal of tissue by local freezing.

cryotherapy Application of cold as means of treatment.

cryptomenorrhoea Apparent amenorrhoea due to obstruction to the flow of menstrual blood.

cryptorchism Failure of one or both testes to descend into the scrotum.

crypts of Lieberkühn Glands found in the mucous membrane of the small intestine. They secrete a mixture of digestive enzymes collectively termed intestinal juice.

crystalloids Substances which will pass through a semi-permeable membrane. They easily crystallize and are readily soluble, *e.g.* salt, sugar; *cf.* colloid.

crystalluria The presence of crystals in the urine.

CSF *See* CEREBROSPINAL FLUID.

cubit, cubitus (1) The forearm. (2) The elbow.

cubital tunnel external compression syndrome Compression of the ulnar nerve on the medical side of the elbow joint causes paralysis and tingling in the hand.

cuirass An external aid to assisted ventilation. Pressure and suction transmitted to chest wall via the device causes it to inspire and expire.

culdoscopy Inspection of internal pelvic organs by passing illuminated instrument through posterior vaginal fornix.

culture Artificial cultivation of tissues, cells or viruses. *C. media*. Substances used as food source for cultures.

cumulative action A term applied to certain drugs which are excreted slowly. After several doses have been given, symptoms of poisoning may arise, *e.g.* mercury, digitalis.

cuneiform Wedge-shaped.

cupping Depression of the optic disc. It is usually pathological and due to raised intraocular pressure.

curare A poison derived from a South American plant. It paralyses motor nerves.

curettage Operation of scraping away tissue with a curette.

curette A spoon-shaped instrument.

curie (CI) Unit of radioactivity.

Curling's ulcer An acute ulcer occurring in the second part of the duodenum following severe burns.

Cushing's disease Due to oversecretion of adrenal corticosteroids secondary to increased anterior pituitary ACTH secretion.

Cushing's syndrome Due to oversecretion of adrenocortical hormones, other than secondarily to anterior pituitary ACTH secretion or treatment with corticosteroid drugs. Characterized by moonface, redistribution of body fat, polycythaemia, hirsutism, acne, amenorrhoea, osteoporosis, glycosuria, hypertension, purpura, muscular weakness and occasionally mental derangement.

cutaneous Pertaining to the skin.

cuticle The layer of flattened cells forming the outer coat of hair.

cutis Dermis.

cyanocobalamin Vitamin B_{12}. A cobalt-containing substance, lack of which interferes with cell division. How it acts is not known.

cyanosis Blue appearance; due to deficient oxygenation of the blood. It occurs in heart failure, diseases of the respiratory tract, and congenital heart disease. *See* BLUE BABY.

cyclamate Salt of cyclohexyl-sulphamic acid. A sweetening agent.

cycle Repeated series of events.

cyclical vomiting Recurrent attacks of vomiting occurring in childhood with headache, and signs of acidosis.

cyclitis Inflammation of ciliary body of eye.

cyclodialysis Drainage of anterior chamber of eye.

cycloplegia Paralysis of the ciliary muscle of the eye.

cyclothymia A type of personality in which there are marked swings of mood from happiness to depression.

cyclotomy Incision through the ciliary body.

cyesis Pregnancy. *Pseudo-c.*: false pregnancy usually due to wish fulfilment.

cyst A tumour containing fluid in membranous sac. *Daughter c.*: One developed from the walls of a large cyst.

cystadenoma Benign growth containing cysts.

cystectomy Removal of urinary bladder.

cystic duct The duct leading from the gall bladder to the common bile duct.

cystic fibrosis A recessively inherited condition characterized by abnormal secretion of the exocrine glands. Typically present in children with recurrent chest infection, malabsorption and failure to thrive. The sweat test shows abnormally high levels of sodium and chloride.

cysticercosis Infection by larval stage of a tapeworm, usually from pork. The parasites may become widespread in the body, invading muscle and nervous tissue and cause serious symptoms, *e.g.* epilepsy.

cystine A sulphur-containing amino acid.

cystinosis A rare inborn error of metabolism of cystine and other amino acids described by Lignac and Fanconi. It is characterized by dwarfism, vitamin D-resistant rickets, anorexia, polyuria, thirst, vomiting and cystine deposits in the tissues.

cystinuria Presence of abnormal amounts of cystine in the urine as occurs, for example, in cystinosis.

cystitis Inflammation of the urinary bladder.

cystocele Hernia of the bladder into the vagina.

cystogram X-ray of urinary bladder.

cystolithiasis Stone in the bladder.

cystometry Measurement of tone of the bladder.

cystoscope An instrument for examining the bladder.

cystostomy Operation of producing an opening from the bladder to the exterior.

cystotomy Incision of the bladder or division of the anterior capsule of the lens of the eye.

cytochromes A number of iron-containing proteins found in cells which form the intermediary link between the electron transport chain, which accumulates hydrogen from oxidation actions taking place in cellular metabolism, and molecular oxygen.

cytogenetics Study of genetics in relation to cytology.

cytology The study of cells.

cytolysis Cell disintegration.

cytomegalovirus Herpes virus causing cytomegalic inclusion-body disease.

cytometer An instrument for counting cells.

cytopathic Abnormality at a cellular level. *C. effect*: death of cells in tissue culture

following viral infection.

cytoplasm *See* CELL.

cytotoxic Substance which is damaging to cells.

cytotoxin Cytotoxic antibody.

cytotrophoblast Inner portion of trophoblast differentiation.

D

dacryadenitis Inflammation of the lacrimal gland.

dacryocystitis Inflammation of the tear sac.

dacryocystorhinostomy Operation to establish a communication between the tear (lacrimal) sac and the nose. It is performed when the tear duct, through which the lacrimal secretion normally drains, is obstructed, thus causing epiphora.

dacryolith Stone in the lacrimal duct.

dactyl A digit of the hand or foot.

dactylitis Non-specific term, usually applied to periostitis of the bones of the digits.

dactylology Talking by the fingers; deaf and dumb language.

Daltonism Red–green colour blindness inherited by a sex-linked recessive trait and therefore much more common in males than females who act as carriers for the gene, *cf.* haemophilia. There are other forms of colour blindness but they are rare.

dandruff Accumulation of desquamated keratinized cells usually in the scalp.

dark adaptation Time required for the physiological readjustment of the eye necessary to permit vision in the dark. This is critically affected by the amount of carotene available to retinal cells, *cf.* light adaptation.

Darwinism Theory of evolution by natural selection as propounded by Darwin.

dB. Decibel.

deaf mute A person who is both deaf and dumb.

deamination The removal of amino (NH_2) group. Occurs in the liver and kidneys by the action of deaminating enzymes which remove the amino groups from amino acids. The reaction produces ammonia which is converted to urea by enzymes in the liver.

death End of life, stopping of body's vital functions. Diagnosis of death depends on absent heart beat and respiration but in a patient receiving basic life support these may not be enough and the concept of brain death is employed. *Brain d.*: absence of electrical activity generated by any centre above the 'brain stem'.

debility Weakness, loss of power.

debridement Thorough cleansing of a wound and excision of the edges.

decalcification Loss or removal of calcium salts from bone.

decapitation The operation of severing the fetal head from the body, very rarely necessary in cases of obstructed labour.

decapsulation Removal of the capsule of an organ, *e.g.* of the kidney.

decerebrate Without brain. Usually applied to experimental situations in which the brain stem of an animal is sectioned, leaving the brain intact but severing the connections with the spinal cord. This results in *d. rigidity* when the limbs are rigidly extended. A similar spasticity may occur clinically as the result of severe brain damage.

decidua Mucous membrane lining the uterus (endometrium) in the thickened and modified form it acquires during pregnancy. Some or all of the decidua is shed with the placenta at birth.

deciduous teeth First dentition or milk teeth.

decompensation Failure of physiological compensation to some stimulus; for example, failure of hypertrophy of a chamber of the heart to overcome obstruction due to a defective valve.

decomposition Putrefaction. Break-down of substances by hydrolytic enzymes.

decompression An operation performed to relieve internal pressure, *e.g.* trephining of the skull. *D. sickness*, otherwise known as 'the bends' or caisson disease: occurs in deep-sea divers and is due to nitrogen in compressed air which at the pressure under which it is breathed goes into solution in the blood but which, at ordinary atmospheric pressure, comes out of solution and forms small bubbles in the tissues.

deconditioning Training to eliminate an unwanted response, reflex or habit. Aversion therapy.

decortication Surgical removal of the outer layer of an organ.

decubitus The recumbent or horizontal position.

decussation (1) An interlacing or crossing of fellow parts. (2) The point at which the crossing occurs. *D. of the pyramids*: the crossing of motor fibres, from one side of the medulla to the other.

deep x-ray therapy *Abbr.* DXT. Treatment of disease, especially malignant disease, by x-rays. They penetrate the tissue and destroy cells which are rapidly multiplying.

defaecation The act of evacuating the bowels.

defeminization Loss of female characteristics.

defibrillator Apparatus which applies electrical impulses to the heart. Designed to stop fibrillation and restore the normal cardiac cycle.

defibrinated Free of fibrin. Plasma that is defibrinated becomes serum.

deficiency diseases Due to an inadequate supply of vitamins in the diet, *e.g.* rickets, scurvy, beriberi.

degeneration Deterioration in structure or function of tissue. When the structural changes are marked, descriptive terms are sometimes used, *e.g.* colloid, fatty, hyaline, etc.

deglutition Act of swallowing.

dehydration Loss of water.

dehydrogenase Enzyme which oxidizes a substrate by removing hydrogen from it.

déjà vu phenomenon Illusion of familiarity when experiencing something new.

deletion Loss of genetic material.

Delhi boil Also known as 'oriental sore'. Cutaneous leishmaniasis.

delirium Extravagant talking, raving, generally due to high fever. *D. tremens*: an acute psychosis usually associated with chronic alcoholism. The patient is disorientated, has hallucinations and is excited. There is a coarse tremor of the fingers, tongue and facial muscles.

delivery Parturition. Childbirth.

deltoid The muscle which covers the prominence of the shoulder and abducts the arm.

delusion A false idea, entirely without foundation in the facts of the environment.

demarcation The marking of a boundary. *Line of d.*: red line which forms between dead and living tissue in gangrene.

dementia A reduction in a previously attained level of intellectual and emotional development. May occur in children as a result of inborn errors of metabolism. In adults is classified as presenile, before the age of 65, and senile, after the age of 65. Commonest varieties are *Alzheimer's d.* and *multi-infarct d.*

demography The study of the human population and its societies.

demulcents Agents which protect sensitive surfaces from irritation.

demyelinating diseases A group of diseases, of which multiple sclerosis is the most common example, where the major visible pathological

lesion is the destruction and loss of myelin sheaths round nerve fibres.

denaturation Alteration in the tertiary structure of a polymer (*e.g.* protein) as the result of the action of heat or chemicals rendering the molecule less soluble.

dendrites Branching cytoplasmic projections of a cell.

dendritic ulcer Ulcer occurring on the cornea as a result of infection by the herpes simplex virus.

denervated Deprived of nerve supply.

dengue A virus disease of the tropics, transmitted by mosquitoes and characterized by fever, headache, limb pains and rash.

Denis Browne splints A number of splints designed to correct congenital deformity, as that of the hip, bear this surgeon's name. His padded metal splints to correct congenital talipes equinovarus are widely used.

dental Pertaining to the teeth. *D. caries*: destruction of the teeth by the action of microorganisms. Holes in the teeth. *D. cyst*: cyst, occurring at the root of a tooth, usually sterile and containing cholesterol. *D. formula*: formula indicating the number of each type of teeth: incisors, canines, premolars and molars. The numbers are written for the upper and lower jaws on one side thus:

$$i\frac{2}{2}; c\frac{1}{1}; p\frac{2}{2}; m\frac{3}{3}$$

dentate   Tooth-shaped.

dentine   The substance which forms the body of a tooth. *See* TEETH.

dentition   Teething. *See* TEETH.

denture   A set of artificial teeth.

deodorant   Substance which prevents or masks unpleasant smells.

deoxidation   Removal of oxygen from a chemical compound.

deoxyribonucleic acid (DNA) Formed from nucleotides containing the sugar deoxyribose and one of four bases, adenine, cytosine, guanine and thymine, which are arranged in chains to give a series. The genetic information of the cell is stored in the DNA molecule in the form of a three base code which has been deciphered by molecular biologists. A gene is envisaged as a chain of base triplets. DNA is capable of self-replication. In the model proposed by Crick and Watson a helix of one strand of DNA is complementary to a second helix to which the bases are paired adenine–thymine, cytosine–guanine; thus when the DNA is dupli-

cated the two helices separate and each becomes a template for the complementary pair.

depersonalization   A neurotic state when a person feels that he has in reality no existence but is only an onlooker at his own behaviour and actions.

depilatory   An agent for removing superfluous hairs from the body.

depletion   Act of emptying; bleeding; purging.

deposit   A sediment.

depot injection   Quantity of a drug, several times a single dose, injected in slowly absorbable form.

depressant   An agent reducing functional activity.

depressed fracture of the skull Fracture in which the damaged area of bone is depressed below the level of the surrounding bone.

depression   A feeling of gloom due to disappointment, loss or failure. In *reactive d.*, due to stress, the patient does not lose touch with reality. *Severe d.* is a psychotic state and there is usually a predisposition to it in the person's make-up. He then loses all touch with reality and needs expert help. *Involutional d.* occasionally occurs at the menopause. In all types of depression there is a risk of suicide.

de Quervain's disease   Stenosing tenosynovitis; a fibrous thickening of the tendon sheath usually of the abductor pollicis longus.

Derbyshire neck Term used to describe a swollen neck due to goitre. Once common in parts of Derbyshire because of local iodine deficiency in the soil and water.

derma Dermis.

dermatitis Inflammation of the skin. The numerous causes may be of external or internal origin. *D. herpetiformis*: blistering disease of the skin associated with gluten sensitivity and characterized by intense itchiness. There is an eosinophil polymorphonuclear leucocytosis. *See also* COELIAC DISEASE.

dermatoglyphics Study of skin ridge patterns.

dermatographia *See* DERMOGRAPHIA.

dermatologist Medical specialist in diseases of the skin.

dermatology The science of skin and its diseases.

dermatome Instrument for cutting a skin graft.

dermatomycosis A skin disease caused by a fungus.

dermatomyositis A rare disease classified as a 'collagen disease' characterized by weakness and muscle tenderness and frequently associated with an erythematous rash.

Occasionally the myocardium is affected. The cause is unknown.

dermatophytes Fungi which grow on the skin.

dermatosis Any skin disease.

dermis Specialized connective tissue supporting the epidermis and the epidermal appendages (hair follicles, sweat glands).

dermographia The production of weals on the skin, resembling urticaria, on gently stroking the skin.

dermoid cyst A cyst containing epithelial substances, especially hair, teeth and sebaceous material.

Descemet's membrane Lining membrane behind the cornea of the eye.

descending colon The part of the large intestine running from the splenic flexure to the sigmoid colon in the left of the abdominal cavity.

desensitization To remove sensitivity to a substance. A method of treatment used for the allergic state.

desiccation The act of drying.

desmoid Like a bundle. Fibroid tissue.

desquamation Loss of squamous cells from the surface of an epithelium.

detached retina Separation between the neural and pigmented layers of the retina or of the whole retina from the choroid. To conserve sight surgical or laser treatment must be used.

detergent Substance which effectively lowers the surface tension of a fluid.

deterioration A worsening condition.

detoxicated With toxic properties removed.

detritus Accumulation of disintegrated material.

detrusor An expelling muscle.

deuteranomaly Anomalous trichromatic colour vision where red, blue and green are seen, the green imperfectly due to inadequate discrimination in yellow part of the spectrum.

dexter Right. Upon the right side.

dextran A blood-plasma substitute.

dextrin An intermediate product in the conversion of starch into sugar.

dextrocardia Congenital transposition of the heart from the left to the right side of chest.

dextrose Grape sugar. Glucose.

dhobi itch Ringworm, mainly in the inguinocrural region. Also called tinea cruris.

diabetes insipidus Syndrome caused by deficient secretion of antidiuretic hormone (ADH) by the pituitary gland, and characterized by polyuria, the urine being of low specific gravity.

diabetes mellitus Usually diabetes. Syndrome caused by a relative deficiency of insulin. Insulin is secreted by the beta cells of the islets of Langerhans in the pancreas and in some manner facilitate the uptake of glucose by cells. In the absence of insulin there is a failure to utilize glucose which leads to biochemical disturbances resulting in ketosis, electrolyte disturbances, etc. The glucose meanwhile is secreted in the urine together with its water of solution and this results in polyuria; the urine, being loaded with sugar, is of high specific gravity. Rarely the findings in the urine of diabetes mellitus are mimicked by a low renal threshold for glucose or some other sugar (galactose, pentose).

diabetic coma Unconsciousness resulting from extreme ketosis.

diabetic neuropathy Asymmetrical affection of peripheral nerves which is a complication of unregulated diabetes.

diabetic retinopathy Complication of unregulated diabetes; the retina shows microaneurysms of the blood vessels and circular haemorrhages and exudates.

diabetogenic Tending to produce abnormally high blood-sugar levels.

diacetic acid Acetoacetic acid. This is a substance occasionally present in the urine: especially in serious cases of diabetes.

diagnosis The decision as to the nature of an illness, arrived at by clinical assessment of the patient and results of investigations.

diagnostic Confirming a diagnosis. Hence *d. symptom*, *d. sign*, *d. result*.

dialysis Method of separating small molecules (crystalloids) from colloids by placing the mixture in a container made of a membrane which is permeable only to small molecules (semipermeable membrane). The container is placed in water into which the small molecules diffuse leaving the colloids in the container. *Peritoneal d.*: peritoneum is used as porous membrane through which waste products are strained off and then washed away by irrigation fluid.

diapedesis The passage of leucocytes through the walls of blood vessels. It occurs in inflammation.

diaphoresis Perspiration.

diaphoretics Agents which increase perspiration, *e.g.* pilocarpine.

diaphragm The muscular septum separating the chest from the abdomen. *Contraceptive d.* (Dutch cap): female barrier contraceptive consisting of a latex or similar dome inserted in the upper vagina before coitus to prevent sperm from entering the cervix. Usually used with spermicides. Helps prevent sexually transmitted diseases.

diaphragmatic hernia Herniation of abdominal viscera through the diaphragm into the chest. Usually congenital as a result of defective development of the diaphragm.

diaphysis The middle part of long bones; the shaft. *See* BONE.

diarrhoea Frequent loose evacuations of the bowels.

diarthrosis A freely movable joint permitting movement in any direction.

diastase An enzyme which converts starch into sugar with intermediate dextrins.

diastasis Dislocation.

diastole That part of cardiac cycle when the ventricles fill with blood, *cf.* systole.

diastolic Relating to diastole.

diathermy The passage of high-frequency electric current through a tissue. Because of the electrical resistance of the tissue, heat is generated. This is diffuse when large electrodes are used, and as such constitutes a physiotherapeutic aid. Tissues may be cauterized by using a small electrode.

diathesis Constitutional disposition to a particular disease.

dichotomy Division into two parts.

dicrotic Having two beats. Usually applies to secondary pulse wave due to the closure of the semi lunar valves since, when this is marked as in conditions associated with vasodilation, *e.g.* high fever, it gives the impression of a double pulse.

dielectric The non-conducting material separating the conducting surface in an electrical condenser.

diet System of food. Food intake.

dietetics The study of food values.

dietitian Somebody trained in the principles of good diet and their application in health and disease.

Dietl's crisis Severe attacks of renal pain accompanied by scanty, bloodstained urine. Occurs in some cases of movable kidney probably due to kinking of the ureter.

differential blood count The determination of the proportion of each type of white cell in the blood, carried out by microscopical examination. Useful in diagnosis.

differential diagnosis Discrimination between diseases with similar symptoms.

diffraction Dispersion of light by the edge of the iris and colloidal particles in the cornea and lens of the eye.

diffusion The gradual assumption of an even distribution of molecules of gases or fluids within a given volume brought about by their random movement.

digestion Process by which food is rendered absorbable.

digit A finger or toe.

digitalis An extract of foxglove leaves containing a number of alkaloids which affect the heart muscle. The most widely used of these 'cardiac' glycosides is digoxin. The effect on the heart is to slow down the rate of conduction of the cardiac impulse.

dilatation Increase in size, enlargement. The operation of stretching.

dilator An instrument for dilating any narrow passage, as the rectum, uterus, urethra.

dilution Solution in which the ratio between solute and solvent has been reduced usually by the addition of solvent.

dioptre The unit of refractive power of lens. A lens of 1 dioptre has a focal length of 1 metre.

dioxide A compound containing two atoms of oxygen, *e.g.* carbon dioxide (CO_2).

diphtheria Infectious disease caused by Corynebacterium diphtheriae and characterized by the formation of a membranous slough on mucous membranes, usually of the throat. A soluble exotoxin is produced by the virulent strains of C. diphtheriae and may cause damage to the heart muscle and nervous system.

Diphyllobothrium latum Fish tapeworm which may infest humans. The tapeworm absorbs vitamin B_{12} and may cause megaloblastic anaemia.

DIPI *Abbr.* direct intraperitoneal insemination. Surgical introduction of prepared semen into the female pelvis at the time of ovulation. A treatment for some forms of infertility.

diplegia Paralysis of both sides of the body.

diplococci Cocci arranged in pairs.

diploë A cellular osseous tissue separating the two cranial tables.

diploid Having chromosomes in pairs. The paired members are homologous.

diplopagus Conjoined twins, sharing one or more vital organs.

diplopia Double vision.

dipsomania Pathological craving for alcohol.

director Grooved instrument used to guide other instruments.

Disablement Resettlement Officer *See* DRO.

disaccharide A sugar consist-

ing of two monosaccharides.

disarticulation Amputation at a joint.

disc Circular plate. *Intervertebral d.* is a fibrocartilaginous articulating layer between vertebrae. *Optic d.* is the area on the retina where the fibres of the optic nerve collect (blind spot).

discharge Emission of material, *e.g.* fluid, pus, light, electricity, etc.

discission Also called needling. Surgical rupture of the lens capsule of the eye.

disclosing tablet A tablet which produces a colour when in contact with dental plaque.

discrete Separate, distinct; opposed to confluent.

disease A process which disturbs the structure or functions of the body.

disinfectants Substances which destroy microorganisms. Usually for external use and affecting fungi and bacteria. Many are poisonous.

disinfestation Chemical or other treatment to remove parasites from skin or gut.

disjunction Separation of halves of chromosome in cell division.

dislocation Displacement of articular surfaces of bone.

disorientation Loss of the ability to locate one's position in the environment, or the mental confusion seen in psychiatric disorders.

dispensing The preparation of medicines.

disproportion General term to indicate that the ratio between the size of the fetal head and the size of the maternal pelvis is abnormally large.

dissection The separation by cutting of parts of the body.

disseminated Scattered. *D. intravascular coagulation (DIC)*: *see* AFIBRINO-GENAEMIA. *D. lupus erythematosus*: *see* LUPUS ERYTHEMATOSUS (SLE). *D. sclerosis*: *see* MULTIPLE SCLEROSIS.

dissociation Abnormal mental state in which the patient fails to recognize certain, frequently unpalatable, facts relating to himself.

dissolution Decomposition.

distal Situated away from the centre.

distichiasis A double row of eyelashes, causing irritation and inflammation of the eye.

distillation The process of vaporizing a substance and condensing the vapour.

diuresis An increased secretion of urine.

diuretics Drugs which increase the volume of urine secreted.

diurnal Daily.

diver's paralysis *See* CAISSON DISEASE.

diverticulitis Inflammation of a diverticulum.

diverticulosis Presence of numerous diverticula in the intestine.

diverticulum A pouch-like process from a hollow organ, *e.g.* oesophagus, intestine, urinary bladder.

dizygotic twins Twins developed from the simultaneous fertilization of separate ova.

DNA *Abbr.* deoxyribonucleic acid.

DNA viruses Viruses in which the genetic material is DNA, *e.g.* adenovirus, papovavirus, herpes virus and pox virus.

dolor Pain.

dominant (1) A gene which has the same expression, *i.e.* produces the same effect when heterozygous (the two genes making up the pair are different) as when homozygous (the two genes are the same), is dominant with respect to allelic genes, *cf.* recessive. (2) Dominance of the right or left cerebral hemisphere over the other is responsible for left-handedness or right-handedness.

donor Individual from whom tissue or organ is removed for transfer to another, *e.g.* blood transfusion, grafting.

dopa reaction Reaction involving the enzymatic oxidation dihydroxyphenylalanine (dopa) to form the pigment melanin.

Doppler effect Change in wavelength of light or sound

reflected from a moving surface. Doppler ultrasound is diagnostic equipment using the Doppler effect on ultrasound beams. Used to detect flow of blood through vessels, *e.g.* leg veins or umbilical vessels.

Dornier basket Instrument for ensnaring and removing renal calculi causing renal colic.

Dornier lithotryptor Instrument which can destroy certain types of renal calculus without surgery.

dorsal Relating to the back. *D. root*: posterior or sensory root. Nerve root carrying sensory fibres which enter the dorsal part of the spinal cord.

dorsiflexion Bending backwards or in a dorsal direction.

dorsum The back.

double-blind trial Clinical trial in which neither physician nor patient knows whether placebo or treatment is being administered.

double vision *Syn.* diplopia.

douche A shower of water usually used to irrigate a cavity of the body. Hot douche 112°F (44°C); cold douche 60°F (16°C).

Douglas's pouch The peritoneal pouch between the back of the uterus and the front of the rectum.

Down's syndrome (*Syn.* Down syndrome or mongolism) A congenital abnormality with mental subnormality, characteristic facies with slanted eyes, a flattened head, small hands with a short, curved little finger. A tendency to poor vision and cardiac defects. There are two sorts: (1) An extra chromosome 21 giving 47 instead of 46. This sort usually born to older mothers. (2) A trisomy of chromosome 21. More often born to younger mothers and may recur in subsequent pregnancy.

drainage tubes Tubes, made of various materials, which are inserted into operation wounds to allow fluids such as blood to drain from the wound.

drastic Strong, severe.

drip, intravenous The administration into a vein of saline, plasma or blood.

drive In psychology, an urge to satisfy a basic need, such as hunger.

DRO *Abbr.* Disablement Resettlement Officer. Official appointed by the Department of Employment to oversee operation of Disabled Persons Employment Acts.

droplet infection Fine droplets of fluid are expelled from the upper respiratory passages during talking or sneezing, etc. These droplets may carry microorganisms which infect persons inhaling the droplets.

dropsy *See* OEDEMA.

drug A substance used in treating an illness or occasionally in its diagnosis. Drugs may be administered by many routes: oral, transcutaneous, injection (subcutaneous, intramuscular or intravenous), rectal, inhalation. Most drugs require a prescription but some can be bought without, *e.g.* many herbal preparations, simple analgesics, such as aspirin, paracetamol. Drugs of addiction are controlled by the Misuse of Drugs Act 1971. *D. addiction*: a dependence on drugs which is beyond the subject's control. *D. eruption*: rash due to sensitivity to a drug. *D. reaction*: general reaction to a drug. This may include fever, malaise, joint pains, rashes, jaundice, etc. *D. resistance*: Strains of microorganisms resistant to the action of antibiotics. The emergence of these resistant strains is now the largest single problem in the treatment of bacterial infection.

Duchenne muscular dystrophy Pseudohypertrophic muscular dystrophy. A genetically determined abnormality of muscle metabolism (myopathy) first affecting the hip and shoulder girdles.

Ducrey's bacillus Haemophilus ducreyi, the organism causing the venereal disease, chancroid.

duct Passage lined by epithelium.

ductless glands *See* ENDOCRINE.

ductus A duct; a little canal in the body. *D. arteriosus* connects the pulmonary artery and the aorta in fetal life. Occasionally this remains patent.

dumping syndrome Term applied to symptoms whch occasionally follow partial gastrectomy: gastric discomfort, cold sweats and palpitations.

duodenal Belonging to the duodenum.

duodenostomy Surgical establishment of a communication between the duodenum and another structure.

duodenum The first 30 cm of the small intestine, beginning at the pyloric orifice of the stomach.

Dupuytren's contracture Fibrous contracture of unknown aetiology affecting one or both palms and occasionally also the soles of the feet.

dura mater The outer membrane lining the interior of the cranium and spinal column.

dwarf Individual of stunted growth.

dys A prefix meaning bad, difficult, painful, abnormal.

dysaesthesia Alteration of sensation.

dysarthria Impairment of speech.

dyschezia Painful defaecation.

dyschondroplasia Multiple enchondromas. Cartilage is deposited in the shaft of some bone(s). The affected bones, often in the hands and feet, are short and deformed.

dyscoria Abnormality in the shape of the pupil.

dysdiadokinesis Inability to carry out rapid alternating movements, such as rotating the hands. A sign of cerebellar disease.

dysentery Inflammation of the large intestine. There are two kinds of dysentery, bacillary and amoebic, the former due to a bacillus, the latter to the Entamoeba histolytica.

dysfunction Abnormal or impaired function.

dyskinesia Impairment of voluntary movement.

dyslalia Mechanical speech defect; *cf.* dysphasia.

dyslexia A specific difficulty with the written word, not due to any visual defect, which may cause backwardness in learning to read.

dysmelia Absence of part of limbs.

dysmenorrhoea A painful or difficult menstruation.

dyspareunia Painful coitus.

dyspepsia Indigestion.

dysphagia Difficulty in swallowing.

dysphasia Difficulty in speaking.

dysplasia Tissue forming along abnormal lines. *Cervical d.*: abnormal cell development in the stratified epithelium at the squamous–columnar junction of the uterine cervix. *See* CERVICAL INTRAEPITHELIAL NEOPLASIA.

dyspnoea Difficult breathing.

dystocia A difficult labour (obstetric).

dystrophy Defective structure due to shortage of essential factors.

dysuria Painful micturition.

E

ear The organ of hearing. It consists of external, middle and internal ear. The *external e.* comprises the auricle and external auditory canal, and is separated from the middle ear by the tympanic membrane. The *middle e.* is an irregular cavity in the temporal bone. In front it communicates with the eustachian tube which forms an open channel between the middle ear and the cavity of the nasopharynx. Behind, the middle ear opens into the mastoid antrum, and this in turn communicates with the mastoid cells. There are two openings into the inner ear, both of which are covered with membrane. A string of tiny bones, joined together, extends from the tympanum to the foramen ovale of the internal ear. These bones are, from the tympanum: (1) malleus, (2) incus, (3) stapes. The *internal e.* comprises: (1) the organ of hearing or cochlea in which are the endings of the auditory nerve, and (2) the organ of equilibrium or balance consisting of the three semicircular canals, arranged matually at right angles. *E. drum*: the tympanum.

ecchondroma A tumour composed of cartilage.

ecchymosis A bruise; an effusion of blood under the skin.

ECG *Abbr.* electrocardiogram.

Echinococcus One of the species of tapeworm. In its adult stage it infests dogs. In its larval stage it produces hydatid cysts in man.

ECHO virus *Abbr.* enterophathic cytopathic human orphan virus; *see* ADENOVIRUS. May cause benign lymphocytic meningitis and epidemic myalgia (Bornholm disease).

echolalia Repetition of everything said.

eclampsia Convulsions arising from severe toxaemia of pregnancy.

ecmnesia A lapse in memory, the memory before and after the lapse being normal.

ecology Biological study of relationships of organisms with environment.

ECT *Abbr.* electroconvulsive therapy.

ectasis Distension, as in bronchiectasis when the bronchial tubes are dilated.

ecthyma A pustular skin disease, a form of impetigo.

ectoderm The outer layer of the primitive embryo. From it are developed the skin and its appendages, and the nervous system.

ectogenous Originating outside the body.

ectomy A suffix denoting removal.

ectopic Not in the usual place. *E. beat*: contraction of the heart (heart beat) which occurs outside the normal rhythm of the heart. *E. pregnancy*: pregnancy in which the fertilized ovum is not situated in the uterus. The ovum may lie in one of the fallopian tubes, ovary cervix, or in the abdominal cavity. In course of time the gestation sac is apt to rupture, causing profuse haemorrhage into the abdominal cavity and necessitating immediate operation. *E. viscera*: organs (viscus) which are situated in an abnormal place as a result of a developmental anomaly.

ectrodactylia Absence from birth of one or more toes or fingers.

ectropion Eversion of the eyelid.

eczema Inflammation of the skin, acute or chronic. There is redness and vesicles may appear which weep and form crusts.

edentulous Without natural teeth.

EDTA *Abbr.* ethylenediamine tetra-acetic acid. A chelating agent used especially in the treatment of lead poisoning.

Edward syndrome A trisomy of an E group chromosome resulting in 47 autosomes and mental subnormality.

EFAs *See* ESSENTIAL FATTY ACIDS.

EEG *Abbr.* electroencephalogram.

effector nerves Nerve-endings found in muscles, glands, etc. and which effect the functioning of the organ.

efferent Conveying from the centre, *e.g.* the motor nerves which convey impulses from the brain and spinal cord to muscles and glands; *cf.* afferent.

effervescent Bubbling. Giving off small bubbles of gas.

effleurage Movement performed in physiotherapy. The tips of the fingers or the whole surface of the hand are moved along the course of the blood vessels and lymphatics stimulating the circulation and lymphatic drainage.

effort syndrome A form of anxiety neurosis, characterized by symptoms referable to the heart.

effusion Fluid extravasated into serous cavities. *Pleural e.*: fluid in the pleural cavity.

egocentric Self-centred.

ejaculation Forcible, sudden expulsion, especially of semen.

elastin Fibrous protein laid down by fibroblasts in connective tissue ground substance. It is structurally similar to collagen and is found particularly in structures which require to withstand mechanical stresses, *e.g.* walls of large arteries. Contrary to earlier opinion, the fibre is considered to be inelastic.

elastosis Increase in elastic tissue in the skin.

elation A happy and exalted state of mind.

elbow The joint between the arm and forearm. The bones forming the joint are the humerus above and the radius and ulna below.

Electra complex Female equivalent of Oedipus complex.

electrocardiogram (ECG) Recording of electrical events occurring in the heart muscle. The recording is made by attaching electrodes to the skin and amplifying the electrical signal. The oscillations may be recorded by a pen writer. As the amplitude of the signal will increase as its source approaches the receiving electrode, and decrease as the source recedes, the form of the recording is dependent on factors such as the position of the electrodes in relation to the heart, bulk of heart muscle, etc. Each lead shows a characteristic tracing for a normal heartbeat. An impulse starts from the sinoatrial node, and passes through the atrial walls causing the atrial to contract (P wave), passes through the atrioventricular node and A-V bundle (P-Q interval) to excite the interventricular septum (Q wave), left ventricular wall (R wave) and right ventricular wall (S wave) causing the ventricles to contract. This is followed by an interval (S-T interval) before the muscle becomes recharged (T waves) ready for the next cycle which begins after the atria have filled with blood (T-P or diastolic interval).

electrocardiophonography
Recording of sound waves from the heart.

electroconvulsive therapy (ECT) Therapy used especially in depressive mental illness, consisting of passing a low amperage electric current between electrodes placed on the side of the head. Ordinarily this would cause a convulsive motor discharge, but the reaction is 'modified', *i.e.* abolished by general anaesthesia and muscle relaxant drugs administered before the shock is applied.

electrode Conducting surface forming a pole to and from which an electric current may flow.

electroencephalogram (EEG) Recording of electrical events occurring in the brain obtained from signals received by electrodes placed at various points on the head. The signals are amplified and recorded as with the ECG. The wave forms comprise the average effect of the discharges of thousands of nerves in the cerebral cortex and the brain stem and can therefore be interpreted only at a gross level.

electrolysis (1) Separation of ions by placing them in an electric field. (2) Destruction of hair follicles by the passage of an electric current.

electrolytes Substances which ionize in solution.

electromagnetic spectrum Wide range of radiations which are transmitted by photons distributed in a frequency pattern known as electromagnetic waves. The electromagnetic spectrum includes radio waves, light, x-rays and gamma rays.

electromotive force (EMF) The measure of the tendency of an electric current to flow from one point to another. The unit of EMF is the volt.

electromyography (EMG) The recording of electrical events occurring in muscle.

electron A negatively charged atomic particle of mass 0.00055. *E. microscopy*. The use of electrons instead of light to visualize microscopic objects is complex but allows very much greater resolution to be obtained and therefore more details to be seen.

electroretinogram Recording of electrical response of retina to light.

elephantiasis Filariasis. A parasitic disease of the lymphatic vessels, causing great enlargement of the limb or limbs affected. It is chronic, and the skin thickens until it somewhat resembles an elephant's hide. The parasite is the Filaria.

elimination The expulsion of poisons or waste products from the body.

elixir A term sometimes applied to certain preparations containing active drugs with a sweet taste.

emaciation The act of wasting or becoming thin.

emasculation Castration of the male.

embolectomy Removal of an embolus.

embolism Obstruction of blood vessel, usually an artery, by a body, *e.g.* thrombus, fat cells, air, transported in bloodstream.

embolus A blood clot or other foreign body in the bloodstream.

embrocation Lotion for rubbing on the skin.

embryo Animal in process of development from fertilized ovum. *E. transfer*: final stage of *in vitro* fertilization treatment with pre-embryo being placed in uterine cavity. *Pre-e.*: preimplantation stage.

embryology Science of the development of the embryo.

embryoma *See* TERATOMA.

embryopathy Disease in, or damage to, embryo by genetic, viral or other agency.

embryotome Instrument for crushing the fetus.

embryotomy Destruction of fetus.

emesis Vomiting.

emetic Agent that causes vomiting.

emission Discharge, especially of semen.

emmetropia Normal sight.

emollients Softening and soothing applications or liniments.

emotion A response of mind and body to stimuli, such as

anger, hate, pleasure or love.

empathy A form of fantasy when one imagines oneself in someone else's shoes' and feels intensely with that person.

emphysema *Pulmonary e.*: The overdistension of the lungs with air. One form of chronic obstructive airways disease with chronic bronchitis and asthma. *Surgical e.*: air bubbles in the subcutaneous tissues following trauma.

empiricism Treatment founded on experience only, not on reasoning.

empyema Collection of pus in a serious cavity.

emulsion Fine suspension in a fluid of particles of an immiscible fluid, *e.g.* milk is an emulsion of fat in water.

enamel The hard outer coating of the tooth. *See* TEETH.

enarthrosis A ball-and-socket joint. *See* JOINT.

encephalitis Inflammation of the brain. *See* MENINGITIS. *E. lethargica*: encephalitis associated with profound disturbance of sleep rhythm.

encephalocele Protrusion of brain through the skull.

encephalography Also called ventriculography. The radiographic examination of the brain after air, which is radiolucent, has been introduced into the cerebral ventricles. Largely superseded by CT scanning.

encephaloid Resembling the brain.

encephalomalacia Softening of the brain.

encephalomyelitis Inflammation of the brain and spinal cord.

encephalon The brain.

encephalopathy Disease affecting the brain.

enchondroma A tumour of cartilage.

encopresis Faecal incontinence.

encounter group Form of group psychotherapy aimed at improving self-awareness and interpersonal communication.

encysted Enclosed in a sac or cyst.

end organ Collection of cells connected to the peripheral nervous system which act as a transducer, transforming a stimulus into a nerve discharge (receptor) or a nerve discharge into a stimulus, *e.g.* end plate. *See* MOTOR END PLATE.

endarteritis Inflammation of the intima or lining endothelium of an artery.

endemic Occurring frequently in a particular locality.

endocarditis Inflammation of the endothelial lining of the heart.

endocardium The endothelial lining of the heart.

endocervicitis Inflammation

of the mucuous membrane lining the canal of the cervix uteri.

endocolpitis Inflammation of the vaginal epithelium.

endocrine The term used in describing the ductless glands giving rise to an internal secretion. Some of the organs of internal secretion have both an internal and an external secretion, and so may have ducts. The endocrines are: suprarenals, thymus, thyroid, parathyroid, pituitary, pancreas, ovaries and testicles.

endocrinology Science of the endocrine glands.

endoderm Germ layer of embryo composed, as is mesoderm, of cells which have migrated from the surface to the interior of the embryo during gastrulation and from which the alimentary tract is largely derived.

endogenous Produced within the body.

endolymph Fluid of the membranous labyrinth of the ear.

endometrioma Tumour, from tissue like that of the endometrium but found outside it in myometrium, ovary, uterine ligaments, rectovaginal septum, peritoneum, caecum, pelvic colon, umbilicus and laparotomy scars.

endometriosis The presence of endometrioma.

endometritis Inflammation of the endometrium.

endometrium The lining membrane of the uterus.

endoneurium Connective tissue surrounding nerve.

endoplasmic reticulum System of membranes found in the cytoplasm of many cells. *See* CELL.

endorphins· Group of hormones chemically related to opioid alkaloids, probably related to sensations of pleasure, pain responses and hypothalamic function.

endoscope An instrument for the inspection of the interior of a hollow organ.

endothelioma A malignant growth originating in endothelium.

endothelium The lining membrane of serous cavities, blood vessels and lymphatics.

endotoxin An intracellular toxin, *i.e.* retained within the bacteria. When the bacteria are disintegrated the toxin is liberated.

endotracheal Within the trachea.

enema Passage of liquid into the bowel per rectum.

enervating Weakening.

engagement of head Descent of fetal head into the cavity of the pelvis. Normally occurs 2–4 weeks before term in the primigravida. In the multigravida may not occur until labour.

engorgement Vascular congestion.

enophthalmos Recession of the eyeball into the orbit.

enostosis A tumour in a bone.

ensiform cartilage The sword-shaped process at the lower end of the sternum.

Entamoeba histolytica The parasite which causes amoebic dysentery.

enteral In the gastrointestinal tract. *E. feeding*: placing nutrients into the intestine articifially, *e.g.* nasogastric tube or gastrostomy.

enterectomy Excision of part of the intestine.

enteric Refers to intestinal tract. *E. coating*: used for oral drugs to delay release of active substance until after passage through the stomach. *E. fevers*: typhoid and paratyphoid have entry portal in the gut.

enteritis Inflammation of the small intestine.

Enterobius vermicularis Threadworm.

enterocele Hernia containing a piece of bowel.

enterococcus Streptococcus faecalis which occurs as a commensal in the alimentary tract, but is pathogenic in other sites and may cause urinary infections, etc.

enterocolitis Acute inflammation of the ileum, caecum and ascending colon giving

rise to symptoms similar to appendicitis.

enterokinase An activating enzyme of the succus entericus which converts trypsinogen into trypsin.

enterolith Stone in the intestines.

enteroptosis Prolapse of the intestines due to stretching of the mesenteric attachment.

enterostenosis Stricture of the intestines.

enterostomy Surgically established opening between the small intestine and another surface, *e.g.* gastroenterostomy, a connection between the stomach and the small intestine. Enterostomies opening on to the anterior abdominal wall are named according to the part of the small bowel involved, thus jejunostomy, ileostomy.

enterotomy Incision into the small intestine.

enteroviruses Viruses which can be isolated from intestinal tract, *e.g.* poliomyelitis, coxsackie and ECHO viruses.

entropion Inversion of the margin of the eyelid.

enucleation (1) Removal of the nucleus. (2) Removal of a central structure, *e.g.* tumour, without its surrounding structures. Usually only possible with encapsulated structures.

enuresis Incontinence of urine. *Nocturnal e.*: bedwetting at night.

environment The external influences which surround an organism.

enzyme Protein which acts as a catalyst. There are many different kinds of enzyme which increase the reactivity of certain substances (*see* SUBSTRATE) with varying degrees of specificity. Enzymes are essential in order for metabolism to occur at body temperature, since most of the chemical reactions taking place in the body would occur at an imperceptibly slow rate in the absence of enzymes to activate the substrate. The precise mechanism of enzyme action is not yet known.

eosin An acid dye used extensively for staining histological sections.

eosinophil A white blood cell staining with acid dyes. Increased numbers are present in allergic conditions.

eosinophilia (1) Property of being stained by acid dyes such as eosin which combine with basic groups in the tissue. (2) Term used to denote an increase above the normal 2–5 per cent in the numbers of polymorphonuclear leucocytes in the blood which stain deeply with eosin.

ependyma The lining membrane of the cerebral cavities and spinal canal.

ependymoma A tumour arising from ependymal cells.

ephedrine Alkaloid from the plant Ephedra vulgaris which potentiates the action of adrenaline.

ephelis A freckle.

epiblepharon Epicanthus.

epicanthus Projection of the nasal fold to the eyelid.

epicardium Visceral layer of the pericardium.

epicondyle Bony eminence as upon the femoral condyles.

epicranium The integuments which lie over the cranium.

epidemic An infectious or contagious disease attacking a number of people in the same neighbourhood at one time.

epidemiology The study of the distribution of disease.

epidermis The outermost layer of the skin. *See* SKIN.

epidermophytosis An infection of the skin by fungi, the hands and feet being principally affected. Often termed 'athlete's foot' as it is frequently contracted in public gymnasia or swimming baths.

epididymis A long, convoluted tube through which sperm pass between the testis and the vas deferens. It forms a mass at the upper pole of the testis.

epididymitis Inflammation of the epididymis.

epididymo-orchitis Inflammation of the epididymis and testes.

epidural analgesia Form of regional analgesia obtained

by placing anaesthetic agent into the epidural space of the lumbar spine. Used in labour.

epigastrium Surface marking on anterior abdominal wall over region occupied by stomach. *See* ABDOMEN.

epiglottis The flap of cartilage which guards the entrance to the glottis or windpipe. *See* LARYNX.

epilation Removal of hair with destruction of the hair follicle.

epilepsy A disorder of the brain marked by the occurrence of convulsive fits. *Idiopathic e.*: typical epilepsy. In many cases the fit is preceded by a warning or aura. This is usually a sensory disturbance. The two main types are: (1) petit mal, momentary loss of consciousness with no convulsion; (2) grand mal, loss of consciousness, tonic and clonic convulsions. *Jacksonian e.*: local spasm, *e.g.* of one limb or one side of the body, due to irritation of the cerebral cortex. It is important to observe in which group of muscles the movements first commence in order that the cerebral lesion may be located.

epileptiform Like the convulsions of epilepsy.

epiloia Also called tuberous sclerosis. Inherited defect characterized by sebaceous adenoma of the face, multiple gliomas in the brain, and tumours of the heart, kidneys and retina. Fits are the earliest signs of the disease and mental deficiency usually follows.

epimenorrhoea Menstrual periods of frequent recurrence.

epinephrine *See* ADRENALINE.

epineurium The sheath of a nerve.

epiphora An excessive flow of tears.

epiphysis The separately ossified end of growing bone separated from the shaft, diaphysis by a cartilaginous plate (epiphyseal plate). As the bone lengthens more ossified tissue is formed on the diaphyseal side of the epiphyseal cartilage and more cartilage is formed on the epiphysis side. When growth is completed the epiphysis and the diaphysis fuse. *Slipped e.*: this affects the upper femoral epiphysis in late childhood. The cause is unknown.

epiphysitis Inflammation of an epiphysis.

epiploon Omentum.

episcleritis Inflammation of the outer layers of the sclera. *See* EYE.

episiotomy Incision of the perineum just at the end of the second stage of labour, sometimes performed to avoid extensive laceration of the perineum.

epispadias A congenital malformation in which the urethra opens on the dorsum of the penis.

epistaxis Bleeding from the nose.

epithelial casts Filaments of renal epithelium found in the urine in certain diseases, when examined under the microscope. They are chiefly cylindrical, are finely granular, and the cells have large nuclei. If in considerable quantity, they signify nephritis, or some other disease of the kidneys.

epithelioma Tumour of epithelium.

epithelium Sheet of coherent cells forming the lining of tubes, cavities and surfaces, except if derived embryologically from mesoderm, when it is termed endothelium or mesothelium. Epithelia are classified according to thickness of the sheet and the shape or function of the cells composing them. Epithelium may be mucous, keratinizing, simple (one cell thick), stratified (many cells thick), squamous (flat cells), cubical and columnar (tall cells).

epitrochlea The inner round projection at the lower end of the humerus.

epulis Tumour on the gums.

erasion Scraping.

Erb's paralysis The muscles of the upper arm are paralysed due to a lesion of the fifth and sixth cervical nerve roots. May result from excessive traction on the arm during labour. It hangs limply, rotated internally from the shoulder, elbow extended, forearm pronated and palm of hand turned outwards.

erectile tissue Specialized vascular tissue which becomes rigid when filled with blood, *e.g.* penis.

erector A muscle which raises a part.

ergograph An instrument for recording the amount of work done by muscular action.

ergosterol A sterol found in fats and present in the skin which is converted into vitamin D by irradiation with ultraviolet light.

ergotism Poisoning by alkaloids present in the fungus Claviceps purpurea which is found in cereals. One of the alkaloids, ergometrine, is used in obstetrics to control postpartum haemorrhage; another, ergotamine, is used in the treatment of migraine.

erosion Ulceration. *Cervical e.* more commonly ectropion, vaginal epithelium is replaced by columnar epithelium growing down from the cervical canal. *Gastric e.* shallow ulceration of the gastric mucosa, *e.g.* in response to aspirin and related drugs.

Superfically resembles but is not true ulceration.

erotic Pertaining to sexual love.

eructation Flatulency, with passage of gas from stomach through the mouth.

eruption A breaking out on the skin.

erysipelas Acute streptococcal infection of the skin.

erysipeloid Also called erythema serpens (fish-handler's disease). It is caused by Erysipelothrix rhusiopathiae entering a puncture wound in the skin and resembles erysipelas in clinical appearance.

erythema Red skin, due to vasodilation in the dermis. *E. multiforme*: lesions consisting of raised red lesions of varying size and shape which may blister. The cause is unknown but it may represent an abnormal immune response. *E. nodosum*: red tender skin nodules on the legs which may occur in conjunction with certain conditions such as tuberculosis and sarcoidosis.

erythrasma An infection of the skin due to a fungus.

erythroblast Nucleated cell which is normally found in the bone marrow and which gives rise to a mature red blood cell.

erythroblastosis fetalis *See* HAEMOLYTIC DISEASE OF THE NEWBORN.

erythrocyanosis Swelling and blueness of the legs due to vascular spasm.

erythrocyte Red blood cell. *E. sedimentation rate*: *see* ESR.

erythrocytopenia Diminished number of red blood cells.

erythrocytosis *See* POLY-CYTHAEMIA.

erythrodermia Red skin. The whole body surface is involved in an inflammatory vasodilation.

erythropoiesis The manufacture of red blood cells.

Esbach's albuminometer A graduated tube used to estimate the quantity of albumin in urine.

eschar A dry healing scab on a wound; generally the result of the use of caustic. Also the mortified part in dry gangrene.

Esmarch bandage A bloodless method for operations. An india-rubber bandage is tightly applied to the limb, beginning at the extremity, and when it has reached above the point of operation a tourniquet is applied and the bandage removed.

esoteric For the initiate only.

esotropia Converging squint.

ESR *Abbr.* erythrocyte sedimentation rate. The rate at which red blood cells stick together and sediment to the bottom of a graduated tube. The ESR provides a crude index of the circulating globulins since it is by becoming coated with globulins that the red blood cells are enabled to stick together. In infective conditions which cause a rise in blood globulins, *e.g.* rheumatoid arthritis, the rate of erythrocyte sedimentation is increased. Now replaced by blood viscosity measurements.

essentiae Essences; strong solutions of one part volatile oil in five of rectified spirits. Usually given in a few drops on sugar.

essential amino acids Amino acids which the body is unable to synthesize and which must therefore be taken in the diet.

essential fatty acids (EFAs) Polyunsaturated fatty acids not synthesized by the body and therefore required in the diet. Prostoglandin precursors.

essential oil A volatile oil distilled from an odoriferous vegetable substance, *e.g.* oil of cloves.

ethics Moral code based on society's religious and legal background influencing daily actions, *e.g.* between doctor and patient.

ethmoid A bone of the nose through which the olfactory nerves pass.

ethnology The science of the races of mankind.

etiology The science of the causation of disease. *Syn.* aetiology.

EUA *Abbr.* examination under anaesthesia.

eugenics The study and cultivation of conditions that will improve the human race.

eunuch Castrated human male.

euphoria Exaggerated sense of well-being.

euploid Having the normal number of chromosomes.

eustachian tube The canal from the throat to the ear. *See* EAR.

euthanasia A painless death procured by the use of drugs.

evacuation Discharge of excrement from the body. *See* MOTIONS.

evaporating lotions Used to procure local coldness. Lead lotion, or eau-de-Cologne and water, are most common.

eventration Protrusion of the intestines.

eversion Folding outwards.

evisceration Removal of the abdominal contents.

evolution Cumulative alteration in the characteristics of a population occurring progressively during the course of successive generations as opposed to the theory of special creation.

evulsion A tearing apart.

Ewing's tumour Malignant tumour of bone occurring in young adults.

exacerbation An increase in

the severity of symptoms; a paroxysm of disease.

exanthemata Diseases accompanied by specific rashes.

exchange transfusion Transfusion of the newborn in which the infant's blood is removed and replaced by donor blood. This procedure may be necessitated by severe haemolysis of the baby's blood in cases of rhesus group incompatibility (*see* BLOOD GROUPING) when the Rh positive blood from the baby is replaced by Rh negative blood. *Intrauterine e. t.*: may be conducted under ultrasound control via the umbilical vessels before birth.

excipient The substance used as a medium for giving a medicament.

excision A cutting out.

excitability (1) Reaction to a stimulus. (2) A state of being unduly excited.

excitement Increased activity of an organ or organism.

excoriation Abrasions of the skin.

excrement Faecal matter.

excrescence An unnatural protruding growth.

excreta The natural discharges from the body: urine, faeces, sweat.

exenteration Removal of all contents. *E. of orbit*: removal of all the contents of the bony orbit. *E. of pelvis*: removal of pelvic contents and transplant-ation of ureters on to the sigmoid colon.

exfoliation Loss of flakes of material from a surface.

exfoliative cytology Study of cells desquamated from epithelia. *See also* CERVICAL SMEAR.

exhibitionism Extravagant behaviour to attract attention. *Sexual e.*: display of genitalia in public.

exhumation Disinterment of a body.

exogenous Due to an external cause.

exomphalos Umbilical hernia of congenital origin.

exophthalmos Protrusion of the eyeball. May accompany enlargement of the thyroid gland.

exostosis A tumour growing from bone.

exotoxin Toxin released from exterior of an organism; *cf.* endotoxin.

expectorant A drug which increases expectoration.

expectoration The coughing up of sputum.

exploration Operative surgical investigation.

expression (1) Intensity with which the effects of a gene are realized in the phenotype. (2) The act of expulsion. (3) Facial appearance.

exsanguinate To make bloodless.

extension (1) Traction applied to a fractured limb to

hold bones in correct relative position. (2) Unbending of flexed joint as opposed to flexion.

extensor A muscle which extends a part.

external conjugate *See* CON-JUGATE.

external os The opening of the cervix into the vagina.

external cephalic version (ECV) A method of changing the presentation of the fetus to cephalic by manipulation of the uterus through the abdominal wall.

extirpate To remove completely.

extra Latin for outside.

extracapsular Outside a capsule.

extracellular Outside the cells but within the organism. *E. fluid*: fluid, within the organism, not contained in cells.

extract Preparation obtained by removing substances from a part or organ.

extrapyramidal tracts Motor nerve tracts and associated centres which do not directly communicate with the main motor pathway (pyramidal tract). It is a very complex system with many functions, one of which is to regulate muscle tone.

extrasystoles Systolic contraction of the heart the impulse for which originates in a focus other than the sinoatrial

node, and is therefore outside the normal chain of events in the cardiac cycle.

extrauterine gestation Pregnancy outside the uterus. *See* ECTOPIC PREGNANCY.

extravasation Escape of fluid from its proper channel into surrounding tissue.

extremity The end part of any organ. A limb.

extrinsic External. From without.

extrovert Outward turned personality, *cf.* introvert.

exudation Oozing; slow escape of liquid.

eye The organ of vision. *E. strain*: headache due to effort required to focus on near objects when the refractive properties of the lens are defective.

eye teeth The canine teeth.

F

face presentation The advance of the fetus face first into the pelvis during labour. Results from extension of the head for fetal or pelvic reason. May deliver vaginally if chin is anterior in pelvis.

facet A small, smooth, flattened surface of bone.

facial Relating to the face. *F. nerve*: seventh cranial nerve supplying the salivary glands and superficial muscles of the face. *F. paralysis*: paralysis of the muscles of the face caused by injury or disease involving the facial nerves.

facies The appearance of the face, *e.g.* adenoid facies with open mouth and vacant expression.

facultative Able to live under varying conditions.

faecalith Stone-like body composed of compacted faeces.

faeces The discharge from the bowels. Common abnormalities to be noted are (1) Colour: black may indicate the presence of altered blood or the patient may be taking iron. Green stools occur in enteritis, clay-coloured stools in jaundice. (2) Consistency: loose watery stools occur in diarrhoea, hard dry stools in constipation. Foreign bodies such as worms may be present. Unaltered blood may be due to haemorrhoids. Mucus and blood may be due to colitis or intussusception.

Fahrenheit Temperature scale formerly used in the graduation of most clinical thermometers in use in the United Kingdom. Normal body temperature is 37°C (98.6°F).

failure to thrive Poor growth and development of an infant due to dietary restriction, malabsorption or systemic illness.

faint Syncope.

falciform Sickle-shaped. Applied to certain ligaments and other structures.

fallopian tubes Two trumpet-like canals, about 8 cm long, passing from the ovaries to the uterus. *See* UTERUS and SALPINGITIS.

Fallot's tetralogy A group of congenital heart defects consisting of dextraposition of the aorta, right ventricle hypertrophy, intraventricular septal defect and stenosis of the pulmonary artery.

fallout Particulate matter containing radioactive material which falls from clouds containing the debris of atomic explosion.

falx cerebri The fold of dura between the two cerebral hemispheres.

familial Affecting several members of one family. *F. periodic paralysis*: periodic muscular weakness due to acute extracellular potassium deficiency.

family planning Use of contraception to space births or limit family size. *F.p. clinic*: provides contraceptive advice and wide range of services related to reproductive health particularly of women.

fanaticism Zeal for some belief or cause carried to excess.

Fanconi syndrome Inherited disorder in which there is a failure of reabsorption of phosphate, amino acids and sugar by the proximal renal tubules resulting in the appearance of these substances in the urine. The kidneys are also unable to produce an acid urine. The resulting clinical features are thirst, polyuria and rickets followed by chronic renal failure.

fantasy A world of imagination controlled by the whim of the individual.

faradism An induced low frequency asymmetrical alternating current used to stimulate muscle where the nerve supply is intact.

farmer's lung Occupational disease due to inhalation of spores from mouldy hay.

fascia Sheet of connective tissue, *e.g. superficial f.*: connective tissue separating the dermis from underlying structures. *Deep f.*: condensations of connective tissue investing muscles and forming compartments for certain structures.

fascicle A little bundle of fibres.

fat (1) Material extractable by fat solvents such as ether. In this sense it includes a large group of chemicals, *e.g.* steroids, carotenoids and phospholipids. (2) True or neutral fat is a compound of glycerol and a certain group of organic aliphatic acids known as fatty acids. *F. embolism*: *see* EMBOLISM.

Fatal Accident Inquiry *See* CORONER.

fatigue Tiredness.

fatty degeneration Term applied to the appearance of certain cells which as a result of damage take on an appearance of having droplets of fat in their cytoplasm.

fauces The short passage between the back of the mouth and the pharynx.

favism Acute haemolysis caused in sensitive individuals by a substance in the fava bean. Those who are sensitive have a deficiency of glucose-6-phosphate dehydrogenase (G6PD) in their red blood cells.

favus A type of ringworm infection.

febrile Relating to fever.

fecundation Impregnation. Fertilization.

fecundity Power of producing young.

feebleminded Subnormal mentality. No longer an official classification.

feedback treatment Used to help patients modify physiological processes. Can be helpful in muscle tension and raised blood pressure.

Fehling's solution Solution which changes colour on reduction. Formerly used to detect reducing substances (sugars) in the urine.

fel Bile.

Felty's syndrome Syndrome

characterized by leucopenia and enlargement of the spleen associated with chronic rheumatoid arthritis. A generalized hyperpigmentation of the skin is sometimes present. The cause of the syndrome is unknown.

female Applied to the sex that bears young.

femoral artery The artery of the thigh, from the groin to the knee.

femoral canal The small canal medial to the femoral vein. The site of a femoral hernia.

femoral vein Main vein draining blood from the leg. Lies medial to the femoral artery at the groin.

femur The thigh bone.

fenestra A window, term applied to certain apertures.

fenestration Making an artificial window; an operation performed in certain types of deafness.

fermentation Decomposition of organic material by enzymes present in certain organisms. *e.g.* yeasts and bacteria.

fertility Ability to produce young; *cf.* infertility.

fertilization Union of male and female germ cells whereby reproduction takes place.

fester Inflammation, with collection of pus.

fetal WHO approved spelling for foetal.

fetishism Substitution of a symbolic object for the normal goal of union with a member of the opposite sex, as fulfilment of the sexual instinct.

fetor Strong unpleasant smell.

fetus Unborn child. Old spelling, foetus, now replaced. *F. papyraceus*: a fetus which has been retained within the uterus for months after its death, and has undergone a kind of natural mummification.

fever Elevation of body temperature above normal.

fibre A thread-like structure.

fibrillation Uncoordinated contraction of heart muscle. May affect the atria only (atrial fibrillation) or the ventricles (ventricular fibrillation). Because fibrillation prevents efficient contraction of the heart muscle it is rapidly fatal when it affects the ventricles. When only the atria are involved the ventricles beat separately at their own rate.

fibrin Long chain protein which forms a fibrous gel matrix as a basis for a blood clot. It is formed from the soluble plasma protein, fibrinogen, by the action of thrombin. *F. foam*: preparation of human fibrin used as haemostatic pack.

fibroadenoma A tumour composed of mixed fibrous

and glandular elements.

fibroblast Fibrocyte. Branched cell found throughout connective tissue which synthesizes collagen and elastin.

fibrocartilage Cartilage with fibrous tissue.

fibrochondritis Inflamed fibrocartilage.

fibrocystic disease *See* CYSTIC FIBROSIS.

fibroelastosis A rare disorder affecting principally the heart in which an excess of collagen and elastin is formed under the endocardium. This impairs the efficiency of the heart with resultant cardiac enlargement and cardiac failure. Occasionally the heart valves are also involved.

fibroid *See* FIBROMYOMA.

fibroma Benign tumour of fibrous tissue.

fibromyoma A tumour composed of mixed muscular and fibrous tissue. Especially common in the uterus, and commonly spoken of as 'fibroids'.

fibrosarcoma Malignant tumour of fibroblasts.

fibrosis Decomposition of fibrous connective tissue and usually occurring in regions that have been damaged by some trauma.

fibrositis Inflammation of connective tissue, although the term is not only used in this strict sense.

fibula The thin bone on the outer side of the leg.

field of vision The area which can be seen without movement of the eye. *See* PERIMETER.

filament Thread-like piece of fibre.

Filaria Parasitic thread-like worm which may cause lymphatic obstruction. *See* ELEPHANTIASIS.

filiform Thread-like. *F. bougie*: a slender bougie.

filter Device used for removing a certain range of material while allowing others to pass through. The selectiveness of the filter is dependent on its properties. Thus, optical filters made from different types of glass pass only light in certain parts of the spectrum. Fluid filters, according to their pore size, are used to remove viruses, bacteria or other suspended impurities. Gas filters remove certain gases from air passed through them by absorption of the gas onto special material.

filtration Passage through a filter.

filum A structure resembling a thread. *F. terminale*: the tapering end of the enlargement of the lumbar spinal cord.

fimbria A fringe, especially the fringe-like end of the fallopian tube.

fine tremor A sign of thyrotoxicosis. Seen as a slight trembling in the tongue and outstretched hand.

finger One of the digits of the hand.

fingerprinting Method of protein analysis by enzymatic breakdown to peptides followed by two-dimensional separation by chromatography.

first intention A surgical term for aseptic healing of a wound by bringing the edges directly together.

first stage of labour Definition of onset is disputed but includes onset of contractions or cervical ripening. The first stage is completed with full dilatation of the cervix.

fissure A split or cleft. *F. in ano*: small ulcerated cleft in the mucous membrane of the anus.

fistula Pathological communication between two epithelial surfaces or cavities, *e.g.* rectovaginal fistula.

fit Convulsion usually with associated loss of consciousness.

fixation (1) Process used in making permanent preparations of tissues by killing the cells with the least structural distortion. Chemicals such as formaldehyde and gluteraldehyde are fixatives. (2) Focusing the eyes on an object. (3) Psychoanalytically being emotionally attached to another person or object.

flaccid Soft, lacking rigidity.

flagellation (1) Sexual deviation involving whipping, component of sadism or masochism. (2) Form of massage.

flagellum Fine, thread-like structure projecting from surface of certain cells, *e.g.* spermatozoa, which by a lashing movement propels the cell; *cf.* cilia.

flame photometer Apparatus used to measure very small quantities of metals by the brightness of their characteristic flame.

flap A piece of skin cut to fold over a wound or amputation stump.

flatfoot Flattening or total loss of the arches of the foot. It then rests completely on the ground, giving characteristic appearance and walk.

flatulence Distension of the alimentary tract by gas.

flatus Gas in the intestine.

flea The human flea is Pulex irritans. It is wingless and sucks blood, giving rise to irritation and sepsis.

flexion Being bent; the opposite of extension.

flexor A muscle which causes flexion.

flexure A bend. A curvature of an organ, *e.g. hepatic f.*, bend of the colon beneath the liver.

floating ribs The two lower pairs of ribs.

flooding (1) Excessive bleeding from the uterus. (2) A form of behavioural therapy, *e.g.* taking agoraphobics into open spaces.

fluctuation A wavelike motion felt on palpation of an abscess or a cyst containing fluid.

fluke Any of the trematode class of worm.

fluorescein A coal-tar derivative which stains the cornea a vivid green if there is any loss of surface epithelium, *e.g.* in an abrasion or ulcer.

fluorescent screen A screen coated with materials which fluoresce when exposed to x-rays.

fluoridation The addition of fluoride, such as when added to drinking water.

fluorine A halogen element. If added in minute quantities to drinking water it causes a reduced incidence of dental decay. The ideal amount of water is 1 ppm.

fluoroscopy Use of fluorescent screen to view x-ray images.

flutter Rapid regular contraction of the atrial muscle of the heart. The rate reaches about 300 beats per minute. Because of the recovery time required by the ventricular myocardium between successive beats, it only responds to every second or third atrial contraction, *e.g.* 2:1 or 3:1.

See HEART BLOCK.

flying squad Emergency clinical unit which can travel rapidly to domiciliary cases. *Obstetric f. s.*: most commonly called to aid resuscitation following antepartum or postpartum haemorrhage or eclamptic fits before transfer to hospital. Rarely needed in urban practice now as may actually delay transfer to hospital.

focus Point of maximum intensity.

foetor *See* FETOR.

Foley catheter Self-retaining catheter, kept in position by small balloon.

folic acid Pteroyglutamic acid, part of the vitamin B complex found in liver, yeast, spinach, etc. Essential for blood formation.

folie à deux Delusion shared by two persons.

follicle (1) Hair follicle. A pit-like structure in the epidermis in which the hair grows and which receives the duct of sebaceous glands. (2) Ovarian follicle. Also called graafian follicle. A fluid-filled vesicle in the ovary containing a maturing ovum which at ovulation is discharged by rupture of the follicle. The ovaries contain many ripening follicles which are under the control of the pituitary glands, but normally only one ruptures at each ovulation.

The epithelium of the follicle produces oestrogens. After ovulation the follicle becomes a corpus luteum producing progesterone. *F. stimulating hormone* (*FSH*): hormone secreted by the anterior lobe of the pituitary gland. In the female it stimulates the growth of ovarian follicles and the production of oestrogens. In the male it promotes the development of spermatozoa in the testis.

follicular keratosis Hyperkeratosis in the region of hair follicles (phrynoderma) seen in vitamin A deficiency, Darier's disease and a number of uncommon skin conditions.

follicular tonsillitis *See* TONSILLITIS.

fomentation A poultice: hot wet application to the skin.

fomites Articles like clothing or bedding which have been in contact with a patient ill with a contagious disease.

fontanelle A soft space in the skull of an infant before the skull has completely ossified. The anterior fontanelle, or bregma, is where the coronal, frontal and sagittal sutures meet. The posterior fontanelle is where the lambdoid and sagittal sutures meet. The anterior fontanelle should be closed by two years of age. Delay is a sign of rickets.

food poisoning Diarrhoea and/or vomiting from eating infected food. Symptoms may be caused by the preformed toxins of Staphylococcus aureus or Clostridium welchii or from infection by organisms of the Salmonella group or rarely by Botulinus toxin. Infected foods are usually meat products or confectionery containing eggs, which have been allowed to remain in warm rooms. Another source of infection may be the unwashed hands of those handling food.

foot That part of the leg below the ankle. *F. drop*: inability to keep a foot bent at right angles to the leg. The toes and foot drop and walking becomes difficult. Usually due to weakness or paralysis of the muscles which dorsiflex the ankle joint. *F. and mouth disease*: virus disease well known in cattle which occasionally affects man causing blistering and ulceration of the buccal mucosa and similar lesions on the hands and feet especially round the nails.

foramen An opening. *F. magnum*: opening in the back of the skull through which the spinal cord passes. *F. ovale.*: opening between the right and left atria in the fetus which allows oxygenated venous blood from the placenta to pass into the left side of the heart and thus bypass the pulmonary circulation. Normally it closes at birth when the pressure in the left atrium rises. *Optic f.*: where the optic nerve enters the skull. Also *jugular f.*, etc.

forceps Surgical pincers used for lifting and moving instead of using the fingers. *F. delivery*: method of assisting the delivery of an infant by applying special forceps to the head.

forebrain Cerebrum.

foreign body General term to include any material in the body which is not normally found in that site. Usually refers to completely extraneous material, *e.g.* sand in conjunctiva or a peanut in the bronchial tube. May be *iatrogenic f. b.*, *e.g.* IUD, hip prosthesis. *F. b. reaction*: typical tissue response to *f. b.* may include a giant cell reaction.

forensic medicine Medicine in so far as it has to do with the law.

foreskin The prepuce, or skin covering the end of the penis.

formication A sensation as of ants creeping over the body. Used almost entirely to denote tingling sensation in a nerve recovering from pressure or injury, and therefore after nerve injury it is a sign of regeneration.

formula (pl. **formulae**) A prescription. Statement of

constituents which form a compound.

formulary A collection of formulae for medical preparations such as those found in the British National Formulary.

fornix (pl. **fornices**) An arch. Applied to various anatomical structures, but especially to the roof of the vagina.

fossa Little depressions of the body, such as *f. lacrimalis*, the hollow of the frontal bone, which holds the lacrimal gland. *Iliac f.*: concavities of the iliac bones of the pelvis.

fostering Short-term care of a child by a non-adoptive family. Used to provide home environment for child prior to reuniting with natural parents or adoption.

Fothergill's operation Repair of the anterior and posterior vaginal walls and amputation of the cervix.

fourchette A thin fold of skin behind the vulva.

fovea Shallow depression in the retina where there is an absence of rods and a concentration of cones (*see* EYE) and where there are no intervening nerves and blood vessels. It is the site of maximum visual stimulation and the region on which the image is focused when the eyes are fixed on an object.

fracture A break in a bone.

A fracture may be: (1) *Simple or closed f.*, not connected with an external wound. (2) *Compound or open f.*, communicating with the surface. (3) *Greenstick f.*, when the bone is fractured half through on the convex side of the bend as in a green twig. Only seen in children. (4) *Comminuted f.*, where bone is broken into more than two pieces. (5) *Impacted f.*, where one fragment is driven into the other. (6) *Complicated f.*, where fracture is combined with injury to another important structure, *e.g.* artery, nerve or organ. (7) *Pathological f.*, occurring spontaneously in diseased bone. The type of break may be: (1) *Transverse f.*, due to direct violence applied at point of fracture. (2) *Oblique f.*, due to indirect violence when a force applied at a distance causes the bone to break at its weakest point. (3) *Spiral f.*, when a limb is violently rotated. (4) *Depressed f.*, only of skull, when bone is driven inwards. *See* COLLES' FRACTURE, POTT'S FRACTURE, SPLINTS, SPONTANEOUS FRACTURE.

fraenum *See* FRENUM.

fragilitas ossium Abnormal brittleness of the bones.

framboesia *See* YAWS.

free association In psychoanalysis, when the patient gives the first word which a stimulus brings to his mind, or a train of ideas.

Frei test Skin test for lymphogranuloma inguinale in which a small quantity of the heat-inactivated virus is injected into the dermis. If positive a red papule appears in 48 hours at the site of injection.

Freiberg's infarction Sclerosis of the head of the second or third metatarsal with flattening of the articular surface and swelling and tenderness of the affected joint.

fremitus A vibration perceived by palpation, always applied to a vibration in the chest.

frenum A small membranous fold attached to certain organs and acting as a check. *F. linguae*: that under the tongue.

Freudian According to Freud's teaching. He taught that psychological disorders often resulted from unconscious sexual impressions during childhood. These he brought to consciousness through psychoanalysis. Dreams he said were the wish-fulfilment of repressed desires.

friction (1) A circular movement in massage performed with the tips of the fingers or thumb as deeply as possible over joints; the object being to break down adhesions. (2)

The sound heard in auscultation when two dry, roughened surfaces rub together as in pleurisy.

Friedreich's ataxia　Inherited degenerative disease of the nervous system in which the posterior and lateral columns of the spinal cord, the cerebellum and occasionally the optic nerves are involved. The onset is in the first or second decade and the condition is progressive. It is characterized by unsteady gait, clumsiness, weakness and dysarthria together with other neurological disturbances.

frigidity　Lack of sexual desire.

Fröhlich's syndrome　A disorder with obesity, sexual infantilism, disturbances of sleep and temperature regulation and diabetes insipidus due to damage of the pituitary and hypothalamus.

frontal　Relating to the forehead. *F. bone*: one of the bones of the skull. *F. sinus*: see SINUS.

frostbite　Injury of the skin or a part from extreme cold. There is redness, swelling and pain and necrosis may result.

frozen shoulder　Pain and stiffness in shoulder joint limiting mobility, of no known cause.

fructose　Fruit sugar.

fructosuria　Fructose, the sugar present in fruits, may be extracted in large quantity from the urine if a considerable amount of fruit has been eaten. If the urine is tested for sugar the fructose gives a positive result and may lead to a mistaken diagnosis of diabetes mellitus.

frustration　Disappointment experienced by a person who is thwarted and prevented by circumstances from achieving some desired object.

FSH　*See* FOLLICLE STIMULATING HORMONE.

FTA test　*Abbr.* fluorescent treponemal antibody test for syphilis.

fugue　A fleeing from reality as in hysteria. The patient has no recollection of his actions during this time.

full-term　The fetus is said to be at term after developing in the uterus for 40 weeks. Infants born after 38 weeks have similar characteristics and are regarded as full-term medically.

fulminating　Severe and rapid in its course.

fumigation　Sterilization of rooms by disinfectant vapour.

function　The normal special work of an organ.

functional disorder　Subjective sensation of malfunctioning of an organ or organs when there is no evidence of organic disease.

fundus　The enlarged part of a

hollow organ farthest removed from the orifice; thus the fundus oculi is the interior of the eye behind the lens and pupil, visible with an ophthalmoscope; the fundus uteri is the top of the uterus.

fungi (sing. **fungus**) A subdivision of Thallophyta including moulds, mushrooms, rusts, yeasts, etc. Simple plants which lack chlorophyll and are either saprophytic or parasitic. A few fungi cause disease in man. Fungi are used as a source of protein and vitamins, certain enzymes, used in baking and brewing, etc. and antibiotics, notably penicillin.

fungicide Any substance used for the destruction of fungi.

funiculitis Inflammation of the spermatic cord.

funnel chest Also called pectus excavatum. A developmental deformity in which the sternum is depressed and the ribs and costal cartilages curve inwards.

furuncle A boil.

furunculosis The appearance of one or more boils.

fusiform Spindle-shaped.

G

gag An instrument for keeping the mouth open.

gait Manner of walking.

galactagogue An agent that causes an increased flow of milk.

galactocele A cyst of the breast containing milk.

galactorrhoea Excessive flow of milk.

galactosaemia A metabolic disorder characterized by presence of galactose in the bloodstream.

galactose A hexose sugar which, in combination with glucose, forms the disaccharide lactose which is present in breast milk.

gall Also called bile. The secretion of the liver; it accumulates in the gall bladder. *G. bladder*: the membranous sac which holds the bile. *See* BILE DUCT.

gallop rhythm Term applied to a particular cadence heard on auscultation of the heart in cases of severe left ventricular failure when as the result of tachycardia there is summation of the sounds of the atrial contraction and of the blood distending the hypotonic ventricles. This gives a third 'beat' which is heard in diastole.

gallows traction *See* BALKAN BEAM.

gallstone Calculus in the gall bladder. If the stone passes into the cystic or common bile duct there is great pain, and if in the common bile duct, jaundice. *See* COLIC.

galvanism Therapeutic use of

direct electric current, *i.e.* continuous or interrupted. Now rarely used for treatment.

galvanometer Instrument to measure the flow of very small electric currents.

gamete A sexual reproductive cell, *e.g.* sperm, ovum.

gamma rays Electromagnetic waves of extremely short wavelength; similar to x-rays but shorter. Employed for dry, cold sterilization of any articles which would be destroyed by moisture or heat. Also used in radiotherapy.

gammaglobulin Protein fraction of plasma, rich in antibodies against infection.

ganglion (1) A collection of nerve cells forming a semi-independent nerve centre. They are found in the sympathetic nervous system and in other parts of the nervous system. (2) Surgically, a chronic synovial cyst generally connected with a tendon sheath; most common site is back of the hand, near the wrist.

ganglionectomy Excision of a ganglion.

gangrene Massive necrosis of tissue as a result of reduced blood supply. *Dry g.*: this results from severe arterial insufficiency. *Wet g.*: this is due to concurrent interference in the venous drainage. *Gas g.*: infection by anaerobic organ-

isms, *e.g.* Clostridium welchii.

gargle A liquid medicine for washing out the throat.

gargoylism Hurler's syndrome. A defect of skeletal development in which the skull is grossly deformed and the digital bones are bulbous, the hands assuming a claw-like appearance. There is often associated congenital heart disease and intellectual impairment.

gas gangrene *See* GANGRENE.

Gasserian ganglion A ganglion of the sensory root of the fifth cranial nerve, deeply situated in the skull. It is sometimes operated on or injected for the relief of intractable trigeminal neuralgia.

gastrectomy Removal of the stomach.

gastric Relating to the stomach. *G. aspiration*, also called *g. suction*: performed postoperatively after operations on the alimentary tract to prevent dilatation of the stomach. A Ryle's tube is passed and the contents aspirated at frequent intervals or continuously. *G. juice*: the digestive fluid of the stomach. *G. lavage*: washing out the stomach: a procedure used in the treatment of poisoning. *G. ulcer*: ulceration of the mucosa lining the stomach. Acute ulceration may be caused by ingested substances, *e.g.* aspirin. Chronic ulceration may be due to reduced capacity of the epithelium to withstand the acid gastric secretion or to a tumour of the epithelium.

gastrin A hormone released by cells in the wall of the pyloric antrum, when it is distended. This stimulates the secretion of gastric juice by the secretory cells in the rest of the stomach.

gastritis Inflammation of the epithelium lining the stomach.

gastrocele Hernia of the stomach.

gastrocnemius A large muscle of the calf of the leg.

gastrocolic reflex Reflex peristaltic contractions in the colon occurring as a result of filling the stomach.

gastroduodenostomy, gastroenterostomy, gastrojejunostomy The operation of making an artificial passage direct from the stomach to the duodenum or the jejunum.

gastroenteritis Inflammation of the stomach and intestines.

gastrogastrostomy, gastrolysis, gastroplasty Operations for the cure of hourglass contractions of the stomach.

gastrointestinal tract The gut including the mouth, oesophagus, stomach, small and large intestine, rectum and anus and the associated structures.

gastropexy Fixing a displaced stomach to the abdominal wall by surgery.

gastroptosis Downward displacement of the stomach.

gastroscope An instrument for inspecting the cavity of the stomach. It has a light at the end and is passed per oesopohagus.

gastrostomy Making an artificial opening into the stomach through which the patient is fed by pouring nourishment through a tube directly into the stomach. Performed for stricture, usually malignant, of the oesophagus.

gastrulation Embryological term used to describe the complex movements of cells of the embryo in which the cells which give rise to the internal organs migrate inside the embryo.

Gaucher's disease A recessively inherited disorder of lipid metabolism in which cells of the reticuloendothelial system become filled with the phospholipid kerasin. It forms one of the group of conditions known as the lipoidoses or lipid storage diseases.

gauze Open mesh material used in surgical dressings.

gavage Forced feeding.

Geiger counter Machine which detects and registers radioactivity.

gelatin Denatured collagen

obtained by boiling connective tissue.

gemellus (pl. **gemelli**) Twin, the name of two muscles in the buttock.

gene The unit of material of inheritance which consists of deoxyribonucleic acid (DNA). The gene is a part of a chromosome which is responsible for one function *e.g.* the blueprint for the arrangement of amino acids in one protein. The place the gene occupies in the chromosome is known as its locus and variants of the gene which arise by mutation and which occupy the similar position in corresponding chromosomes are known as allelomorphs, *i.e.* genes occupying similar positions are allelic to each other.

general paralysis of the insane Also called GPI. Dementia due to involvement of the brain in syphilis.

generation (1) Reproduction. (2) Specific group of individuals resulting from a mating: thus F_1 generation (first filial generation) offspring resulting from the mating of parental generation (P_1); F_2 generation (second filial generation) offspring resulting from crossing the members of F_1 generation among themselves.

genetic Pertaining to generation. *G. code*: sequence of nucleotides on chromosome by which gene activity is expressed. Three nucleotides (codon) are responsible for activity of each gene and message is transmitted through DNA and RNA systems.

genetics Study of heredity and its variations.

geniculate bodies Posterior nuclei of the thalamus. The fibres of the visual pathway relay in the lateral geniculate bodies.

geniculate ganglion Ganglion of the sensory part of the facial nerve.

genitalia The generative organs.

genome The total genetic information available in a cell, organism or species contained on the chromosomes of cells.

genotype The genetic makeup of an individual, *i.e.* the set of alleles inherited by the individual.

gentian violet An antiseptic dye, used as a paint or lotion, strength 1 in 100 to 1 in 1000.

genu The knee. *G. valgum*: knock-knee, a deformity in which the knees are bent inwards. *G. varum*: bow-legged.

genupectoral position The knee–chest position, the patient resting upon the knees and chest.

geriatrics The study of disease among the elderly.

germ A microbe, bacillus.

German measles *See* RUBELLA.

germicide An agent that destroys microorganisms.

gerontology The study of ageing.

gestation Pregnancy. *G. sac*: the fetus with its enveloping membranes, decidua, etc. The contents of a pregnant uterus.

Ghon focus Small focus of infection found in primary infection by tubercle bacillus.

giardiasis Infection with Giardia intestinalis.

GIFT *Abbr.* gamete intrafallopian transfer. Placement of oocytes and spermatozoa into the fallopian tube in the hope that fertilization and pregnancy will occur. Derivation of *in vitro* fertilization suitable for treatment of women with intact fallopian tubes.

gigantism *See* ACROMEGALY.

Gilliam's operation Operation for uterine retroversion, in which the round ligaments are shortened or sutured to the rectus muscle sheath.

gingival Relating to the gums.

gingivitis Inflammation of the gums.

ginglymus A hinge joint such as elbow or knee.

girdle Band encircling the body. A term used to describe distribution of cutaneous nerve supply to the thorax. *G.*

pain: pain in this distribution.

glabella Triangular space between the eyebrows.

glairy Slimy, albuminous.

gland (1) Cell or collection of cells which produce specialized substance(s) to be secreted outside the organ into the bloodstream (endocrine gland) or on to an epithelial surface (exocrine gland). (2) Term, accepted by common usage, applied to lymph nodes.

glanders A virus disease of horses which is occasionally transmitted to man.

glandular fever *See* INFECTIOUS MONONUCLEOSIS.

glans Bulbous extremity of the penis and clitoris.

glaucoma A disease of the eye with hardening of the globe, due to an increase in the intraocular pressure; acute forms of this disease if untreated may lead to complete loss of sight in a few days.

glenoid A cavity, a term applied to the socket of the shoulder joint.

glioma A tumour composed of neuroglia, nerve connective tissue. It may develop in the brain or spinal cord.

gliomyoma A tumour composed of nerve and muscle tissue.

Glisson's capsule The connective tissue capsule of the liver, enveloping the portal vein, hepatic artery, hepatic ducts.

globulin Group of proteins widely distributed in the body with numerous specialized functions. One group, the gammaglobulins, are antibodies.

globus hystericus Hysterical choking feeling as of a ball in the throat.

glomerulonephritis One of the causes of acute nephritis syndrome. The exact pathogenesis is not known, but lesions in the glomeruli of the kidneys are frequently associated wtih streptococcal infection in the throat or elsewhere.

glomerulus The filtration unit of a nephron. It consists of a coil of fine capillaries apposed to an expansion of urinary epithelium.

glomus tumour Tumour formed from specialized muscle cells which surround blood vessels (pericytes). These are particularly frequent in sites where arteriovenous shunts are situated in the skin, *e.g.* at tips of fingers and toes. Characterized by extreme tenderness.

glossal Relating to the tongue.

glossectomy Surgical removal of the tongue.

glossitis Inflammation of the tongue.

glossodynia Pain in the tongue sometimes associated with trigeminal neuralgia but often of unknown origin.

glossopharyngeal Relating to tongue and pharynx. *G. nerve*: the ninth cranial nerve.

glossoplegia Paralysis of the tongue.

glottis The aperture between the vocal cords in the larynx.

glucocorticoids Steroid hormones, secreted by the adrenal cortex, which control carbohydrate metabolism.

glucose Dextrose. A hexose sugar, *i.e.* containing six carbon atoms, which is widely distributed in nature in disaccharides like sucrose and lactose and polysaccharides such as starch. Glucose is the currency of energy production in metabolism.

glucose tolerance test Test performed in cases suspected of diabetes, occasionally in other instances. A glucose load is taken, usually by mouth, and the concentration of glucose in the blood is estimated at intervals afterwards.

glue ear Accumulation of fluid in middle ear. The commonest cause of deafness in children.

glue sniffing *See* SOLVENT ABUSE.

gluteal Pertaining to the buttock.

gluten A protein constituent

of certain cereals which acts as an antigen in coeliac disease.

gluteus *G. maximus, G. medius, G. minimus*: the three large muscles of the buttock.

glycaemia Presence of sugar in the blood.

glycerin Clear, viscous fluid produced as a byproduct in the manufacture of soap.

glycine An amino acid.

glycogen A polysaccharide composed of hexose sugars connected in branching chains. *G. storage disease*: inherited disorder in which there is a deficiency of enzyme(s) involved in the breakdown of glycogen. As a result the tissues of the body become infiltrated with glycogen.

glycogenesis The formation of glycogen from glucose.

glycogenolysis Breakdown of glycogen.

glycolysis Breakdown of glucose.

glycoside Substance which on hydrolysis yields a sugar, usually glucose, and one or more other substances.

glycosuria Sugar in the urine.

gnathic Relating to the jaw or cheek.

goblet cells Pear-shaped cells in certain epithelia which secrete mucin.

goitre Enlargement of the thyroid.

Golgi apparatus Microscopic system consisting of a number of membrane-surrounded vacuoles. It is involved in secretion.

gonadal dysgenesis Failure of development of gonads. Usually due to chromosome abnormalities. *See* TURNER'S SYNDROME.

gonadotrophic Promoting the activity of the gonads.

gonadotrophins Hormones which stimulate the gonads, *e.g.* FSH, LH.

gonads Reproductive glands: ovary of the female, testis of the male.

gonococcus The microbe causing gonorrhoea. It is a Gram-negative intracellular diplococcus. *See* BACTERIA.

gonorrhoea Venereal disease caused by the gonococcus. May be transmitted to the newborn as it passes through an infected birth canal (ophthalmia neonatorum), and to children by means of infected towels and linen.

Goodpasture syndrome Pneumonitis with haemoptysis followed by glomerulonephritis and uraemia.

gouge A grooved instrument of steel used to scoop out dead bone.

gout Inherited defect of purine metabolism in which uric acid is in excess in the tissues. During acute attacks it is characterized by painful swelling of a joint, classically the big toe.

GPI *Abbr.* general paralysis of the insane.

graafian follicles *See* FOLLICLE.

Graefe's knife Scalpel used in ophthalmic surgery.

graft To induce union between tissues which are normally separate. The parts may be transferred from one place to another in the same individual (autograft) or from one individual (donor) to another (recipient) of the same species (homograft) or of a different species (heterograft).

gram (g) Metric unit; 30 g equivalent to 1 oz avoirdupois approximately.

Gram's stain Bacteria which resist decolorization by alcohol after staining with methyl violet and Gram's solution are termed Grampositive, *e.g.* staphylococci, pneumococci. Those which are decolorized by alcohol are termed Gram-negative, *e.g.* E. coli, gonococci.

grand mal *See* EPILEPSY.

granular Composed of grains or granulations. *G. layer*: region in keratinizing epithelia where the cytoplasm of the cells appears granular.

granulation tissue Newly formed vascular connective tissue formed at surface of wounds.

granule Small particle or grain.

granulocyte A polymorphonuclear white blood cell having a granular cytoplasm. Granules may be basophilic, acidophilic (eosinophilic) or neutrophilic.

granuloma A tumour composed of granulation tissue.

graph A diagrammatic record of given information.

gravel A popular term for small concretions formed in the kidney or bladder.

Graves' disease *See* HYPERTHYROIDISM.

gravid Pregnant.

Grawitz tumour A malignant epithelial tumour of the kidney.

greenstick fracture *See* FRACTURE.

grey matter Tissue of the CNS in which are situated numerous cell bodies of nerves, dendritic processes, glial cells, etc.

Griffith's types Strains of Streptococcus pyogenes classified according to surface antigens.

grippe Influenza.

groin Junction of the thigh and abdomen.

grommet Small, plastic tubular device inserted into the tympanic membrane of the ear. It acts as an artificial eustachian tube and is designed to prevent the accumulation of fluid in the middle ear. It is extruded spontaneously after a time. *See also* GLUE EAR.

growing pains Pain of uncertain origin which may accompany phases of rapid growth in children. There is a danger of overlooking acute rheumatism.

growth hormone (GH) Anterior pituitary hormone involved in growth; deficiency may result in dwarfism and excess in gigantism or acromegaly. *G.h. test*: GH levels normally drop with raised blood sugar but this does not occur in acromegaly.

guaiacum Sometimes used to detect presence of blood in the urine.

guar Natural fibre which may be prepared in the form of a drink. Impedes sugar absorption and helps stabilize diabetic control.

Guillain–Barré syndrome Acute infective polyneuritis in which there is both motor and sensory loss. The most characteristic feature is the great rise of protein content while the cell count of the cerebrospinal fluid remains normal.

guillotine An instrument for excising the tonsils.

guinea worm Nematode worm which may infest man. The female migrates into the subcutaneous tissues.

gullet The oesophagus.

gumboil Abscess in periodontal tissues.

gumma A soft tumour occurring in the tertiary stage of syphilis. This may ulcerate. The characteristics of a gummatous ulcer are: a vertical, punched-out edge; healthy surrounding tissues; the base formed by a 'washleather' slough; it is painless and very slow to heal. *See* SYPHILIS.

gustatory Pertaining to taste.

gut The intestine.

Guthrie test Screening test on babies for several inborn errors of metabolism including phenylketonuria.

gynaecology The study and practice of the management and treatment of disorders affecting female organs, *e.g.* ovaries, uterus, vagina.

gynaecomastia Enlargement of the breasts in a male.

gyrus (pl. **gyri**) A convolution, such as the convolutions of the brain.

H

habit Constant and often involuntary action established by frequent repetition.

habitat The natural abode of an animal or plant.

haem (1) Prefix pertaining to blood. (2) Tetrapyrrollic ring containing an atom of ferrous iron. When combined with protein globin forms haemoglobin.

haemagglutinin Antibodies present in the blood which combine with red blood cells of a different blood group and cause agglutination. *See* BLOOD GROUPING.

haemangioma Abnormal growth of blood vessels.

haemarthrosis Effusion of blood into a joint cavity.

haematemesis Vomiting blood.

haematin The oxidized product of haem.

haematinic A substance which increases the amount of haemoglobin in the blood, *e.g.* iron.

haematocele A swelling or cyst containing blood.

haematocolpos Collection of menses in the vagina due to the presence of a septum.

haematocrit Packed cell volume (PCV). It is a measurement of the proportion of the circulating blood occupied by red blood cells.

haematology The study of the blood.

haematoma A swelling composed of blood. A bruise.

haematometra Accumulation of blood in the uterus.

haematomyelia Haemorrhage into the spinal cord.

haematoporphyrin *See* PORPHYRINS.

haematorrhachis Haemorrhage into the extramedullary region of the spinal cord.

haematosalpinx Distension of the fallopian tube with blood.

haematoxylin Basic dye prepared from logwood. It stains acid groups in tissue, particularly nucleic acids, and is much used in histology.

haematozoa Protozoan parasites in the bloodstream.

haematuria Blood in the urine.

haemochromatosis Also known as 'bronzed diabetes'. An inherited defect in the metabolism of iron with resultant deposition of iron in tissues thus interfering with their function. Diabetes mellitus, hyperpigmentation of the skin and cirrhosis of the liver are associated clinical features.

haemoconcentration Concentration of the blood.

haemocytometer Instrument to measure the average diameter of red blood cells.

hacmodialysis Passage of circulating blood through dialysing apparatus, *e.g.* artificial kidney, to restore normal balance of chemical components.

haemoglobin Respiratory pigment in red blood cells composed of an iron-containing group (haem) and a complex protein (globin). In combination as haemoglobin it has the property of forming a reversible combination with oxygen.

haemoglobinometer Instrument to measure the amount

of haemoglobin in the blood.

haemoglobinuria Haemoglobin, freed by lysis of red blood cells, in the urine.

haemolysin Agent causing the breakdown of the red cell membrane.

haemolytic Having the power to destroy red blood cells. *H. anaemia*: resulting from destruction of red cells as in forms of poisoning, or by the action of antibodies. *H. disease of the newborn*: jaundice in a rhesus-positive infant caused by red cell destruction by anti-rhesus antibodies generated in the rhesus-negative mother's circulation during pregnancy. *See* BLOOD GROUPING.

haemopericardium Blood in the pericardium.

haemoperitoneum Blood in the peritoneal cavity.

haemophiliac A person suffering from haemophilia.

haemophilias A group of conditions with a congenital and inherited tendency to haemorrhage because of impaired blood clotting mechanism. Haemophilia A, factor VIII deficiency, and haemophilia B (Christmas disease), factor IX deficiency, are both X-linked disorders which appear in males but are carried by females of the family.

haemophilic arthropathy Joint damage which occurs in haemophiliacs caused by

bleeding into joints.

Haemophilus influenzae Bacterium often isolated among organisms causing secondary infection in virus diseases of the respiratory tract. They do not cause influenza.

haemophthalmia Haemorrhage into the eye.

haemopoiesis The process of formation of the blood cells, particularly the red blood cells. In the fetus, haemopoiesis occurs in the spleen and liver, in the adult, in the bone marrow.

haemopoietin Complex of vitamin B_{12} and intrinsic factor which stimulates haemopoiesis.

haemoptysis Coughing up blood.

haemorrhage A flow of blood. It may be: *arterial h.*:, occurring in spurts, and bright red in colour; *venous h.*:, occurring in a steady stream and dark in colour; *capillary h.*:, oozing from a large wound surface. Haemorrhage may be (1) *primary h.*:, at time of injury; (2) *reactionary h.*:, within 24 hours of injury due to a rise in the blood pressure; (3) *secondary h.*:, usually within 7–10 days of injury, due to sepsis. Haemorrhage may be *visible h.* or *concealed h.*, into one of the cavities of the body and not appearing at the surface. The symptoms of concealed haemorrhage are pallor of skin and mucous membranes, quick, sighing respiration, rapid, small, weak pulse, restlessness, subnormal temperature, coldness, sweating and collapse. *Inevitable h.*: bleeding due to placenta praevia.

haemorrhagic disease of newborn Widespread haemorrhage in newborn babies due to a deficiency of vitamin K which is required for the synthesis of the clotting factor prothrombin. Because vitamin K deficiency is common, most newborn babies in the UK are given prophylactic injections of vitamin K immediately after birth.

haemorrhoidectomy Surgical removal of haemorrhoids.

haemorrhoids Varicose rectal veins.

haemostasis The prevention of haemorrhage or the measures taken for its arrest.

haemostatic An agent to arrest a flow of blood.

haemothorax Escape of blood into the cavity of the chest.

hair ball Also called trichobezoar. It is a rare cause of intestinal obstruction. Persons swallowing hair are frequently feeble-minded.

hair follicle *See* FOLLICLE.

half-life The time in which the total radiation emitted by a radioactive substance is reduced by decay to half its original value. It is a constant for each isotope and is independent of the quantity.

halitosis Foul breath.

hallucination The patient perceives something for which there is no sensory stimulus, *i.e.* the sights and sounds are entirely imaginary; *cf.* delusion.

hallucinogen Drug causing hallucinations.

hallux The big toe. *H. rigidus*: literally a rigid big toe caused by destruction and ankylosis of the metatarsophalangeal joint. *H. valgus*: displacement of the big toe towards the other toes.

halogens Non-metallic elements of the series fluorine, chlorine, bromine, iodine. They are anionic in solution and combine with metals to form salts.

hamartoma A term used to classify tumours arising from the overgrowth of developing tissues. Benign lesions such as vascular naevi and neurofibromas.

hamate bone One of the wrist bones.

hammer toe A deformity of a toe in which there is permanent dorsal flexion of the first phalanx and plantar flexion of the second and third phalanges.

hamstrings Muscles traversing more than one joint, usually the muscles and tendons traversing the popliteal region.

handicapped Having a defect in physical or mental development which interferes with daily activities.

Hand–Schüller–Christian disease Granulomas containing cholesterol are found affecting chiefly the skull; the orbit and pituitary gland may be affected. The aetiology is unknown. General symptoms may include hypercholesterolaemia, splenomegaly, eczema, polyuria and exophthalmos.

hangnail Skin in nail fold that may overgrow the nail.

haploid Having a set of unpaired chromosomes in the nucleus, characteristic of gametes, *i.e.* sperm cells, ova.

hapten Substance which itself cannot induce antibody production but is antigenic when combined with a protein.

hard chancre *See* CHANCRE.

harelip Defect of development in which there is a failure of fusion between the central and lateral maxillary buds leaving a fissure in the upper lip. It is frequently associated with various degrees of cleft palate.

Hartmann's pouch A pouch at the neck of the gall bladder in which gallstones may become impacted.

Hartmann's solution A saline solution containing sodium lactate. Used in acidosis and also in severe haemorrhage before blood is crossmatched for transfusion.

Hashimoto's disease A chronic thyroiditis due to autoimmunity to thyroglobulin. It causes myxoedema.

hashish Extract of Indian hemp.

haustrations Sacculations of colon seen on x-ray.

haversian canals The minute canals which permeate bone. *See* BONE.

hay fever Allergic rhinitis caused by exposure of sensitized respiratory epithelium to certain pollens.

headache Pain in the head.

Heaf test A method used for testing immunity to tuberculosis before doing BCG.

healing Any procedure which cures. The repair of broken tissue.

health A state of well-being with mind and body functioning at their optimum.

heart A hollow muscular organ situated in the anterior chest to the left of the midline. It pumps the blood round the circulatory system and is derived from a modification of blood vessels and is thus lined by endothelium (endocardium), folds of which form the heart valves. The heart muscle is modified to conduct electrical impulses. The heart is contained in a serous membraneous bag known as the pericardium. *H. block*: state of partial or complete prevention of the passage of the cardiac impulse through the atrioventricular bundle. *See also* ELECTROCARDIOGRAM. *H. murmurs*: adventitious sounds heard on auscultation of the heart resulting from altered haemodynamics, in which the flow of blood through the heart becomes turbulent and exceeds a certain critical velocity. These conditions may occur when there is narrowing or incompetence of valves, abnormal communications between chambers of the heart, or where there is a hyperdynamic circulation as in hyperthyroidism and severe anaemia. *H. sounds*: the first heart sound 'lub' is due to the closure of the right and left atrioventricular valves which occurs at the beginning of the ventricular contraction (*systole*). The second sound 'dup' is due to the closure of the aortic and pulmonary valves. Very occasionally a third sound is heard due to rapid filling of the atria. *Abnormal h. s.* may be due to exaggeration or distortion of the normal sounds, *e.g.* 'splitting' of the components of the first or second sounds or the production of adventitious new sounds. *See* HEART MURMURS. *H. transplant*: see TRANSPLANT.

heartburn Burning sensation at lower end of the oesophagus, due to acid regurgitation from the stomach.

heart–lung machine Machine used in cardiac surgery to oxygenate the blood.

heat exhaustion Condition caused by great heat when patient has rapid pulse, dyspnoea and abdominal cramp due to excessive sweating and loss of sodium chloride.

heat stroke Hyperpyrexia due to failure of temperature-regulating mechanisms of the body.

hebephrenia *See* SCHIZOPHRENIA.

Heberden's nodes Small bony nodules which form at the sides of the finger joints in osteoarthritis.

hedonism Excessive devotion to pleasure.

Hegar's dilators A series of graduated metal bougies for dilating the cervix and uterus.

Hegar's sign Spongy feel of the cervix in pregnancy.

Heimlich's manoeuvre Rapid squeezing of the upper abdomen to dislodge foreign body obstructing the pharynx.

Hela cells Malignant squamous epithelial cells originating from carcinoma of cervix uteri. Used as medium for growth of viruses in tissue culture.

heliotherapy Treatment by exposure to sunlight.

helium An inert gas, used in certain respiratory tests.

helix Literally twisted. Used to describe (1) the configuration of certain molecules, *e.g.* DNA, keratin, and (2) the outer rim of the external ear.

Heller's operation Division of muscle between stomach and oesophagus in cases of dysphagia in cardiospasm.

helminthagogue Medicine to expel worms.

helminthiasis Infestation with worms.

helminthology Study of worms.

hemeralopia Partial blindness: patient is not able to see in bright daylight.

hemianopia Loss of sight in half of the visual field.

hemiatrophy Atrophy of one side of the body only.

hemiballismus Violent athetoid movements resembling throwing action of one side of the body due to brain damage.

hemicolectomy Surgical removal of half the colon, thus right or left hemicolectomy.

hemicrania Headache on one side of the head. *See* MIGRAINE.

hemiparesis Paralysis of one side of the body.

hemiplegia Paralysis of one side of the body. The lesion is in the opposite side of the brain.

hemispheres Usually cerebral hemispheres, the two sides of the forebrain.

hemizygous Genetic constitution of male as regards sex-linked traits.

Henoch's purpura A form of syndrome caused by sensitivity reaction of the vascular endothelium. Blood leaks out of the damaged vessels causing purpuric spots in the skin and other variable symptoms according to which organs are affected. In the *Henoch type* there is abdominal pain. The *Schönlein type* is associated with joint involvement. Often both types coexist.

hepar The liver.

heparin A sulphur-containing polysaccharide which is stored by mast cells. It has the property of preventing blood from clotting, *i.e.* it is an anticoagulant.

hepatectomy Excision of the liver.

hepatic Relating to the liver. *H. coma*: coma resulting from the effect on the brain of toxins which are normally metabolized by the liver. Occurs in advanced liver failure. *H. flexure*: the right-hand bend of the colon, under the liver. *H. portal system*: system of veins which carry the blood from the intestine to the liver so that, with the exception of neutral fats, all the materials absorbed from the gut go straight to the liver.

hepatitis Inflammation of the liver due to infection or chemical toxicity. *Infective h.*: a virus disease spread by faecal–oral route. *H. B virus* spread by blood contact or inoculation (*serum h.*). These are the main forms of *viral h.* and the latter has a longer incubation period. In either disease hepatocellular jaundice and hepatic failure may develop. *Toxic h.* may result from chemical exposure, *e.g.* to carbon tetrachloride.

hepatization Conversion into a liver-like substance. A term used to describe the lungs in lobar pneumonia.

hepatocele Hernia containing hepatic tissue.

hepatolenticular degeneration *See* WILSON'S DISEASE.

hepatoma Neoplasm of liver cells.

hepatomegaly Enlargement of the liver.

hepatosplenomegaly Enlargement of both the liver and spleen.

hereditary Transmitted from one's ancestors.

heredity The transmission of genetic characteristics.

hermaphrodite Abnormality of development in which an individual has tissue capable of producing both male and female gametes. It is associated with ambiguity of secondary sexual characteristics and the individual is generally sterile.

hermetic Protected from the air. Airtight.

hernia Protrusion of an organ from its normal position, most common in the case of the bowel. *Inguinal h.* is through the inguinal canal, and *femoral h.* through the femoral ring. *Scrotal h.* is hernia descending into the scrotum, and *umbilical h.* is hernia at the navel. A hernia not amenable to manipulation is termed *irreducible*. If the blood supply to this is interfered with it is termed *strangulated h. H. cerebri*: protrusion of the brain through a wound in the skull. *Ventral h.*: hernia of the ventral surface of the body such as an *umbilical* or *incisional h.*: the latter is through an old scar.

hernioplasty Operation for hernia when the weak structures are repaired.

herniorrhaphy Operation to repair a hernia.

herniotomy Dividing the constricting band of a strangulated hernia and returning the protruding part.

heroic Severe treatment of the kill-or-cure type.

herpangina Mild epidemic throat infection in children. Vesicles and later ulcers on and around tonsils, probably caused by coxsackie viruses.

herpes Vesicular eruption due to infection by a virus. *H. simplex* virus may reside in epidermal cells without causing any reaction but under certain circumstances, for example associated with a cold, an immunological reaction to the virus occurs with blistering and ulceration of the skin known as 'cold sores'. *H. zoster* virus is closely related, if not identical with, the chickenpox virus and attacks sensory nerves producing pain and vesiculation in the distribution of the nerves (shingles).

herpetic Relating to herpes.

herpetiform Resembling herpes.

Hess's test Test used in the differential diagnosis of purpura. A cuff is inflated on the arms so that the veins are obstructed, thus raising the pressure in the capillaries. If the capillaries are weak blood seeps out forming small purpuric spots when the cuff is released.

heterogeneous Differing in kind or in nature.

heterograft *See* GRAFT.

heterologous Derived from a different species.

heterophoria Latent squint. A squint which develops only when the patient is tired or in ill health.

heterotropia Squint.

heterozygous Having two different allelomorphs in the corresponding loci of a pair of chromosomes, *cf.* homozygous. The phenotype of the heterozygote may correspond to one allelomorph (dominant gene) or may be intermediate between the two alleles.

hiatus An opening or space. *H. hernia*: hernia of the stomach through the diaphragm at the oesophageal opening.

hibernation Winter sleep. Artificial hibernation (hypothermia) is now widely employed in surgery.

hiccough (hiccup) Repeated spasmodic inspiration associated with sudden closure of the glottis which gives rise to the characteristic 'hic' sound. It may be produced by irritation of the diaphragm but in most cases the cause is unknown.

hidradenitis Inflammation of the sweat glands.

hidrosis Sweating.

hilar Relating to the hilum.

hilum Site at which the pedicle of an organ is attached.

hindbrain Embryological component which becomes the medulla and cerebellum.

hip The upper part of the thigh. *H. joint*: ball and socket joint between the head of the femur and the acetabulum. *Congenital* *dislocation of h.j.*: abnormality of development in which the head of the femur does not articulate with the acetabulum.

Hippocrates Greek physician (400 BC) regarded as the founder of medicine as a science.

Hirschsprung's disease Developmental abnormality in which there is a defect in the nerve supply to part of the terminal colon which acts as an obstruction and results in dilatation and hypertrophy of the more proximal segment (congenital megacolon).

hirsuties Abnormal growth of hair.

His, bundle of *See* ATRIO-VENTRICULAR BUNDLE.

histamine An organic base which is released from tissues, especially mast cells, following injury. It increases the permeability of blood vessels and thus acts as the initiator of the inflammatory reaction.

histidine An amino acid.

histiocyte Macrophage-like cell in connective tissue.

histochemistry Study of the distribution of enzymes and chemicals in tissues by means of special staining methods.

histogenesis The differentiation of tissues.

histology The morphological study of tissues.

histolysis Degradation of tissue.

HIV *Abbr.* human immunodeficiency virus. *See also* AIDS, ARC.

hives Urticaria.

hobnail liver The gross appearance of a cirrhotic liver.

Hodgkin's disease A neoplasm of lymphatic tissue, *i.e.* the lymphocyte–histiocyte system. Clinical features of the disease are lymph node enlargement, splenomegaly, anaemia and fever.

Holger–Nielsen method A method of artificial respiration used occasionally if the face is too badly injured for the mouth-to-mouth method.

Holmes' syndrome Disturbance, especially of space perception, after cerebral palsy.

Homan's sign Physical sign of deep vein thrombosis in the leg. Pain is felt in the calf when the toes are dorsiflexed.

homeostasis Maintenance of a stable system.

homeothermic Maintaining constant body temperature.

homicide Killing a person.

homoeopathy Medicine worked on the system of cures such as those started by Hahnemann. Homoeopathic medicines are mostly given in infinitesimal doses.

homogeneous Having the same nature.

homograft *See* GRAFT.

homolateral On the same side. Ipsilateral.

homologous Of the same type. Identical in structure.

homosexuality Attraction towards members of one's own sex. *See also* BISEXUAL.

homozygous Having the same gene in the corresponding loci on paired chromosomes; *cf.* heterozygous.

hookworm *See* ANKYLOSTOMA DUODENALE.

hordeolum A stye on the eyelid.

hormone A substance produced in one organ, which excites functional activity at a distant site. *H. replacement therapy*, or HRT, is the use of a hormone or combination of hormones to counteract the hormone imbalance during and after the climacteric.

Horner's syndrome Unilateral small pupil, ptosis and vasodilatation of the cheek with absence of sweating, due to damage to the sympathetic nerves in the neck.

horseshoe kidney Developmental abnormality of the kidney in which the left and right kidneys are joined.

host Organism on which a parasite lives.

hourglass contraction A condition of the uterus in prolonged labour. *See* RETRACTION.

hourglass stomach A stomach divided by a constriction or spasm into two separate cavities seen after a barium meal x-ray. It may be due to a temporary spasm or the result of fibrosis of a gastric ulcer.

housemaid's knee Prepatellar bursitis.

Houston's folds Three oblique folds in the mucous membrane of the rectum.

humanized milk *See* MILK.

humerus The bone of the upper arm.

humidity Moisture. State of being moist.

humour A fluid, thus *aqueous h.* and *vitreous h.* of eye.

hunger pain A symptom of peptic or duodenal ulcer. The pain is relieved on taking food.

hunger stools Frequent small greenish stools passed by underfed infants.

Huntington's chorea Inherited defect which results in the onset in middle age of chorea and progressive dementia. *See also* CHOREA.

Hurler's syndrome *See* GARGOYLISM.

Hutchinson's teeth A condition of the upper central permanent incisors: the cutting edge is smaller than the base, and therefore the teeth are peg-shaped. The edge is deeply notched, a sign of congenital syphilis.

hyaline Transparent like glass. Hyaline cartilage is smooth and pearly. It covers the articular surfaces of

bones. *H. membrane*: eosinophilic material found lining
the alveoli of premature and
other babies causing reduced
pulmonary surfactant with
hyaline membrane disease.
Main cause of respiratory distress syndrome.

hyaloid membrane The glassy
membrane which encloses the
vitreous humour of the eye.

hybrid Offspring resulting
from gametes which are genetically unlike.

hydatid Cyst formed by the
larvae of certain tapeworms.

hydatidiform mole Cyst
formed from the degener-
ation of the chorion. It may
give rise to chorionepi-
thelioma.

hydragogue Substance which
attracts water, *i.e.* it is os-
motically active.

hydramnios Excess of amniotic fluid.

hydrarthrosis Collection of
fluid in a joint.

hydrate Combination with
water.

hydroa aestivale Form of
porphyria in which the skin is
sensitive to light. Blisters result from exposure to the sun.

hydrocarbon A compound
formed of hydrogen and
carbon.

hydrocele Swelling containing clear fluid. Most often
applied to watery swelling of
scrotum.

hydrocephalus Excess of

cerebrospinal fluid causing
pressure on the brain.

hydrocortisone The major
glucocorticoid secreted by the
adrenal.

hydrolysis Breakdown of
complex substance(s) with the
addition of water to give
simpler substances.

hydrometer An instrument
for determining the specific
gravities of liquids.

hydrometra Collection of
fluid in the uterus.

hydronephrosis Distension of
the pelvis and calyces of the
kidney due to obstruction to
the ureter. Prolonged back
pressure results in atrophy of
the renal substance.

hydropathic Relating to cure
by means of water; as by
baths.

hydropericardium Fluid in
the pericardial sac, *i.e.* pericardial effusion.

hydroperitoneum Peritoneal
effusion, *i.e.* ascites.

hydrophobia *See* RABIES.

hydropneumothorax Fluid
and air in the pleural cavity.

hydrops Oedema. *H. fetalis*:
generalized oedema associated with severe haemolytic
anaemia in the fetus due to
Rhesus incompatibility.

hydrosalpinx Distension of
the fallopian tube by clear
fluid.

hydrotherapy Use of water in
treatment.

hydrothorax Fluid in the cavity of the chest.

5-hydroxytryptamine (5-HT) Serotonin. Substance which acts as a chemical transmitter in brain synapses. It is also elaborated by argentaffin cells of the gastrointestinal tract and stimulates smooth muscle.

hygiene The science of the preservation of health.

hygroma Cyst in the neck resulting from abnormal development of the lymphatic system.

hygrometer An instrument for measuring the moisture in the atmosphere.

hygroscopic Having the property of absorbing moisture from the air, *e.g.* common salt.

hymen A fold of membrane at the entrance to the vagina.

hymenotomy Incision of hymen.

hyoid Shaped like a V; the name of a bone at the root of the tongue.

hyper Prefix denoting excessive, above, or increased.

hyperacidity Excess acid.

hyperactivity Overactivity.

hyperaemia Excess of blood in a part.

hyperaesthesia Excess of sensitiveness in a part.

hyperalgesia Excessive sensibility to pain.

hyperasthenia Great weakness.

hyperbaric A pressure greater than atmospheric pressure.

hyperbilirubinaemia Excess of bilirubin in the blood. Normal level of serum bilirubin is less than 20 μmol/litre.

hypercalcaemia Excess of calcium in the blood.

hypercapnia Excess of carbon dioxide in the blood.

hyperchlorhydria Excess of hydrochloric acid in the gastric juice.

hyperchromia Excessively coloured.

hypercholesterolaemia Excess of cholesterol in the blood.

hyperemesis Excessive vomiting. *H. gravidarum*: of pregnancy.

hyperexcitability Ease of excitation as of a nerve or muscle fibre.

hyperextension Extension beyond the normal range of a joint.

hyperflexion Flexion beyond the normal range.

hyperglycaemia Excessive sugar in the blood; occurs in diabetes mellitus.

hypergonadism Excessive secretion of sex hormones causing precocious puberty and premature fusion of the epiphyses.

hyperhidrosis Excess of perspiration.

hyperkalaemia Excess of potassium in the blood.

hyperkeratoses Lesions on

the skin in which there is excessive production of keratin.

hyperkinesis Excessive movement.

hyperlipaemia Familial increase in serum triglycerides with abdominal crises and liability to early coronary artery atheroma.

hypermetropia Long sight, a visual affection. The opposite of myopia. Corrected by wearing a biconvex lens.

hypermnesia An exaggeration of memory involving minute details of a past experience. It may occur in mentally unstable individuals after a shock.

hypermotility Increased motor activity.

hypermyotonia Increase in muscle tone.

hypernatraemia Excess of sodium in blood.

hypernephroma Malignant tumour of kidney.

hyperonychia Thickening of the nails.

hyperostosis Hypertrophy of bony tissue.

hyperparathyroidism Excessive secretion of parathormone, usually from an adenoma of one of the parathyroid glands.

hyperphagia Eating to excess.

hyperphoria Elevation of one visual axis above the other.

hyperpiesis *See* HYPERTENSION.

hyperpituitarism Excess secretion of hormones from the anterior pituitary, especially somatotrophin or growth hormone. *See* ACROMEGALY.

hyperplasia Excessive growth of tissue.

hyperpnoea Overbreathing.

hyperpyrexia High fever, arbitrarily above 40.5°C (105°F).

hypersecretion Excessive secretion.

hypersensitive Excessive sensitivity.

hypersplenism A condition in which there is enlargement of the spleen associated with inhibition of maturation of cells in the bone marrow. It is thought that the spleen secretes some inhibitory factor.

hyperstimulation, ovarian Result of excessive gonadotrophin (FSH) therapy to induce ovulation. Risk of high multiple birth, cystic ovarian enlargement, ascites, pleural and pericardial effusion. *See* SUPEROVULATION.

hypertension Blood pressure above the normal limits, *i.e.* above 140/95 resting BP. Hypertension may be primary or essential, i.e. cause unknown, or secondary to arterial obstruction, renal disease, endocrine disturbances and other factors.

hyperthermia Raised body temperature.

hyperthymia An overactive

state of mind with a tendency to perform impulsive actions.

hyperthyroidism Excessive secretion of thyroid hormones.

hypertonia Excessive tonicity, as in a muscle or an artery.

hypertonic High tone. (1) Increased tone of muscle. (2) Having a higher osmotic pressure than body fluids; *cf.* isotonic, hypotonic saline.

hypertrichosis Excessive growth of hair, or growth of hair in unusual places.

hypertrophy Increase in size in response to demand on the structure; *cf.* hyperplasia.

hyperventilation Over-breathing.

hypnosis Condition resembling sleep in which conscious control of behaviour is reduced. The state is brought about voluntarily in the subject by 'suggestion'.

hypnotic (1) Relating to hypnotism. (2) Drug producing sleep.

hypo Prefix denoting below.

hypoaesthesia Diminished sense of feeling in a part of the body.

hypocalcaemia Diminished amount of blood calcium.

hypochlorhydria Deficiency of hydrochloric acid in the gastric juice.

hypochondria An anxiety state about health, the patient suffering from many imaginary ills.

hypochondriac Person suffering from many and varied ills for which no organic cause may be found.

hypochondrium Surface anatomy nomenclature relating to the region of the anterior abdominal wall beneath the ribs.

hypochromic Deficient in colour. Usually applies to red blood cells in which there is a reduced haemoglobin content, hence *anaemia*.

hypodermic Beneath the skin; used of injections.

hypofibrinogenaemia Condition in which there is a deficiency of fibrinogen in the blood.

hypogastric Pertaining to the hypogastrium.

hypogastrium Lower median abdominal region.

hypoglossal Beneath the tongue. *H. nerves*: twelfth pair of cranial nerves.

hypoglycaemia Deficiency of sugar in the blood.

hypogonadism Defective development of the ovaries or testicles.

hypokalaemia Reduced potassium content of blood.

hypomania Mild form of the affective disorder, mania, in which there is abnormal elation of mood and great energy.

hypomotility Decreased movement.

hyponatraemia Reduction of blood sodium concentration.

hypoparathyroidism Diminished function of parathyroid glands.

hypophoria Depression of one visual axis below the other.

hypophosphataemia Reduced inorganic phosphate content of blood.

hypophosphatasia Abnormally low amount of alkaline phosphatase in the blood. *Congenital h.*: inherited deficiency of alkaline phosphatase in the bone cells. As a result there is a failure of the bones to calcify adequately, the serum calcium concentration may rise and there may be anorexia, vomiting and wasting. The amount of alkaline phosphatase in the serum is greatly reduced.

hypophysectomy Operation to remove the pituitary gland.

hypophysis cerebri Pituitary gland.

hypopiesis *See* HYPOTENSION.

hypopituitarism Condition resulting from insufficiency of pituitary secretion.

hypoplasia Tendency to grow to a size smaller than normal.

hypoproteinaemia Too little protein in the blood.

hypoprothrombinaemia Deficiency of prothrombin in blood.

hypopyon Pus in the anterior chamber of the eye.

hyposecretion Too little secretion.

hypospadias Malformation of lower wall of the urethra, so that the urethra opens on the undersurface of the penis.

hypostasis Deposit: passive congestion.

hypostatic pneumonia Due to congestion at bases of lungs, often caused by allowing elderly patients to lie flat on their backs for long periods.

hypotension Low blood pressure.

hypothalamus A special area of grey matter in the floor of the third ventricle of the brain. Linked with the pituitary gland and also with the thalamus and the autonomic nervous system.

hypothenar eminence Prominence on the palm below the little finger.

hypothermia State of being abnormally cold. Occurs following exposure and in cold weather among those not able to heat their homes adequately. A disease of social deprivation. *Artificial h.*: technique used in conjunction with major heart surgery, etc., in which the blood is cooled by passing it through a heat exchanger. The body temperature is lowered to about 29.44°C (85°F), at which level the oxygen requirements of tissues, especially the brain cells, are greatly reduced. This enables the circulation to be stopped for a time.

hypothesis A suggested explanation of some happening or phenomenon.

hypothrombinaemia Deficiency of thrombin in the blood.

hypothyroidism Insufficiency of thyroid secretion.

hypotonia Deficient tone, especially of muscle.

hypotonic (1) Lacking in tone. (2) Of salt solution: having an osmotic pressure less than that of physiological saline (0.9 per cent NaCl).

hypovitaminosis Suffering from lack of vitamins in food intake.

hypoxia Lacking oxygen.

hystera The uterus or womb.

hysterectomy Surgical removal of the uterus. There are many varieties. *Abdominal h.*: through an abdominal incision. *Total h.*: complete removal. *Subtotal h.*: cervix left in place. *Vaginal h.*: removal through the vagina. May be combined with removal of ovaries, fallopian tubes and surrounding tissues for malignant disease or with vaginal repair procedures for prolapse or urinary incontinence.

hysteria A functional neurosis in which there is a reaction, never fully conscious on the part of the patient, to obtain relief from stress by the exhibition and experience of symptoms of illness.

hysterography Radiological examination of uterus.

hysteromyomectomy Excision of uterine fibroid.

hysteropexy Suturing of the uterus to the abdominal wall to prevent prolapse.

hysterosalpingography X-ray examination of uterus and fallopian tubes following the introduction of a contrast medium.

hysterotomy Incision into the uterus. The term usually excludes caesarean section.

hysterotrachelorrhaphy Repair of a lacerated cervix uteri.

I

iatrogenic Applied to disorder resulting from treatment.

ichthyosis Also called fish-skin disease. Inherited defect of keratinization in which the skin is dry and scaly. The so-called acquired ichthyosis is similar in appearance but due to defective nutrition.

icterus Jaundice.

idea A mental image.

identical twins Monozygotic twins, *i.e.* derived from the same fertilized ovum.

identification (1) Recognition. (2) Psychiatric emotional attachment to an individual resulting in transposition of behavioural characteristics.

idiopathic Without apparent cause.

idiosyncrasy Individual character or property. Generally used in connection with unusual or unexpected response to drugs.

ileitis Inflammation of the ileum. *Regional i.*: Crohn's disease. Characterized by localized regions of non-specific chronic inflammation of the terminal portion of the ileum. Occasionally other parts of the intestine are also affected. The cause is not known.

ileocaecal valve Valve at the junction of the large and small intestines.

ileocolitis Inflammation of ileum and colon.

ileocolostomy Surgical anastomosis between the ileum and the colon.

ileoproctostomy Surgical anastomosis between the ileum and the rectum.

ileorectal Relating to the ileum and the rectum.

ileostomy Fistula constructed so that the ileum opens on the anterior abdominal wall to act as an artificial anus.

ileum The lower portion of the small intestine between the jejunum and the caecum. *See* BOWEL.

ileus Obstruction of the bowel. Paralytic ileus is

caused by paralysis of the muscle. It may be a complication of abdominal operations, particularly if the bowel has been extensively handled. It may also be due to peritonitis.

iliac crest The crest or highest portion of the ilium. *I. spine*: the tubercle at the anterior end of the iliac crest.

iliococcygeal Relating to the ilium and the coccyx, *e.g. i. ligament*: ligament passing between the ilium and the coccyx.

ilium The upper part of the innominate bone.

illegitimate Born out of wedlock.

illusion A deceptive appearance. The misinterpretation of a sensory image.

image A mental picture of an external object. *I. intensifier*: apparatus to increase brightness of fluoroscopic image in x-ray screening.

imbalance Lack of balance.

immobility The state of being fixed.

immune response Immunological reaction to antigenic stimulus.

immune thrombocytopenic purpura (ITP) Purpuric rash and other features of thrombocytopenia due to autoimmune antiplatelet antibodies.

immunity State of resistance to infection due to the presence of antibodies capable of combining with antigen(s) carried by the infecting organism and thus damaging the invader or neutralizing enzymes or toxins released by the organism. As well as viruses, bacteria and other parasites, the body regards cells from a different individual, *i.e.* different genotype, as infecting organisms. Hence the difficulties of homografting kidneys, etc.; *see* GRAFT. In a wider, and less common, usage of the term, immunity implies all mechanisms, such as impermeability of the skin, antiseptic properties of sebum, disinfection of food by stomach acid, etc. which enable the body to resist infection.

immunization Process of increasing the state of immunity, either by contact with the infecting organism or some variant of it, which is *active i*. In *passive i*. there is receipt of antibody. Active immunization is the principle behind vaccination against smallpox, inoculation against diphtheria, tetanus, etc. Passive immunization is temporary: the fetus is passively immunized by antibodies from the maternal blood and these enable the newborn baby to resist infection for about 6 weeks after birth.

immunoassay Quantitative estimation of proteins, *e.g.*

hormones, by serological methods.

immunocompromised A state of being susceptible to infection because of deliberate immunosuppression or disease involving the immune system.

immunoelectrophoresis Analysis of antigens by combination of electrophoresis and immunodiffusion.

immunofluorescence Microscopic demonstration of antigens and antibody by fluorescent dye technique.

immunogenic Generating an immune response.

immunoglobulins Group of globulins able to react as antibodies.

immunology Scientific study of immunity.

immunosuppression Deliberate inhibition of normal immune response, especially to permit successful organ grafting.

impaction Wedging or jamming together, e.g. impacted fracture where the bony fragments are jammed together. Impacted wisdom tooth, where there is insufficient room in the jaw to accommodate the erupting tooth, which becomes jammed.

impalpable Not capable of being felt.

imperforate Completely closed.

impetigo Acute infection of the skin. Most commonly

caused by the staphylococcus or streptococcus.

implantation The act of setting in; grafting. *Dermoid i.*: cyst due to the accidental implantation of epidermis into the dermis.

implants Pellets of drugs such as testosterone which are inserted under the skin from where they are slowly absorbed.

impotence Absence of power or desire for sexual intercourse. Inability to perform the sexual act.

impregnation The act of becoming pregnant; the fertilization of an ovum by a spermatozoon.

in extremis At the point of death.

in situ In position.

in utero Within the uterus.

in vitro Literally, within the glass, *i.e.* in the test tube as opposed to in life; *cf.* in vivo. *I.v. fertilization* (IVF): the 'test tube baby' technique for treating infertility due to tubal blockage or other causes. Oocytes are removed from the ovarian follicles usually after superovulation, incubated with prepared sperm and if fertilization occurs pre-embryos are replaced in the uterus. *See* EMBRYO TRANSFER, SUPEROVULATION.

in vivo In the living body.

inanition Exhaustion from want of food.

inarticulate (1) Without joints. (2) Unable to speak clearly.

incarcerated Imprisoned. Term applied to a hernia which cannot be reduced.

incest Sexual intercourse between near relatives.

incidence Occurrence, such as of a disease.

incipient Beginning.

incision Act of cutting into with a sharp instrument.

incisors Chisel-shaped cutting teeth at the front of the mouth. *See* DENTAL FORMULA.

inclusion bodies Extraneous material found in the cytoplasm of cells. The term does not include material in phagocytosis or pinocytosis vacuoles and is almost exclusively applied to bodies formed by accumulations of virus material.

incoherent Disconnected.

incompatible Incapable of admixture, *e.g.* incompatible transfusion.

incompetence Incapable of natural function, *e.g.* aortic incompetence in which the aortic valve of the heart does not close adequately with the result that blood leaks back into the left ventricle.

incontinence Absence of voluntary control over the passing of urine or faeces.

incoordination Inability to perform harmonious muscle movements.

incrustation Forming of a scab on a wound.

incubation Literally to hatch. *I. period*: time between infection and the appearance of symptoms when it is assumed the infecting organisms multiply.

incubator Apparatus used to provide optimum conditions for incubation. Incubators are used for many purposes. (1) Premature babies. (2) Culture of viruses, bacteria and other organisms. (3) To allow enzyme reactions to proceed at optimum temperatures.

incus A small anvil-shaped bone of the middle ear. *See* EAR.

index (1) The forefinger. (2) The ratio of measurement of any quantity in comparison with a fixed standard.

indication Circumstances determining a particular form of treatment.

indicator Substance showing a chemical reaction by its change in colour.

indigenous Native to a particular place.

indigestion Failure of the digestive powers; dyspepsia.

indolent Slow to heal.

induction (1) Influence of one embryonic tissue in modifying the development of another. (2) In obstetrics, the artificial production of labour.

induration Hardening of tissue.

industrial disease A disease due to a person's occupation, such as silicosis found among silica workers, etc.

industrial dermatitis Contact dermatitis due to material used in industrial processes.

inebriety Habitual drunkenness.

inertia (1) Resistance to change in motion. (2) In psychiatry, extreme apathy. (3) *Uterine i.*: sluggish contraction of the uterus during labour.

infant Baby less than one year old.

infanticide Murder of an infant.

infantile eczema Type of eczema affecting infants and children.

infantile paralysis Anterior poliomyelitis, *see* POLIOMYELITIS.

infantilism Persistence of childish ways in an adult.

infarct Region of tissue affected by ischaemic changes due to the blocking of the principal artery supplying the part.

infection A disease or disease process due to a pathogenic organism. *Cross-i.*: the communication of a disease from one patient to another. *Droplet i.*: in the fine spray which is ejected from the mouth on talking, sneezing or coughing. *Wound i.*: postoperative infection in a surgical incision.

infectious disease A communicable disease.

infectious mononucleosis Glandular fever. Probably a virus infection and characterized by malaise, pyrexia, muscle pains, sore throat, enlargement of the lymph glands and the spleen and an increase in the numbers of mononuclear white blood cells. Occasionally there is enlargement of the liver, jaundice and a rash. *See* PAUL-BUNNELL TEST.

inferior Lower. *I. vena cava*: the chief vein of the lower part of the trunk of the body.

inferiority complex A feeling of unjustified inferiority which may show itself by overconfident or aggressive behaviour.

infertility The inability to reproduce includes failure of conception and recurrent abortion and occurs in at least 17 per cent of UK couples. It affects both males and females although the underlying cause may be a defect in either such as anovulation, tubal blockage or defective spermatogenesis. No cause is found in the majority of cases.

infestation The invasion of the body by parasites such as lice.

infiltration Penetration of tissue by fluid, cells or other material.

inflammation The vascular response to tissue damage. It consists of dilatation of blood vessels, increased permeability of vessels to the passage of serum into the tissue and the diapedesis of leucocytes into the site of the damage.

inflation Blown out and expanded by air or gas.

influenza Virus infection affecting the epithelium of the respiratory tract.

infra Below.

infrared Electromagnetic waves with longer wavelength than visible red light, *i.e.* photons with a lesser frequency than the lower end of the visible spectrum. Because it is easily absorbed, *i.e.* not reflected, by bodies, infrared radiation transfers heat to the absorbing material and is used therapeutically for this purpose.

infundibulum (1) A funnel-shaped orifice or passage. (2) Outgrowth of floor of brain forming part of the pituitary gland.

infusion (1) Fluid allowed to flow into a vein (intravenous infusion) or a muscle (intramuscular infusion) by a gravity feed. (2) Crude extract of material using boiling water, *e.g.* tea is an infusion of tea leaves.

ingestion Taking in of food or other substances.

ingrowing toe nail Lateral parts of a nail growing into the nail bed often causing discomfort and infection.

inguinal Pertaining to the groin. *I. canal*, about 4 cm in length, lies in the groin, and is occupied in the male by the spermatic cord, and in the female by the round ligament, with their corresponding vessels and nerves.

inhalation Volatile medicinal substance which is inhaled.

inherent Existing or abiding in a person, *e.g.* an inherent property or quality.

inhibition Literally restraint. The term is used ubiquitously to imply the prevention of some activity, thus psychological inhibition, enzymatic inhibition, nerve inhibition, etc.

initial Pertaining to the beginning.

injected Congested.

injection Introduction of material under pressure into tissues.

innate Inborn, congenital.

innervation The supply of nerves or the conveyance of nervous impulses to or from a part. *Reciprocal i.*: one set of muscles contracts whilst those opposing it relax.

innocent Not malignant.

innocuous Harmless.

innominate artery The large artery which arises from the arch of the aorta and divides

into the right common carotid and right subclavian arteries.

innominate bone Bone forming anterior walls and sides of the pelvic cavity.

innoxious Not harmful.

inoculation Introduction of microorganisms into tissues or culture media, etc.

inorganic Mineral as opposed to living material or its products. The distinction at a refined level is not obvious.

inquest A judicial inquiry into the cause of death. *See also* CORONER.

insecticide A preparation for destroying insects.

insemination Introduction of semen into the vagina. *Artificial i.*: injection of semen into vagina or uterus. The semen may either be from the legal husband (AIH) or from a donor (AID).

insertion The attachment of a muscle to the part it moves.

insidious Literally, cunning. Usually applies to onset of disease in which there are no perceptible signs or symptoms.

insight An awareness of one's own mental state and behaviour.

insomnia Sleeplessness.

inspiration The act of breathing in.

inspissated Thickened by evaporation.

instep The longitudinal arch of the foot.

instillation Pouring in drop by drop.

instinct An inherited organization of perception, feeling and action, *e.g.* the sight of something which threatens life arouses the emotion of fear and the instinct to flee.

insufflation Blowing into a structure.

insula Small part of the cerebral cortex lying deeply in the lateral sulcus.

insulation Material preventing loss of or access to internally situated structure of heat, light, electrical current, water, etc.

insulin A polypeptide hormone, secreted by the beta-cells of the islets of Langerhans in the pancreas, which exerts control over the metabolism of glucose in the body. Acts to lower blood sugar levels by stimulating uptake, utilization of glucose by cells, and conversion and inhibition of breakdown of glycogen. Deficiency results in diabetes mellitus and insulin injections provide replacement therapy. Available in several short-acting and long-acting forms.

insulinoma Adenoma of islets of Langerhans.

integument The skin.

intellect Reasoning power whereby we can think logically.

intelligence Certain mental ability involving reasoning and recognition of pattern, etc. as distinct from memorization of information or other mental functions. *I. quotient (IQ)*: a measure of intelligence expressed as a figure where the average is 100. *I. tests*: tests not based on a person's knowledge but on his ability to reason.

intensive care unit (ICU) Specialized hospital ward where acute illnesses are treated.

intention tremor Tremor which occurs only during active movement.

inter Prefix meaning 'between' (Latin) and used with many medical terms, such as *intercostal*, between the ribs; *intermittent* fevers, in which there are regular pauses between the attacks.

interarticular Between the joints.

intercellular Between cells, *e.g.* intercellular fluid.

intercourse Communication. *Sexual i.*: coitus.

intercurrent Occurring between. *I. infection*: an infection occurring in a patient already suffering from some other one.

interferon Material elaborated by cells which interferes with the synthesis of nucleoprotein. It thus tends to limit the multiplication of viruses within the cell.

intermittent Occurring at intervals. When applied to the pulse, signifies that some of the beats of the heart fail to reach the wrist. *I. claudication*: literally intermittent limping, due to ischaemia of the muscles of the legs.

internal Inside. *I. os*: the junction of the cavity of the cervix uteri with that of the body of the uterus. *See also* UTERUS. *I. podalic version*: version of the fetus by inserting one hand into the uterus, bringing a foot down and so changing the presentation to breech. Most commonly used to deliver second twin.

interosseous Between two bones.

interphase Period of cell cycle between two successive cell divisions.

interstitial Between parts, *i.e.* in connective tissue. *I. keratitis*: manifestation of congenital syphilis consisting of inflammation of the cornea.

intertrigo Eczematous condition of deep crevices or folds of skin, due to retention of perspiration.

intertrochanteric Between the trochanters.

interventricular Between the ventricles.

intervertebral Between the vertebrae.

intestinal malabsorption *See* MALABSORPTION SYNDROME.

intestinal obstruction Obstruction to the passage of food or faeces through the intestine. It may be due either to a physical blockage or to the absence of peristalsis.

intestines The alimentary canal from the stomach to the anus.

intima Inner coat of arteries consisting of endothelium and its elastic fibre attachment to the connective tissue of the mesial or middle layer.

intolerance Constitutional incapacity to endure or benefit by a remedial agent.

intra Prefix meaning within (Latin).

intra-abdominal Within the abdominal cavity.

intra-articular Within the capsule of a joint.

intracellular Within a cell.

intracranial Pertaining to the interior of skull.

intradermal In the dermis.

intradural Within the dura mater.

intragastric In the stomach.

intrahepatic Within the liver.

intralobular Within a lobule.

intramedullary In the bone marrow.

intramuscular Inside a muscle, *e.g.* intramuscular (IM) injection.

intranasal Within the nasal cavity.

intraocular fluids The fluids inside the eye, such as the aqueous and vitreous humours. The aqueous humour is constantly being formed from the ciliary body and is drained through the canal of Schlemm. If this circulation is impaired the *i. f. pressure* may rise. *See* GLAUCOMA. The normal pressure is 20–25 mmHg.

intraosseous Within a bone.

intraperitoneal Pertaining to the peritoneal cavity.

intrathecal Pertaining to the lumen of a sheath or canal, usually meaning the spinal canal.

intratracheal Inside the trachea. Thus *i. cannula*. Those used for the administration of anaesthetic are known as endotracheal tubes.

intrauterine Within the uterus. *I. death (IUD)*: cessation of fetal life between 28 weeks gestation and delivery. *I. device (IUD)*: Plastic or copper-coated plastic device of varying shapes inserted into the uterus through the cervix to prevent conception. Exact method of action not known. Copper may help its effectiveness. Previously called intrauterine contraceptive device (IUCD).

intravenous Pertaining to the lumen of a vein. *I. infusion*: running fluid into a vein over a period of time through an indwelling needle or catheter. *I. injection*: injecting drugs directly into a vein or into an already indwelling needle or catheter.

intrinsic Inherent, peculiar to a part. *I. factor*: factor present in normal gastric juice which enables the absorption of cyanobalamin (vitamin B_{12}) to take place. It is probable that it is an enzyme.

introitus Opening into a viscus. Usually refers to the external opening of the vagina.

introspection State of mental self-examination.

introvert An individual whose attention centres on himself rather than on outside things. Opposite to an extrovert.

intubation Insertion of a tube into a passage or organ, especially tracheal intubation.

intussusception Condition in which part of the intestine is drawn into a more distal part.

inunction Putting ointment on the skin.

invagination Forming a pouch.

invasion Onset.

inverse Opposite.

inversion Turning upside down or inside out.

involucrum New bone forming around dead bone.

involution (1) A turning in. (2) The shrinking of the uterus and surrounding structures after labour. The uterus, from weighing 0.9 kg at labour shrinks in 8 weeks to the weight of 56 g. Arrest of this process is called sub-involution.

involutional melancholia Severe depressive illness in the elderly which usually responds well to antidepressant treatment.

iodism Iodine poisoning.

ion An atom or group of atoms carrying an electrical charge. *I. exchange resin*: high molecular weight polymers with attached ions that will exchange for others in surrounding tissues. Given orally or rectally.

ionization The process of becoming electrically charged.

ionizing radiation High energy radiation capable of producing ions in materials exposed to it.

ipsilateral On the same side.

IQ *See* INTELLIGENCE QUOTIENT.

iridectomy Cutting off a piece of the edge of the iris to make an artificial pupil to the eye.

iridocele Protrusion of a portion of iris through a wound in the cornea.

iridocyclitis Inflammation of the iris and uveal tract.

iridoplegia Paralysis of the muscle which constricts or dilates the pupil.

iridotomy An incision into the iris.

iris The coloured circle surrounding the pupil of the eye.

iritis Inflammation of the iris.

irradiation Exposure to electromagnetic waves or atomic particles (alpha, beta and gamma rays, neutrons).

irreducible Incapable of being retuned to its proper place by manipulation; usually term applied to a hernia.

irrigation Washing out.

irritant Agent causing irritation, *i.e.* resulting in a response.

ischaemia Diminished supply of blood to a part.

ischaemic contracture Volkmann's contracture. Permanent shortening of muscle by fibrosis.

ischium The lower and hind part of the innominate bone.

islets of Langerhans Endocrine cells scattered in groups or islands within the pancreas. *See also* INSULIN.

isoantibodies Terminology used to distinguish types of antibody in the circulation capable of acting against red blood cells. Isoantibodies are specific for individual red cell antigens, *e.g.* AB or rhesus antigens.

isolation The act of setting apart; an isolation room or ward is one kept for contagious or infectious diseases, and the doctor and nurse have to follow strict rules to prevent the spread of the disease.

isomers Substances having the same chemical composition but unlike physical or chemical properties owing to a difference in the relative positions of the atoms within the molecules.

isometric Of equal length. Static.

isotonic Having the same tone. *I. solutions.*: these have the same osmotic pressure as physiological saline, 0·9 per cent NaCl.

isotopes Differing forms of the same element with different atomic weights but the same chemical properties. *Radioactive i.*: isotopes with radioactive properties, emitting alpha, beta or gamma radiation. Used to diagnose and treat disease.

isthmus The neck or constricted part of an organ.

itching Sensation of irritation of the skin which commonly causes scratching.

itis Suffix meaning inflamed, *e.g.* dermatitis, inflammation of the skin.

ITP *Abbr.* immune thrombocytopenic purpura.

IUD (1) *See* INTRAUTERINE DEATH. (2) *See* INTRAUTERINE DEVICE.

IVF *See* IN VITRO FERTILIZATION.

J

Jacksonian epilepsy *See* EPILEPSY.

Jacquemier's sign Blueness of the vaginal walls seen in early pregnancy.

jaundice A syndrome characterized by increased levels of bile pigments in the blood and tissue fluids. These pigments are taken up by the tissues giving rise to a yellow colour of the sclera, skin and mucous membranes. The causes of jaundice are generally classified as obstructive, hepatocellular and haemolytic. Excessive destruction of red blood cells (haemolysis) may be secondary to inherited abnormalities in their metabolism (spherocytosis), or infection, *e.g.* malaria or lysis in antigen-antibody reactions, *e.g.* rhesus incompatibility, or other causes. *Hepatocellular j.*: includes conditions such as infective hepatitis, a virus disease affecting the liver; toxic damage to the liver cells, *e.g.* acute yellow atrophy, and other conditions which reduce the efficiency of the liver in excreting bile pigments. Obstruction to any portion of the biliary tree may result in jaundice. The commonest cause of obstruction is gallstones.

jaw bone Either maxilla or mandible.

jejunectomy Excision of jejunum or part of it.

jejunostomy Making an artificial opening into the jejunum.

jejunum   That portion of the small intestine which lies between the duodenum and the ileum. *See* BOWEL.

jerk   A sudden contraction of muscle.

jigger   A tropical sand flea (Dermatophilus penetrans) which is parasitic in man, burrowing into the toes. Another name is chigoe.

joint   Point of contact of two or more bones. An articulation.

jugular   Relating to the neck. *J. veins*: two large veins in the neck which convey most of the blood from the head.

joint   Classified according to structure and movement allowed. *Fibrocartilaginous j.* with moderate movement, *e.g. intervertebral j. Fibrous j.* with little movement, *e.g.* symphysis pubis, *sacroiliac j. Synovial j.* with cartilaginous surfaces lubricated by synovial fluid allows wide range of movement limited only by shape of surfaces, *e.g. hip j.* which is ball and socket shape with full range of movement. *Interphalangeal j.*: hinge shape with movement in one direction only.

Jung   The founder of one school of psychoanalysis.

jurisprudence, medical   *See* FORENSIC MEDICINE.

justo major   Generally and equally enlarged pelvis.

justo minor   Generally and equally contracted pelvis.

juxtaglomerular apparatus   Group of cells forming cuff round afferent renal arteriole at its entry to Bowman's capsule, which probably acts as a stretch receptor to control release of renin when arteriolar tension falls.

juxtaposition   Placed alongside or next to.

K

kala-azar   Visceral leishmaniasis. A disease caused by the protozoon *Leishmania donovani* which is transmitted from man to man by sandflies. The parasite is found in reticuloendothelial cells in the liver, spleen, bone marrow and occasionally lymph nodes and causes fever, anaemia and enlargement of the spleen.

karyotype   The chromosome pattern of a cell or picture thereof. In somatic cells the normal pattern is diploid (two sets), in gametes it is haploid (one set). Male karyotype is 46 autosomes with X and Y sex chromosomes; female is 46 XX. Chromosomal abnormalities are reflected in karyotype. *See* DOWN'S SYNDROME, KLINEFELTER'S SYNDROME.

Kayser–Fleischer rings   Brownish pigmented rings

seen in the cornea of patients with Wilson's disease.

Kell factor An uncommon blood group factor. Anti-Kell antibodies may cause cross-matching problems and haemolytic disease.

Keller's operation Operation to correct hallux valgus.

keloid Overgrowth of connective tissue arising in scars.

keratectasia Protrusion of the cornea.

keratectomy Surgical removal of part of the cornea.

keratin Fibrillar protein made from closely bonded polypeptide chains. It is produced by epithelial cells and imparts great strength to keratin-containing structures, such as horns, hooves and hair, and protective covering of the skin.

keratitis Inflammation of the cornea.

keratolytics Agents which break down keratin, *e.g.* salicylic acid.

keratoma A callosity or horny overgrowth.

keratomalacia Abnormal softening of cornea which may lead to ulceration and blindness. Occurs in association with vitamin A deficiency.

keratome Scalpel used in ophthalmic surgery.

keratometer Instrument for measuring corneal astigmatism.

keratoplasty Corneal graft.

keratosis Thickening of the horny layer of the skin.

kerion A term for crusted ringworm.

kernicterus Many areas of the brain, particularly the basal ganglia, central cerebellar nuclei, the medulla and hippocampus are stained yellow with bilirubin. The brain cells are damaged. A complication of haemolytic jaundice of the newborn.

Kernig's sign A sign of meningitis. It consists of an inability to extend the knee joint when the thigh is flexed at right angles to the trunk.

ketogenic diet Diet with high fat content.

ketonaemia Ketone bodies in the blood.

ketone Chemical compounds containing carbonyl radicle (C=O), *e.g.* acetone.

ketonuria Ketone bodies in the urine.

ketosis The presence of ketonaemia and ketonuria. May result in situations where fat is metabolized for energy, *e.g.* starvation, diabetes mellitus or with dehydration.

ketosteroids Steroid substances which contain carbonyl radicles. Many of the breakdown products of steroid metabolism are excreted in the urine as ketosteroids.

kidneys Bilaterally situated upper abdominal viscera the function of which is to secrete urine. *Artificial k.*: apparatus through which blood is passed and allowed to dialyse (*see* DIALYSIS) across a membrane, usually a coiled tube, placed in a warm bath of saline. This process allows waste products and other materials to be removed from the blood and simulates the function of the kidneys. *Ectopic k.*: kidney which is abnormally situated in the abdominal cavity. *K. failure*: renal failure is basically the inability of the kidneys to do their job. There may be a number of different reasons for this and renal failure is usually classified as extrarenal and renal. Extrarenal causes are: severe haemorrhage or burns, dehydration or other causes of a prolonged and severe drop in blood pressure so that the blood flow to the kidneys is too low for them to function. Renal causes are classed as acute, *e.g.* acute nephritis, and chronic renal failure which may be the end result of a large number of widely different kidney diseases.

Kienboeck's disease An atypical osteochondritis affecting the semilunar bone of the wrist.

Killian's operation For suppuration in the frontal sinus. Removal of part of frontal bone to allow complete drainage.

kilogram One thousand

grams, equivalent to 2·2 lb.

Kimmelstiel–Wilson syndrome Nephrotic syndrome associated with diabetes mellitus.

kinaesthesis The sense of muscular movement.

kinematics The study of motion.

kineplasty A plastic amputation with the object of making the stump useful for locomotion.

kinesis Movement. Usually applied to cells migrating in response to a stimulus.

kinetics The study of movement or change.

Kirschner wire Wire used in orthopaedic surgery to apply skeletal traction to a fractured bone.

kiss of life Mouth-to-mouth artificial respiration.

Klebsiella Genus of bacteria.

Klebs–Loeffler bacillus The bacillus of diphtheria. Also known as Corynebacterium diphtheriae.

kleptomania Obsessional neurosis which is manifested by compulsive stealing.

Klinefelter's syndrome Syndrome resulting from nondisjunction of the X chromosome with the result that the individual inherits an extra X chromosome and has an XXY complement of sex chromosomes. The patient is sometimes of low intelligence and may have eunuchoid characteristics.

Klumpke's paralysis Paralysis of the flexor muscles to the wrist and fingers caused by injury to the eighth cervical and first dorsal nerves.

knee The joint between femur and tibia.

kneecap Patella.

knee–elbow position *See* GENUPECTORAL.

knee-jerk A jerk of the leg elicited by tapping on the patellar tendon when the knee is flexed. May be absent or exaggerated in diseases of the nervous system.

knock-knee Genu valgum.

knuckle Dorsal aspect of a phalangeal joint.

Koch's bacillus Mycobacterium tuberculosis.

Kock–Weeks bacillus Microorganism causing acute conjunctivitis.

Köhler's disease Osteochondritis affecting the scaphoid bone in the foot which becomes compressed and sclerotic. It occurs in children.

koilonychia Spoon shaped nails found in iron deficiency anaemia.

Koplik's spots Small white spots to be found on the inner surface of the cheeks in measles, often before the skin rash appears.

Korsakoff's syndrome A confusional state especially as to recent events due to brain injury or toxic causes such as chronic alcoholism. Confabulation is used by the patient in an attempt to cover the memory defect.

kraurosis vulvae Degenerative condition of the vulva.

Krebs citric acid cycle *See* CITRIC ACID CYCLE.

Krukenberg's tumour A secondary carcinoma in the ovary diagnosed before the primary which is usually gastrointestinal.

Küntscher nail An intramedullary nail used to fix fragments of fractured long bone in alignment.

Kupffer cells Reticuloendothelial cells which line the sinusoids of the liver.

Kveim test Intradermal test for sarcoidosis by injection of splenic extract from known sarcoidosis patient.

kwashiorkor Syndrome characterized by wasting, oedema, anaemia and enlargement of the liver and due to lack of adequate protein in the diet. Occurs most commonly when a child is weaned from the breast.

kyphoscoliosis Combined anteroposterior deformity (kyphosis) and lateral curvature (scoliosis) of spine.

kyphosis Anteroposterior curvature of the spine causing humpback deformity.

L

labia majora (sing. **labium**). Two large folds at the mouth of the pudendum; also called the *labia pudendi*.

labia minora Two smaller folds within the majora; called also the nymphae.

labial Relating to the lips or to the labia.

labile Unstable.

laboratory A place where scientific experiments and investigations are carried on.

labour The progress of the birth of a child. There are three stages. (1) The dilatation of the cervix. (2) The passage of the fetus through the canal and its birth. (3) From the birth of the child to the expulsion of the placenta.

labyrinth The internal ear made up of the cochlea and three semicircular canals. *Membranous l.*: with the *bony l.* of the petrous temporal bone.

labyrinthitis Inflammation of the labyrinth.

laceration A lacerated wound with torn or irregular edges; not clean cut.

lacrimal (lachrymal) Relating to tears and the glands which secrete them.

lacrimation Flow of tears.

lactalbumin The albumin of milk. A protein.

lactase An enzyme of the succus entericus which converts lactose into glucose.

lactate A salt of lactic acid.

lactation The process or period of suckling.

lacteals The lymphatic vessels, which convey the chyle from the intestinal canal.

lactic acid An acid produced by the fermentation of lactose.

lactiferous ducts The canals of the mammary glands.

lactifuge Reduction of milk secretion.

lactobacillus A non-pathogenic Gram-positive bacterium.

lactogenic Promoting the flow of milk. *L. hormone.*: prolactin. A hormone released from the anterior pituitary which causes milk production following parturition. *See* PROLACTIN.

lactose A disaccharide sugar, composed of glucose and galactose, which occurs in milk.

lacuna A space.

Laennec's cirrhosis The commonest type of cirrhosis of liver and frequently attributable to damage to the liver by high consumption of alcohol.

laevulose *See* FRUCTOSE.

lambdoid Like Greek letter λ, chiefly applied to the suture between the occipital and parietal bones.

lamellae Thin sheets of tissue, *e.g.* bone.

lamina A thin layer.

laminectomy Excision of

vertebral laminae. Allows removal of a prolapsed intervertebral disc (slipped disc).

Lancefield's groups A classification of streptococci into groups of which group A includes the common pathogenic haemolytic streptococcus.

lancet A sharp pointed surgical instrument.

Langerhans' islets Small area of special cells in the pancreas, secreting insulin. *See* INSULIN and DIABETES.

lanolin Purified wool-fat. Used as the basis for various ointments.

lanugo hair Thin unmedullated hair. Often fetal.

laparoscope Endoscope for examining the abdominal cavity.

laparotomy Operation involving the opening of the abdominal cavity, usually as an investigative procedure.

laryngeal Relating to the larynx. *L. stridor*: gasping respiration due to spasm of the glottis.

laryngectomy Removal of the larynx.

laryngismus stridulus Laryngeal spasm.

laryngitis Inflammation of the larynx.

laryngology Study of diseases of the larynx.

laryngopharynx The lower part of the pharynx.

laryngoscope Instrument for examining a larynx.

laryngospasm Spasm of the glottis.

laryngostenosis Stricture of the larynx.

laryngotomy Cutting into the larynx for the insertion of a tube.

laryngotracheobronchitis Acute viral inflammatory disease affecting the respiratory tract. Often occurs during influenza epidemics and affects principally young children. A cause of croup.

larynx The upper part of the windpipe from which the voice sounds proceed.

laser (Light Amplification by Stimulated Emission of Radiation.) Source of intense monochromatic light which can be delivered in large but precise amounts to very small areas. Used especially in ophthalmology for detached retina, and experimentally.

Lassa fever A viral fever usually contracted in tropical Africa. Incubation time is up to two weeks. Resembles enteric fevers with oropharyngeal ulceration. High mortality and infectivity. Strict isolation required.

lassitude Feeling of weakness, a frequent feature of debilitating diseases such as anaemia.

latent Not visible, lying hidden for a time. *L. period*: incubation time.

lateral On the side; *cf.* medial. *L. meniscus:* cartilage between femur and tibia on the outside of the knee. *L. position:* lying on the side. This position, favoured by some obstetricians, may be adopted by the mother during delivery.

laughing gas Nitrous oxide gas. An anaesthetic.

lavage Washing out.

laxative A mild purgative.

lead poisoning Usually occurs in children due to excessive lead in atmosphere or chewing cots and toys covered with paint containing lead. The symptoms and signs include malaise, colic, peripheral neuropathy, and sometimes encephalitis. Pallor is often marked and a blue line on the gums is characteristic.

leather-bottle stomach Loss of elasticity in the stomach wall resulting from infiltration of neoplastic cells. *Syn.* linitus plastica.

lecithin A phospholipid.

leech Aquatic worm which is able to suck blood from the skin. May be used medically to reduce haematoma.

leg Anatomically the part of the lower limb from knee to ankle. *White l.:* condition caused by venous thrombosis in the lower limb. Sometimes seen after childbirth.

Legionella haemophila Caus-

ative organism of legionnaire's disease. May be spread from droplet infection from contaminated cooling and air-conditioning systems.

legionnaire's disease An atypical pneumonia first described after an outbreak at a convention of the American Legion in Philadelphia in 1976. Usually responds to erythromycin, but can be fatal.

Leishman–Donovan body Eosinophilic bodies representing rounded forms of *Leishmania donovani* found in the cells parasitized in kala-azar.

leishmaniasis *See* KALA-AZAR.

lens Transparent refractile tissue of the eye which focuses the image on the retina.

lente insulin Slowly absorbed insulin preparation.

lenticular Pertaining to a lens.

lentigo A freckle.

leontiasis ossea A localized form of fibrous dysplasia of bone, causing deformation of the face.

leproma Swelling in the skin found in certain cases of leprosy.

leprosy Hansen's disease is an endemic disease of the tropics. It is of low infectivity and is caused by *Mycobacteria leprae*. Leprosy is a notifiable disease in the UK.

leptomeningitis Inflammation of the pia mater and arachnoid coverings of the brain, distinguished from pachymeningitis, in which the dura mater is the seat of inflammation.

Leptospira Type of spirochaete; notably *L. icterohaemorrhagae* which causes Weil's disease.

Leriche syndrome Obstruction to the flow of blood at the lower end of the aorta giving rise to intermittent claudication, and pain in the buttocks in association with impotence.

lesbian Homosexual woman.

lesion Any injury or morbid change in the function or structure of an organ.

lethal Deadly, fatal.

lethargy Drowsiness.

leucine An amino acid.

leuco, leuko Prefix meaning white (Greek).

leucocyte A white blood cell.

leucocythaemia Abnormally increased numbers of white cells in the blood.

leucocytolysis Destruction of leucocytes.

leucocytosis Increased numbers of white cells in the blood.

leucoderma A condition in which there are patches of skin which are defectively pigmented, and consequently pale in colour.

leuconychia Curved white lines on the fingernails showing interrupted nutrition.

leucopenia Diminution of the number of white cells in the blood.

leucopoiesis Formation of white blood cells.

leucorrhoea A whitish mucoid discharge from the vagina.

leucotomy Transection of nerve fibres passing to and from a lobe of the brain. Usually *prefrontal l.*: an operation undertaken to relieve certain types of mental disorder in which the prefrontal lobes are surgically isolated from the rest of the brain.

leukaemia A disease of blood-forming organs, characterized by increase of white cells of the blood. *Lymphatic l.*: where large numbers of primitive lymphocytes appear in the blood. *Myeloid l.*: where primitive polymorphonuclear leucocytes appear in large numbers. *Monocytic l.*, *eosinophilic l.*: as for the other forms, but exhibiting monocytes and eosinophils respectively. *See* BLOOD.

leukoplakia A smooth glazed white state of the tongue which may precede cancer of that organ. A similar condition of the vulva is also found in women and may be malignant.

levator A muscle which lifts up a part. *L. ani*: muscle of the pelvis which plays an important part in keeping pelvic viscera in position. *L. palpebrae superioris*: muscle which raises the upper eyelid.

levulose Fruit sugar or fructose.

libido The drive to obtain satisfaction through the senses. Term sometimes used for sexual desire.

Libman–Sachs endocarditis Endocarditis in which the valves of the heart are damaged. The disease is associated with systemic lupus erythematosus.

lice *See* PEDICULOSIS.

lichen (1) Subdivision of Thallophyta, which are organisms formed from a symbiotic association of algae and fungus, and found on rocks, trees and bare areas. (2) A term used in dermatology roughly descriptive of the appearance of certain eruptions such as *l. simplex* (*see* LICHENIFICATION), and *l. planus*. The latter has a characteristic appearance consisting of an eruption of diamond-shaped flat violaceous papules.

lichenification Also called lichen simplex. Thickening of the epidermis caused by constant friction. Often it occurs on the skin in sites exposed to habitual rubbing or scratching, from which it inherits the original name of neurodermatitis.

lid retraction A sign of hyperthyroidism in which the upper eyelids are raised so as to expose the sclera above the cornea.

lie of fetus The position of the fetus in the uterus is termed its lie, *i.e.* transverse lie, vertical lie.

Lieberkühn's glands Tubular glands of the small intestine, which secrete the intestinal juice.

lien The spleen.

lienculus An accessory spleen.

ligament A tough band of fibrous tissue connecting together the bones at the joints.

ligation The application of a ligature.

ligatures Threads of silk, wire, catgut, fascia, nylon, etc., used to tie arteries, stitch tissue, etc.

light adaptation The contraction response of the pupil of the eye to light incident on the retina. Also termed light reflex, *cf.* dark adaptation.

lightning pains Shooting, cutting pains felt in some cases of tabes dorsalis.

limbus Literally a border; applied to the junction between the sclera and cornea.

liminal At the threshold of perception.

linctus A syrup. Usually applied to a cough mixture.

linea alba The white line down the centre front of the abdomen. It is formed by the tendons of the abdominal muscles.

linea nigra A pigmented line seen in pregnant women running in midline from above the umbilicus to the symphysis pubis.

lineae albicantes *See* STRIAE GRAVIDARUM.

lingual Relating to the tongue.

liniment A liquid preparation for application to the skin with friction.

linitus plastica *See* LEATHER-BOTTLE STOMACH.

linolenic acid A constituent of vegetable fats, essential for health.

lint Loosely woven cotton material, having one side smooth and the other rough. The smooth side is applied next to the skin.

lipaemia Presence of excess of fat in the blood.

lipase Enzyme which splits the esters of fatty acids. *See* FAT.

lipoatrophy Loss of subcutaneous fat. A complication which may arise in sites of insulin injections.

lipochondrodystrophy Gargoylism or Hurler's syndrome.

lipodystrophy A disorder of

fat metabolism which most commonly affects women, who show little fat above the waist but are obese about the buttocks and legs.

lipoidosis General term for diseases of fat metabolism.

lipoids Substances, *e.g.* lecithin, which resemble fats, in being dissolved by organic solvents such as alcohol and ether. They occur in living cells.

lipoma Tumour of fat cells.

lipotrophic substances Substances which mobilize fat from the liver.

Lippes loop One type of intrauterine device (IUD).

liquor amnii The watery fluid by which the fetus is surrounded.

liquor folliculi Fluid in a graafian follicle.

liquores Solutions of active substances in water, *e.g.* liquor calcis saccharatus, limewater.

listeria A type of bacteria which can cause listeriosis in humans.

lithagogues Drugs which expel or dissolve stones.

lithiasis Formation of stone.

litholapaxy Operation for crushing a stone in the bladder and removing the fragments at the same sitting.

lithopaedion A calcified fetus in the abdominal cavity.

lithotomy Operation of cutting into a bladder to remove

a stone. *L. position*: patient supine with thighs and knees flexed. The hips must be abducted.

lithotrite An instrument for crushing stones in the bladder. It is passed through the urethra.

lithotrity Operation of crushing a stone in the bladder.

lithuria Passing gravel or crystals of uric acid with the urine.

litmus A blue pigment turned red by acids. *L. paper*: paper impregnated with litmus; used for testing urine and gastric secretion. A red litmus paper is turned blue by an alkali.

litre (l) 1000 ml or 1.7598 pints or 35.196 fluid ounces.

Little's disease Spastic paraplegia or diplegia of infants due to birth injury or faulty development of the brain.

Littré's hernia A femoral or inguinal hernia containing a Meckel's diverticulum or appendix.

liver Large organ occupying the upper right portion of the abdomen. It has many important functions including the secretion of bile, the manufacture of serum albumin and the storage of glycogen, etc.

livid Bluish in colour.

LMP *Abbr.* last menstrual period.

LOA *Abbr.* left occipito-anterior presentation of fetus.

lobar Pertaining to a lobe.

lobe Rounded division of an organ.

lobectomy Excision of a lobe.

Lobo's disease Keloid tumours of the legs induced by fungus infection.

lobule Small lobe.

localized Limited to a certain area; not widespread.

lochia The vaginal discharge following delivery. For the first day or two is almost pure blood, but in normal cases becomes rapidly brown and then paler and ceases in a few weeks.

locked twins A condition of twins at delivery when some part of one absolutely prevents the birth of the other by causing complete impaction.

lockjaw *See* TETANUS.

locomotor ataxia Impaired gait in walking. A chronic disease due to degeneration of parts of the spinal cord and nerves. *See* TABES.

loculated Divided into many cavities.

locum tenens A practitioner who temporarily takes the place of another.

loin The lateral portion of the back between the thorax and pelvis.

longevity Long life.

longsighted *See* HYPERMETROPIA.

LOP *Abbr.* left occipitoposterior presentation of fetus.

LP *Abbr.* lumbar puncture.

lordosis Undue curvature of the spine with the convexity forwards; an exaggeration of the normal curve of the lumbar part of the spine.

lotion A medical solution for external use.

louse A type of insect. *See* PEDICULUS.

Lovset's manoeuvre An obstetrical manoeuvre used to deliver breech presentations with extended arms.

low back pain *See* LUMBAGO.

lower uterine segment That portion of the uterus between the cervix and the lower end of the body which develops during late pregnancy. Most caesarean sections are done through this portion.

LSD *Abbr.* lysergic acid, a hallucinogen.

'lub-dup' Heart sounds. The first sound is heard when the atrioventricular valves close, the second on closure of the semilunar valves.

lubricant Any substance, such as an oil, which makes a surface slippery.

lucid Clear.

Ludwig's angina An acute inflammatory condition in the sublingual and submaxillary regions.

lumbago Low back pain, thought to be due to spasm of the lumbar muscles and associated with injuries to the lumbar spine, *e.g.* lumbar spondylosis and prolapsed in-

tervertebral disc.

lumbar Pertaining to the region of the loins and the spinal segments between thoracic and sacrum. *L. puncture*: the operation of tapping the cerebrospinal fluid in the lumbar region. *L. sympathectomy*: operation to remove the sympathetic chain in the lumbar region to obtain vasodilatation in the lower limbs.

lumen The cavity inside a tube.

lumpectomy Surgical removal of a lump, usually in the breast without more extensive surgery, *e.g.* mastectomy. Used as a definitive procedure with radiotherapy.

lungs The two organs of respiration, situated in the right and left sides of the cavity of the chest.

lunula White crescent at the root of the nail.

lupus erythematosus A disorder classed with the so-called collagen diseases. A localized form may affect the skin of exposed regions. The generalized form is known as systemic *l. e.* (SLE). The clinical manifestations of the disease are very varied. The criterion of diagnosis is the detection of antinuclear factor (ANF) by immunofluorescent techniques. Antibodies to DNA may also be found. LE cells may be present but are found in other diseases as well as SLE.

lupus vulgaris Tuberculosis affecting the skin.

luteinizing hormone (LH) Hormone of the anterior pituitary gland stimulating ovulatory disruption of a follicle and the formation of corpus luteum in the ovary. It then stimulates androgen secretion from Leydig's cells.

luteotrophin *See* LUTEINIZING HORMONE.

luteus Yellow (Latin). *See* MACULA LUTEA and CORPUS LUTEUM.

luxation Dislocation of a joint.

Lyme disease An acute inflammatory disease spread by the bite of a tick living on deer. First reported in Lyme, Connecticut but now seen in the UK.

lymph That part of the blood plasma which has passed through the walls of the capillaries, bathing the tissue cells, giving them nourishment and taking away waste products. It is also found in the lymphatic vessels and serous cavities.

lymphadenitis Inflammation of the lymphatic glands.

lymphadenoid goitre *See* HASHIMOTO'S DISEASE.

lymphangiectasis Dilated state of lymphatic vessels.

lymphangioma Tumour arising from the endothelial cells lining the lymphatic vessels.

lymphangioplasty An operation for the relief of lymphatic obstruction.

lymphangitis Inflammation of lymphatic vessels.

lymphatic leukaemia *See* LEUKAEMIA.

lymphatics Small vessels pervading the body, and containing lymph.

lymphocytaemia Increase of lymphocytes in the bloodstream.

lymphocytes One of the normal varieties of white blood cells.

lymphocytosis Excess of these cells in the blood: found in leukaemia, whooping cough, tuberculosis and lymphadenoma.

lymphocytopenia Deficiency of lymphocytes.

lymphogram Method of demonstrating the lymphatic system following the injection of contrast medium opaque to x-rays.

lymphogranuloma inguinale Sexually transmitted disease due to a virus.

lymphoid Having the character of lymph. *L. tissue*: adenoid tissue.

lymphoma Tumour of lymphatic tissue.

lymphosarcoma A sarcoma originating in lymphatic tissue.

lysine *See* AMINOACIDS.

lysins Antibodies able to dissolve cells. Haemolysins, those able to dissolve red blood cells. Bacteriolysins, those able to dissolve bacteria.

lysis Dissolution.

lysosomes Intracellular vesicles produced probably by the Golgi apparatus in which are segregated a number of hydrolytic enzymes. *See* CELL.

M

McBurney's point On the line from umbilicus to anterior superior iliac spine, at the outer edge of rectus muscle; corresponds to base of the appendix, and pressure here may cause tenderness depending on the position of the appendix.

McMurray's test Test for torn cartilage of the knee joint. The knee is flexed and then extended while held in forced external or internal rotation to test for respectively torn medial or lateral meniscus.

maceration The softening of a solid by soaking it in a liquid; or of a fetus which has died some time before delivery.

Mackenrodt's ligaments Also called transverse cervical or cardinal ligaments. One of the chief supports of the uterus.

macro Large (Greek).

macrocephalus A fetus with an abnormally large head.

macrocheilia Excessively large lips.

macrocytes Abnormally large cells, present in the blood in certain types of anaemia.

macrodactyly Enlargement of the fingers.

macroglobulinaemia Syndrome associated with presence in blood of abnormal globulins of high molecular weight, characterized by multiple haemorrhages, dyspnoea and fatigue, especially in elderly men.

macroglossia Hypertrophy of the tongue.

macromastia Abnormally developed breasts.

macrophages Wandering scavenger cells which form part of the reticuloendothelial system. Their function is to engulf tissue debris and foreign particles. In connective tissue they are termed histiocytes and in the blood they are known as monocytes. The engulfment of material is termed phagocytosis.

macroscopic Visible to the naked eye.

macrostomia Rare abnormality of development of the mouth due to non-fusion of the mandibular and maxillary processes.

macula A spot discolouring the skin. *M. lutea*: central spot of the posterior surface of the retina, just lateral to the optic disc marked by a small depression, and where vision is most acute.

maculopapular A rash having both macules and papules.

Magendie, foramen of An opening in the roof of the fourth ventricle through which the cerebrospinal fluid passes into the subarachnoid space.

magnetic resonance imaging (MRI, NMI or NMR) Imaging technique using computer analysis of the signals a tissue produces in response to a strong magnetic field.

main en griffe Claw-like deformity of hand.

mal Sickness. *M. de mer*: sea sickness. *Grand m.*: major epilepsy. *Petit m.*: minor epilepsy.

malabsorption Reduced ability to absorb substances in the food from causes such as intestinal hurry, loss of absorbing surface as in extensive bowel resections, and diseases affecting the bowel wall including tropical sprue, coeliac disease and idiopathic steatorrhoea. *M. syndrome*: syndrome produced by malabsorption which is characterized by some or all of the following features: diarrhoea, loss of weight, abdominal dis-tension, anaemia, tetany and vitamin deficiencies.

malacia Pathological softening.

maladie de Roger Term sometimes used to describe small ventricular septal defects which do not give rise to symptoms unless some secondary disorder, such as bacterial endocarditis, supervenes.

maladjustment A state of being not in line as with a badly set bone. In psychology, development which is not acceptable to the society in which the individual lives.

malaise A general feeling of illness or discomfort.

malalignment Faulty alignment of fragments of a fracture or occasionally used of teeth.

malar Relating to the cheekbone.

malaria Tropical disease caused by parasite transmitted by Anopheles mosquitoes. There are four varieties of human malaria due to infection respectively by *Plasmodium vivax m.* (benign tertian), *Plasmodium ovale m.* (benign tertian), *Plasmodium falciparum m.* (malignant tertian) and *Plasmodium malariae m.* (quartan). Clinical features are periodic attacks of shivering followed by headache, vomiting, fever and profuse sweating.

malformation Deformity.

malignant Virulent, fatal, usually of a tumour. A *m. tumour* or *growth* is one which if not totally removed will spread and cause similar growths in other parts of the body until the patient dies, *e.g.* carcinoma, sarcoma. *m. exophthalmos*: exophthalmos occurring in the absence of any marked evidence of hyperthyroidism. Proptosis is extreme and there is progressive oedema and swelling of the lids and later ulceration of the cornea, diplopia and blindness. *M. hyperpyrexia*: usually an inherited disorder in which an abnormal reaction to certain anaesthetic drugs leads to a rapid rise in body temperature. *M. hypertension*: hypertension associated with papilloedema and evidence of renal failure. *M. pustule*: anthrax contracted from cattle, causing gangrenous carbuncle.

malingering Shamming sickness.

malleolus The projection of the ankle-bone. The inner malleolus is at the lower extremity of the tibia, the outer one at the lower extremity of the fibula.

mallet finger Deformed finger with flexion of distal phalanx. Usually due to rupture of a long extensor tendon where it is inserted on the distal phalanx.

malleus A hammer-shaped bone of the middle ear. *See* EAR.

malnutrition A state of undernourishment.

malocclusion Failure of the teeth to close properly on biting.

Malpighian corpuscle Mesh of capillaries which act as a filtering coil for blood passing through the kidneys.

malposition Any position other than occipitoanterior during labour.

malpractice Unethical, inappropriate or negligent dealing with or treatment of a patient by doctor, nurse or other professional.

malpresentation Any presentation, other than the vertex, of the fetus during labour.

malrotation of gut Abnormality of development in which the intestine becomes fixed to the mesentery in an abnormal way. This makes the gut liable to volvulus.

maltase An enzyme of the succus entericus which converts maltose into glucose.

maltose A disaccharide, composed of two molecules of glucose.

malunion Faulty union of divided tissues, as of the fragments of a broken bone.

mammae The breasts, or milk-supplying glands.

mammaplasty Plastic surgery on the breasts particularly to reduce the size of very heavy breasts.

mammary Relating to the breasts.

mammilla The nipple.

mammography A technique to demonstrate tissue changes in the breast: xero-radiography is frequently used for this technique.

Manchester repair A type of gynaecological operation for uterovaginal prolapse. Consists of anterior colporrhaphy, cervical amputation with shortening of transverse cervical ligaments and posterior colporrhaphy. *Syn.* Fothergill's repair.

mandible The lower jaw.

mania Pathological combination of elation and energy. The patient is uncontrollably excited.

manic depressive psychosis A mental illness when intense excitement alternates with depression.

manipulation Handling, rubbing and working with the hands to procure some healing result. Also forced movements of joints to re-establish a normal range of movement.

mannerism Habitual expression or actions of an individual which are characteristic of him/her. Under stress they may become exaggerated.

manometer An instrument for measuring the pressure of gases and liquids.

Mantoux test Test of the body's reaction to antigenic material prepared from tubercle bacilli. This material, called tuberculin, is injected intradermally in serial dilutions (1.0 TU; 10.0 TU; 100 TU in 0.1 ml isotonic saline). A localized inflammatory reaction within 48 hours signifies a positive response.

manual Done by hand.

manubrium sterni The uppermost part of the sternum.

manus Latin for hand.

MAOI Monoamine oxidase inhibitor. A drug used in some types of depression. Hypertensive crises can occur if the patient eats certain foods including cheese, broad beans, yeast extract, etc.

maple syrup urine disease A recessively inherited inborn error of metabolism. A diet free from leucine, isoleucine and valine is needed as these amino acids are not metabolized and lead to brain damage. There is a characteristic urinary odour. May be diagnosed antenatally.

marasmus Progressive emaciation.

marble bone disease Familial osteosclerosis. *See* ALBERS-SCHÖNBERG'S DISEASE.

Marfan's syndrome Syndrome due to abnormal development characterized by spider digits (*see* ARACHNODACTYLY), hypertonus, high-arched palate, dislocation of lenses and various cardiac anomalies, particularly atrial septal defect and coarctation of the aorta.

marihuana *See* CANNABIS.

Marion's disease Contracture of the bladder neck, giving rise to difficulty in passing urine.

marrow The soft substance which fills the medullary canal of a long bone and the small spaces in cancellous bone. The red cells of the blood are formed in the bone marrow. *M. puncture*: investigative procedure involving the aspiration of marrow cells, usually by puncturing the sternum or iliac crest with a needle. *M. transplantation*: a treatment for blood dyscrasias involving return of healthy donor marrow to the circulation after total body irradiation to destroy marrow malignancy in the recipient.

marsupialization Old method of treating mesenteric cysts by opening the cavity on to the external abdominal wall, thus making a sort of kangaroo pouch.

masochism Self-torture from which a sexual pleasure may be derived.

massage Manipulation and rubbing of body designed to promote blood flow.

masseter Powerful muscle which lifts the mandible, thus closing the jaws.

mast cells Cells found in the blood and the tissues which store histamine which is released when the cells are damaged. They are distinguishable by their content of basophilic granules.

mastalgia Breast pains.

mastectomy Surgical removal of the breast. *Radical m.*: the breast is removed together with the lymph glands of the axilla and the pectoral muscle.

mastication Chewing.

mastitis Inflammation of the breast.

mastodynia Pain in the breasts often in the premenstrual phase.

mastoid Literally, breastlike. The *m. process* is the projecting portion of the temporal bone behind the ear; it contains numerous air spaces including the *m. antrum*.

mastoidectomy Excision of the inflamed cells.

mastoiditis Inflammation of the mastoid cells.

masturbation Manipulation of the genitalia to produce sexual excitement.

materia medica Branch of medical study dealing with the nature and use of drugs,

i.e. pharmacology and therapeutics.

matrix Continuous medium
in which structures are em-
bedded.

matter Any substance. Pus is
sometimes referred to as matter. *Grey m.*: the nerve cells
or non-medullated nerve
fibres. *White m.*: medullated
nerve fibres which are en-
veloped by a white sheath.

maturation Ripening; the
process of becoming fully developed.

maxilla The upper jawbone.

maxillary Pertaining to the
maxilla.

MCHC *Abbr.* mean cell
haemoglobin concentration.

MCV *Abbr.* mean cell
volume.

ME *Abbr.* myalgic encephalomyelitis. *See* BENIGN.

mean The average.

measles Morbilli. An infectious disease common in
children. Incubation period
10–12 days. Early symptoms
are those of a cold, sore
throat, cough and rise in temperature, Koplik's spots. The
rash appears on the fourth
day, about the neck and behind the ears, gradually
spreading to the rest of the
body and extremities. Re-
covery occurs about the
seventh or ninth day. Most infectious period is before the
rash appears. *German m.*:
rubella.

meatus An opening into a
passage.

mechanics of labour The
series of forces which act
upon the fetus while it is
being driven through the birth
canal, with the resistance to
those forces, and the resulting
effects of both upon the attitude and movements of the
fetus.

Meckel's cartilage Part of the
articular surface of the jaw.

Meckel's diverticulum A
small blind protrusion occasionally found in the lower
portion of the ileum.

meconium A black sticky
substance voided from the
bowels of an infant during
the first day or two after its
birth.

media (1) Nutrient fluids for
the culture of organisms or
tissues. (2) The middle layer
of blood vessels.

medial On the inside, *cf.*
lateral (on the outside); towards the median line.

median In the middle. *M.
line*: an imaginary lon-
gitudinal line dividing the
body down the centre. *M.
nerve*: one of the nerves of the
arm.

mediastinoscopy Endoscopic
examination of the media-
stinum.

mediastinum The space in
the chest between the two
lungs. It contains the heart,
glands and important vessels.

medical jurisprudence *See* FORENSIC MEDICINE.

medicament Any medicinal drug or application.

medication A medicine given to a patient. *Preoperative m.*: one given before an operation as a basal anaesthetic.

medicinal Pertaining to the science of medicine or to a drug.

medicine (1) The treatment of disease. (2) A drug used to prevent or treat disease.

medicochirurgical Relating to both medicine and surgery.

Mediterranean anaemia *See* THALASSAEMIA.

medium Material to nourish cultures of tissues, cells and microorganisms.

medulla Latin for marrow. *M. oblongata*: the lowest part of the brain where it passes through the foramen magnum and becomes the spinal cord. It contains the vital centres which govern circulation and respiration. *See* BRAIN.

medullary Relating to the marrow.

medullated nerve fibre Nerve fibre surrounded by a sheath of myelin.

medulloblastoma Malignant tumour, from embryonic cells of neuroepithelial origin, occurring in the cerebellum.

megacephaly An abnormally large head.

megacolon Enlargement and dilatation of the colon. *Con-*

genital m.: Hirschsprung's disease.

megakaryocytes Large bone marrow cells which produce the blood platelets.

megaloblast Large, nucleated primitive red blood cell. They occur in the peripheral blood when there is a defect of red blood cell maturation in the bone marrow, as for example in vitamin B_{12} deficiency.

megolomania Insanity with delusional ideas of personal greatness.

meibomian cyst Chalazion.

meibomian glands Sebaceous glands of the eyelids.

Meig's syndrome Fibroma of the ovary associated with pleural exudate.

meiosis Successive divisions of diploid cell to yield haploid gametes. The gametes (spermatozoa, ova) must have their chromosome number reduced by half in order to compensate for the doubling which occurs by fertilization.

melaena Black tarlike stools, due to the presence of blood which has undergone changes in the alimentary tract. The blood is often from a gastric or duodenal ulcer.

melancholia A state of profound depression in which there is often a slowing down of all mental and physical functions, feeling of guilt and self-denigration. Suicide is a possibility.

melanin Black pigment formed by the polymerization of quinonoid molecules. It is widely distributed in nature and is the skin pigment of man.

melanoma A tumour composed of melanocytes, the cells which are responsible for the production of melanin.

melanosis Black spots in the tissues.

melanotic Black.

melatonin The pineal gland hormone. Probably psychoactive and neuroactive.

membrane A thin lining. *M. bone*: bone arising from dermal connective tissues as opposed to bone arising from cartilage.

menarche The age at which menstruation begins.

Mendel's laws Two laws of inheritance promulgated by Mendel. The first states that allelomorphs segregate, *see* MEIOSIS; and the second that independent assortment of alleles occur. The second law is subject to the genes being situated on separate chromosomes since it depends on the independent behaviour of chromosome pairs during meiosis. When two or more genes are located on the same chromosome the alleles are said to be linked.

Mendelson's syndrome Inhalation of regurgitated gastric contents when the cough reflex is suppressed, *e.g.* when under anaesthesia or drunk, causing considerable pulmonary damage and bronchospasm.

Ménière's disease Giddiness resulting from disease of the internal ear or the equilibrating mechanism of the brain.

meningeal Pertaining to the meninges.

meninges The membranes surrounding and covering the brain and spinal cord. They are, from without: the dura mater, the arachnoid, the pia mater.

meningioma Tumour derived from the meninges.

meningism Syndrome characterized by symptoms and signs of meningitis but occurring in the absence of any causative organism. Probably a non-specific inflammatory reaction of the meninges to circulating toxins or some other trauma.

meningitis Inflammation of the meninges due to infection by organisms. Acute bacterial or viral meningitis is characterized by fever, headache, vomiting, backache and development of a stiff neck. Stupor, coma and convulsions may follow. A more insidious onset is sometimes seen in tuberculous meningitis. There may be a rash in meningococcal meningitis in infants.

meningocele Protrusion of meninges from a bony defect usually in the spine, *e.g.* spina bifida.

meningococcus A micro-organism, the cause of cerebrospinal fever.

meningoencephalocele A meningocele containing nerve tissue may be classed as meningoencephalocele if it contains brain, or *meningomyelocele* if it contains spinal cord.

meniscectomy Removal of a semilunar cartilage from the knee joint.

meniscus (1) A semilunar cartilage. (2) A lens. (3) The crescent-like surface of a liquid in a narrow tube.

menopause Cessation of menstruation. Ovulation stops and reproductive life ends. It usually occurs between 40 and 50 years of age and is associated with alterations in hormonal balance which sometimes produce troublesome symptoms such as hot flushes, etc.

menorrhagia Excessive menstrual bleeding.

menses The menstrual flow.

menstruation Monthly discharge of uterine mucosa with resultant bleeding which occurs in the absence of pregnancy in sexually mature females.

mental (1) Pertaining to the mind. (2) Pertaining to the chin.

mentoanterior, mentoposterior Types of face presentation. *See* FACE PRESENTATION.

mesarteritis Inflammation of the middle coat of an artery.

mesencephalon The midbrain.

mesenchyme Embryonic connective tissue which forms bone, cartilage, connective tissue and blood, etc.

mesenteric Pertaining to the mesentery.

mesentery A fold of the peritoneum enveloping and suspending the intestines.

mesmerism Hypnosis.

mesoappendix The mesentery of the appendix vermiformis.

mesocolon The fold of the peritoneum attached to the colon.

mesoderm Germ layer of cells which have migrated from the surface of the developing embryo during gastrulation and which is situated between the ectoderm and the endoderm. The mesoderm gives rise to muscle, blood and connective tissues, etc.

mesonephroma Malignant tumour of ovary, whose structure resembles that of renal glomeruli and tubules.

mesosalpinx Peritoneal fold enclosing the fallopian tube and continuous with the broad ligaments.

mesothelioma Malignant tumour of mesothelial cells most commonly affecting the pleura.

mesothelium General term applied to the epithelium lining serous cavities.

mesovarium A short peritoneal fold connecting the ovary to the posterior layer of the broad ligament.

metabolic Pertaining to metabolism. *M. disorders*: disorders in which there is interference with the normal processing of substances by the body. This includes a very extensive list of conditions, congenital or acquired, including diabetes mellitus; renal failure, hepatic failure, etc.

metabolism Chemical process taking place in living cells which may be divided into constructive or building-up processes (anabolism), and destructive or breaking-down processes (catabolism) *Inborn errors of m.*: disorders due to an inherited defect in metabolism such as albinism, phenylketonuria, Wilson's disease and mucoviscidosis, etc.

metacarpals The five bones of the hand joining the fingers to the wrist.

metacarpophalangeal Relating to the metacarpus and phalanges.

metamorphosis Transformation.

metaphase *See* MITOSIS.

metaphysis Part between the shaft, diaphysis, and the end, epiphysis, of the long bones.

metaplasia Term applied to the apparent transformation of adult tissues.

metastasis Transfer or spreading of a disease from one organ to another which is remote. A malignant growth spreads in this way.

metatarsalgia Pain in the fore part of the foot.

metatarsals The five bones of the foot between the tarsus and toes.

meteorism Distension of the intestines by gas.

methaemoglobin Haemoglobin which has been altered so that the iron which it contains is in the oxidized state (F^{3+}). In this state the haemoglobin cannot take up oxygen. The abnormal haemoglobin may be excreted in the urine (methaemoglobinuria).

methionine A sulphur-containing essential amino acid. It acts as a donor of methyl ($-CH_3$) groups in reactions known as transmethylations.

metra The womb.

metre A measure of length, containing 100 cm, or 1000 mm, and equal to 39.370 in.

metric system System of weights and measures employing the metre and the

173

gram as standard units which are multiplied or divided by powers of ten.

metritis Inflammation of the womb.

metropathia haemorrhagica Excessive menstrual bleeding due to excess of oestrogens.

microbe Microorganism. *See* BACTERIA, VIRUS.

microbiology Study of micro-organisms.

microcephalic Having an abnormally small head.

micrococci *See* BACTERIA.

microcyte A small red blood cell.

microcythaemia Anaemia in which the red blood cells are diminished in size as in iron deficiency anaemia. It is usually termed microcytic anaemia.

microglia Certain type of lymphocyte found in nervous tissue.

micrognathia Abnormally small jaw due to defective development of the mandible. Occasionally it is associated with congenital laryngeal stridor due to lack of tone in the arytenoepiglottic folds.

microgram (μg) One-millionth part of a gram.

micrometre (μm) A millionth part of a metre.

microorganism Any microscopic plant or animal.

microphthalmos Abnormal smallness of the eyes.

microscope An instrument which magnifies minute objects invisible to the naked eye.

microsomes These are the broken-up fragments of intracellular membranes. *See* CELL. When a tissue is homogenized and the resultant material separated by density gradient centrifugation a number of fractions can be isolated, *e.g.* the fraction containing mitochondria, the fraction containing lysosomes, etc. One of these fractions contains remnants of membranes and is called the microsomal fraction.

Microsporum Genus of fungi some species of which are parasitic to man. They are able to digest keratin and thus live in the hair and on the skin surface.

microsurgery Fine surgery requiring an operating microscope.

microtome An instrument for cutting fine sections for microscopic examination.

micturition The act of passing urine.

midbrain Small part of the brain between the forebrain and hindbrain.

midriff The diaphragm.

midwife A woman who is trained to conduct confinements.

midwifery The art and science of the conduct of pregnancy, labour and the puerperium.

migraine Paroxysmal attacks of headache, usually with nausea and often preceded by disorders of vision. Migraine is usually unilateral.

Mikulicz's disease A syndrome consisting of the following triad: symmetrical enlargement both of the salivary glands, and the lacrimal glands with narrowing of the palpebral fissures. Also parchment-like dryness of the mouth. The cause is unknown.

miliaria Prickly heat. Due to obstruction to the ducts of the sweat glands.

miliary Like millet seed. Thus *m. tuberculosis* is an acute form of infection in which the tissues are studded with small tubercles so as to resemble a mass of millet seeds.

milium Small white lumps in the skin, frequently on the eyelids.

milk The secretion of mammary glands. The average composition is:

	Human milk	Cow's milk
	%	%
Protein:		
lactalbumin	1.4 ⎱2	0.75 ⎱4
casein	0.6 ⎰	3.25 ⎰
Fat	4.0	4.0
Carbohydrate	6.0	4.0
Salt	0.2	0.7
Water	87.8	87.3

Human milk is neutral or slightly alkaline. Cow's milk is usually slightly acid by the time it reaches the consumer. Specific gravity 1.026 to 1.036.

milk teeth Primary dentition. *See* TEETH.

Miller–Abbott tube A double-bore rubber tube which is passed via the mouth into the duodenum so that intestinal suction can be applied in obstruction of the upper intestinal tract.

millicurie (mCi) Unit of radioactivity, one-thousandth of a curie.

milligram (mg) One-thousandth part of a gram.

millilitre (ml) One-thousandth part of a litre. It is almost equivalent to a cc.

millimetre (mm) One-thousandth part of a metre.

Milroy's disease Lymphangiectasis of the lymphatics of a limb. A pathological dilatation of the lymphatic vessels usually as a result of defective development.

Milwaukee brace Body splint used to correct scoliosis or spinal curvature.

miner's anaemia *See* ANKYLOSTOMA DUODENALE.

miner's nystagmus Nystagmus due to insufficient light striking the retina. The eye compensates for moving so that the maximum number of rods are exposed to the light, a process akin to the method of seeing faint stars by not looking directly at them since the macula lutea has more cones and fewer rods than the retina. Cones are less sensitive to light than rods but are essential for colour vision. *M.n.* occurs in partial blindness due to disease of the eye.

miosis Abnormal contraction of pupils of the eye of less than 2 mm.

miscarriage *See* ABORTION.

missed abortion *See* ABORTION.

Misuse of Drugs Act (1971) Statute aimed at controlling manufacture and distribution of addictive drugs. 'Controlled' drugs include morphine, opium, heroin, cocaine, cannabis and pethidine.

mitochondria Small membranous bodies which occur in the cell cytoplasm. They have a complex internal structure of folded membranes and harbour a great number of enzymes, particularly those connected with oxidative metabolism and the production of energy.

mitosis The usual process of nuclear division which occurs when a cell divides, *cf.* meiosis. Before division the cell reduplicates its chromosomes by synthesizing DNA chains complementary to those contained in the cell, *see* DEOXYRIBONUCLEIC ACID. This process takes place dur-

ing the so-called interphase. The phases of nuclear division are prophase, metaphase, anaphase and telophase.

mitral valve Valve of the heart between the left atrium and the left ventricle. Disease of this valve may give rise to mitral stenosis when there is narrowing of the orifice of the valve or mitral regurgitation or incompetence when the valve fails to close properly.

mittelschmerz Pain occurring at the time of ovulation which may be associated with a slight loss of blood vaginally.

MNS blood group system Groups are characterized by possession of one or both antigens M and N. In English population 28 per cent possess M, 22 per cent N, 50 per cent M and N; 55 per cent have antigen S, usually in association with M.

modiolus Central axis of the cochlea.

molality Solution strength expressed as the number of moles of solute to 1 kg of solvent.

molar teeth The grinding teeth. *See* DENTAL FORMULA.

molarity Solution strength expressed as the number of moles of solute dissolved per litre of solution.

mole (1) Hairy, pigmented raised area of skin. (2) In obstetric practice, a tumour composed of coagulated blood, fetal membranes and the embryo; due to haemorrhage into a gestation sac, and followed sooner or later by abortion. *Carneous* or *fleshy m.*: when mole is retained in utero for some time, the fluid part of the blood-clot becomes absorbed, leaving solid fleshy masses, in the midst of which traces of the embryo may or may not be found. *Hydatidiform* or *vesicular m.*: neoplastic degeneration of the chorion in the early weeks of pregnancy, resulting in the death of the embryo and the conversion of the chorionic villi into beadlike cysts or vesicles which may attain the size of a grape. Two prominent symptoms are (*a*) undue enlargement of the uterus for the period of amenorrhoea; (*b*) a watery pink discharge which may contain vesicles. No fetal parts are felt and no fetal heart heard, and the uterus feels softer than in a normal pregnancy. As soon as diagnosed the uterus should be emptied. The villi may become malignant and locally invade the wall of the uterus. It is then known as *invasive m.* or chorioadenoma destruens. If metastasizing it is a chorioncarcinoma or chorionepithelioma. (3) The molecular weight of a substance in grams.

molecule A combination of atoms forming a definite substance. Thus one atom of sodium with one atom of chlorine forms one molecule of sodium chloride.

molluscum contagiosum A virus disease affecting the skin.

Mönckeberg's sclerosis Sclerosis of the medium and small arteries with extensive degeneration of the middle muscle lining, with atrophy and calcareous deposits in the muscle cells.

mongolism *See* DOWN'S SYNDROME.

Monilia *See* THRUSH.

monitoring Automatic recording of physiological functions, *e.g.* pulse, blood pressure.

monoamine oxidase inhibitors (MAOIs) Drugs stimulating nervous system by inhibiting monoamine oxidases and causing pressor amines to accumulate in brain tissue. If foods containing these (*e.g.* cheese, yeast extract, broad beans, etc.) are taken concurrently, reaction may be severe or even fatal.

monocular Relating to one eye only.

monocytes Largest white cells found in the blood. They are macrophages of the reticuloendothelial system.

monocytosis Term employed when moncytes comprise more than 8 per cent of the total white cell count.

monograph Book on one subject only.

monomania A neurosis where the patient has fixed ideas on one particular subject.

mononeuritis multiplex Rare form of peripheral neuritis in which there is selective involvement of isolated nerves.

mononuclear With one nucleus.

mononucleosis Increased proportion of mononuclear white cells in the blood. *See* INFECTIOUS MONONUCLEOSIS.

monoplegia Paralysis of one limb.

monorchid, monorchis Having only one testicle.

monosaccharides Simplest sugars, *e.g.* glucose.

Monro's foramen Interventricular foramen. The communication between the two lateral ventricles and the third ventricle of the brain.

mons veneris The eminence just over the os pubis in women.

Montgomery's follicles Small prominences about the nipple, which become more evident during pregnancy and lactation. *See also* AREOLA.

Mooren's ulcer Basal cell carcinoma affecting the cornea.

morbid Diseased, disordered, pathological.

morbilli Measles.

morbus Latin for disease.

Morgagni, hydatids of Small translucent cysts arising from the embryonic pronephros which occur attached by pedicles to the fimbriated end of the fallopian tubes or to the epididymis in the male.

morgue A public mortuary.

moribund Dying.

morning sickness *See* VOMITING OF PREGNANCY.

Moro reflex Present in the neurologically intact neonate it is the extension of limbs following startling.

morphine An alkaloid obtained from opium, used as a sedative or anodyne.

morphoea Scleroderma affecting the skin only. Patches of atrophic, depigmented skin overlie connective tissue which has lost its elasticity.

morphology The study of shape and structure of living organisms.

mortality Death. The annual death rate in this country is the number of registered deaths × 1000 divided by the mid-year population. The *infant m. rate* is the number of deaths of infants under 1 year × 1000 divided by the number of registered live births. The *maternal m. rate* is the number of deaths of women ascribed to pregnancy or childbearing × 1000 divided by the number of registered live and stillbirths.

mortuary A place where dead bodies are kept.

morula Early stage in development of fertilized ovum.

mosaic In genetics a term applied to individuals made up of cells of different genetic constitution.

motile Able to move independently.

motions The evacuations of the bowels. *See* FAECES, STOOLS.

motor end-plate An accumulation of nuclei and cytoplasm of muscle fibres at the termination of motor nerves.

motor nerves Nerves carrying motor neurone fibres. Motor neurones carry impulses from the central nervous system to the effector organ; *cf.* sensory nerves.

motor neurone disease Disease of unknown cause characterized by the degeneration of the anterior horn cells of the spinal cord, the motor nuclei of the cranial nerves and corticospinal tracts.

motor root The ventral root of the spinal cord; *cf.* dorsal root.

mould *See* FUNGI.

moulding The alteration in shape of the infant's head produced by the pressure it is subjected to while being driven through the birth canal.

mountain sickness Disorder resulting from lack of oxygen at high altitudes.

movements (fetal) *See* QUICKENING.

MRI *Abbr.* magnetic resonance imaging.

MS *Abbr.* multiple sclerosis.

MSS *Abbr.* Multiple Sclerosis Society.

mucilage Aqueous solutions of gums or starch.

mucin Term loosely used for mucopolysaccharide and protein compounds (mucoprotein).

mucocele A cyst distended with mucus, as of the gall bladder or lacrimal sac.

mucoid Resembling mucus.

mucolytic Substance which reduces the viscosity of mucus.

mucopurulent With mucus and pus.

mucosa A mucous membrane.

mucous membrane A surface which secretes mucus. The lining of the alimentary canal, air passages, and urinogenital organs: merges into true skin at the various orifices of these canals.

mucous polypus A small outgrowth from the mucous surface of the cervix uteri or of the nose.

mucoviscidosis *See* CYSTIC FIBROSIS.

mucus Viscous fluid containing mucoprotein, *see*

MUCIN. It is secreted by special mucus-producing cells in mucous epithelia.

multigravida Pregnant woman who has previously had two or more pregnancies.

multilocular Having many locules.

multipara A woman who has had more than one child.

multiple myeloma Neoplasm of plasma cells which infiltrate and replace the bone marrow. Characteristic features are anaemia, bone pains and large quantities of circulating globulins of an abnormal type which may be excreted in the urine. *See* BENCE-JONES PROTEIN.

multiple pregnancy Twins, triplets, or any larger number of fetuses gestated together by one mother.

multiple sclerosis (MS) *Syn.* disseminated sclerosis. A demyelinating disease of the brain and spinal cord. It may affect the optic nerves causing optic neuritis or nerves which move the eyes causing double vision. Often starts in young adults and may follow a progressive or benign course. Bladder function is often affected. Sensation and stability of the limbs may be a problem.

mumps Acute virus-mediated parotitis. Occasionally the testes or ovaries may be involved.

Munchausen syndrome Persistent production of a fake medical history by a patient in order to receive attention.

murmur Abnormal sound on auscultation of heart. *See* HEART SOUNDS.

Murphy's sign If continuous pressure is exerted over an inflamed gall bladder while the patient takes a deep breath, it causes him to 'catch' the breath just before the zenith of inspiration.

muscle Specialized tissue composed of highly contractile cells. There are three varieties of *m.* in the body: (1) striated, voluntary; (2) smooth, involuntary; and (3) cardiac.

muscular atrophy *See* PERONEAL MUSCULAR ATROPHY.

muscular dystrophy A group of conditions also known as myopathies in which there is degeneration of groups of muscles without apparent nerve involvement. *See also* DUCHENNE MUSCULAR DYSTROPHY.

musculospiral nerve A nerve of the arm.

mutagen Agent known to produce mutation.

mutant A gene which has undergone a mutation, or an individual possessing characteristics due to such a gene.

mutation Relatively permanent alteration in the coding of part of the chromosomal deoxyribonucleic acid. These alterations are infrequent and occur at random but their frequency can be greatly increased by radiation. Mutations occurring in gametes, *i.e.* spermatozoa or ova, or their precursors are important since they may produce an inherited change in the characteristics of the individual developing from them, *see* MUTANT. Mutations in a body cell (somatic mutations) are transmitted to the clone of cells to which it gives rise.

mute Without the power of speech. Dumb.

mutilation Destruction or removal of an organ. Has profound psychological consequences.

myalgia Pain in the muscles.

myalgia, epidemic Bornholm disease. Characterized by sudden onset of fever and intercostal or diaphragmatic pain. It is thought to be caused by a virus.

myasthenia Debility of the muscles. *M. gravis*: disorder characterized by abnormal fatigue of striated muscle (*see* MUSCLE), with rapid recovery after rest. The cause is not known but appears to be some form of biochemical disturbance affecting the transmission of the impulse from the nerve-ending to the motor end-plate. Striking improvement in muscle power follows

the administration of neostigmine. Occasionally *m. gravis* is associated with hyperplasia of the thymus.

myatonia Lack of muscle tone.

mycelium The filaments of fungus forming an interwoven mass.

mycetoma Also known as Madura foot. A tropical disease due to infection with a vegetable parasite akin to that of actinomycosis. The part affected, most commonly the foot, becomes the seat of chronic inflammatory swelling with formation of ulcers and sinuses.

Mycobacterium A genus of bacteria. *M. leprae* causes leprosy, *M. tuberculosis*, tuberculosis.

Mycoplasma A genus of microorganism. Their pathogenicity is disputed but they are probably causative of primary atypical pneumonia and are associated with genital tract infection.

mycosis Disease caused by a fungus.

mycotoxins Toxic substances produced by fungi.

mydriasis Increase in the size of the pupil of the eye.

mydriatics Drugs which dilate the pupil of the eye, *e.g.* atropine, homatropine.

myelin Phospholipid–protein complex which invests the larger nerve fibres. It is produced by Schwann cells which appear to wrap coils of their cell membrane round the fibres. The coils condense to form myelin.

myelitis Inflammation of the spinal cord.

myelocele *See* MENINGO-MYELOCELE.

myelocyte Bone marrow cell.

myelogram Radiograph of the spinal cord.

myeloid Like marrow. *M. tissue*: tissue giving rise to the cellular elements of the blood, *e.g.* red cells, white cells and platelets.

myeloma *See* MYELOMATOSIS.

myelomatosis Multiple myeloma. The marrow cavity is filled with abnormal plasma cell production. Leads to anaemia, thrombocytopenia or immunosuppression.

myelopathy Any neurological disorder rising from disease of the spinal cord.

myelosclerosis Replacement of bone marrow by fibrous tissue.

myocardial Pertaining to the muscle of the heart. *M. infarction*: a heart attack. Destruction of heart muscle following occlusion of cardiac vessels Death may result from cardiac arrest or arrhythmia. Intense pain resembles angina pectoris.

myocarditis Inflammation of the myocardium.

myocardium The heart muscle.

myofibrils Thread-like structures bound together to form muscle fibres, probably essential contractile elements of muscle.

myogenic Originating from muscular tissue.

myoglobin A specialized haemoglobin found in muscle which has slightly different dissociation characteristics from that in the blood so that oxygen is transferred from the blood to the muscle.

myoma Any tumour composed of muscular tissue.

myomectomy Removal of a myoma; usually referring to a fibroid from the uterus.

myometrium Uterine muscle.

myopathy Any primary disease of muscle.

myope A shortsighted person. Myopic, pertaining to shortsightedness.

myopia Shortsightedness; corrected by wearing a biconcave lens.

myosarcoma A malignant tumour of muscle.

myosin Muscle protein, part of the actomyosin complex.

myosis Contraction of the pupil of the eye.

myositis Inflammation of a muscle. *M. ossificans*: may follow stretching of an injured muscle, its fibres and haematoma are replaced by cancellous bone. The condition can be prevented by resting the injured muscle.

myotics Drugs which cause the pupil to contract.

myotomy Cutting through a muscle.

myotonia Tonic muscular spasm. *M. atrophica* or *dystrophica*: a hereditary disorder characterized by wasting of the muscles of the face, neck and limbs associated with cataract, frontal baldness in men and gonadal atrophy. *M. congenita*: Thomsen's disease. A dominantly inherited disorder in which the only symptom is the slow relaxation of muscles after contraction which makes it difficult, for example, for the patient to relax his grasp.

myringa The tympanic membrane of the ear.

myringitis Inflammation of the tympanic membrane of the ear.

myringoplasty Operation to reconstruct a chronically perforated tympanic membrane.

myringotomy Incision of the tympanic membrane of the ear, performed when the presence of pus is suspected in the middle ear.

myxoedema Syndrome due to hypothyroidism and characterized by dry atrophic skin, swelling of the limbs and face and retardation both physical and mental. The metabolic rate is diminished and the patient dislikes the cold intensely. There is usually loss of hair in the frontal and pubic regions and the outer third of the eyebrows.

myxoma Tumour of connective tissue containing mucoid material.

myxosarcoma A malignant myxoma.

myxoviruses The influenza group of viruses.

N

nabothian follicles Cystic swellings on the cervix caused by closure of glandular crypts in the columnar endocervical epithelium as an ectropion or erosion is covered with squamous epithelium by a process of metaplasia.

NAD *Abbr.* nothing abnormal detected.

naevus (pl. **naevi**) Mole (Latin). Usually applied to *cellular n.*, a small skin lesion resulting from the proliferation of naevus cells which are thought to be related to melanocytes, *see* MELANOMA. Naevus is also a general term for congenital skin lesions, *i.e.* birth marks, resulting from abnormalities in the development of superficial blood vessels, lymphatics, etc.

NAI *Abbr.* non-accidental injury. *See* BATTERED BABY SYNDROME.

nail Horny plate found at the tip of finger or toe.

nape Back of the neck.

napkin rash Rash in the napkin area due to irritation of the skin by ammonia produced by bacteria which ferment the urea in the urine.

narcissism An abnormal love of oneself: named after Narcissus, who fell in love with his own reflection.

narcoanalysis Psychoanalysis practised with the patient in a state of basal narcosis. Founded on the principle that the unconscious (subconscious) thoughts are less likely to be suppressed if the patient is rendered drowsy.

narcolepsy A condition characterized by sudden attacks of sleep occurring repeatedly during the day.

narcosis A state of unconsciousness produced by the use of narcotics.

narcotic A drug which produces unconsciousness, *e.g.* paraldehyde, the barbiturates.

nares The nostrils.

nasal Relating to the nose.

nasogastric tube A tube passed by the nostril, pharynx and oesophagus to the stomach to allow drainage of the stomach contents or parenteral feeding via the stomach.

nasolacrimal Relating to the nose and lacrimal apparatus.

nasopharyngeal Pertaining to the nasopharynx.

nasopharynx The space between the posterior nares, the base of the skull, the soft palate, the upper end of the oesophagus, and the epiglottis.

nates The buttocks.

natural childbirth A school of opinion concerning childbirth which advocates the minimum of medical interference with the process of delivery which is considered to be a normal physiological process.

nausea A feeling of sickness.

navel The umbilicus, the point of connection of the umbilical cord.

navicular The boat-shaped tarsal bone.

nebula A cloud or mist. Term applied to filmy corneal opacities.

nebulizer A device to produce a mist of dispersed fluid and may contain drugs to enter the lungs and air passages. Usually used in asthma.

neck Narrow part near the end of an organ. *Derbyshire n.*: goitre. *Wry n.*: torticollis.

necropsy Examination of a body after death.

necrosis Death of tissue.

necrotic Relating to necrosis.

needle-holder Spring-loaded forceps for holding surgical needles.

needling Perforation with a

needle especially in cataract. *See* DISCISSION.

negativism A state of mind in which the ideas and behaviour of an individual are in opposition to those of the majority and contrary to suggestion.

negligence Lack of care and attention expected from a doctor or nurse that results in damage to a patient.

Neisseria Genus of diplococci. *N. gonorrhoeae* causes gonorrhoea; *N. meningitidis* causes epidemic cerebrospinal meningitis.

Nelaton's line Line from the anterior superior iliac spine to the tuberosity of the ischium.

nematodes Worms including roundworms, threadworms and eelworms. Some of these are parasitic to man, *e.g.* hookworm.

neoarthrosis A new joint.

neocortex Cerebral cortex excluding hioppocampal formation and piriform area.

neonatal Relating to the first four weeks of life. *N. mortality*: death rate in the first 28 days of life.

neonate Newborn infant in the first month of life.

neoplasm A tumour. An abnormal local multiplication of some type of cell. A neoplasm may be either *benign* if it shows no tendency to spread, or *malignant* if the growing cells infiltrate surrounding

tissues and invade other parts of the body.

nephrectomy Removal of kidney.

nephritis Inflammation of the kidney. The term nephritis is used to describe a large number of widely differing conditions affecting the kidney largely because of the unsatisfactory nature of most classifications of renal disease. The classification given here should be taken only as an explanatory guide: (1) Localized renal inflammation: (*a*) pyelonephritis: infection arising usually from the urinary tract and characterized by the presence of pus and pathogenic organisms in the urine. One or both kidneys may be involved. (*b*) *focal n.*: usually a stage in a renal infection (often chronic) characterized by haematuria. The infection is blood-borne, *e.g.* bacterial endocarditis. (2) Diffuse, non-suppurative, bilateral renal disease is responsible for three broad renal syndromes: (*a*) *acute n.*: characterized by facial oedema, oliguria, haematuria, proteinuria and hypertension. The most common cause of this syndrome is acute *glomerular n.* (*type I n.*); (*b*) nephrotic syndrome; (*c*) chronic renal failure. The end result of a great number of widely different diseases affecting the kidneys.

nephro- Pertaining to the kidney.

nephroblastoma Wilms's tumour. A neoplasm of the kidney which occurs in children.

nephrocalcinosis A complication of hyperparathyroidism in which calcium becomes deposited in the renal tubules.

nephrocapsulectomy Operation to remove the kidney capsule.

nephrolithiasis Stone in the kidney.

nephrolithotomy Removal of a stone from the interior of the kidney.

nephroma Tumour of the kidney.

nephron The basic unit of the kidney. Each kidney contains about a million nephrons but not all of these are working at any one time. Each nephron consists of a filtering mechanism (the glomerulus) and a long tubule which is specialized in various regions to reabsorb substances from the urine which pass through it. The modified filtrate of the blood plasma which is thus produced is collected in the renal pelvis and leaves the kidney in the ureter.

nephropexy Stitching a movable kidney into a firm position.

nephroptosis Downward displacement of the kidney.

nephrosclerosis Renal disease secondary to hypertension.

nephrosis A term originally introduced to describe a group of patients with nephrotic syndrome in whom the lesion was thought to be in the tubules. Since then it has undergone several changes of meaning. In present usage it is applied to cases of nephrotic syndrome in which there is no obvious renal lesion and which respond well to steroid treatment.

nephrostomy Surgical opening into the kidney to drain it.

nephrotic syndrome A syndrome characterized by proteinuria, hypoproteinaemia and oedema. There are many causes of this condition including subacute glomerular nephritis (*type II nephritis*), diabetic nephropathy, amyloid disease, systemic lupus erythematosus, poisons (*e.g.* mercury), thrombosis of the renal veins and nephrosis.

nephrotomy Cutting into the kidney.

nephroureterectomy Excision of kidney and ureter.

nerve A bundle of fibres, conveying the impulses of movement and sensation to and from the organs. *See* MOTOR NERVES, SENSORY

NERVES, VASOMOTOR. *N. root:* each spinal nerve arises from the spinal cord by two roots. The dorsal root carries the sensory fibres and the ventral root the motor fibres.

nervous Pertaining to the nerves. *N. system: see* CENTRAL NERVOUS SYSTEM.

nettle rash Urticaria.

neural Relating to nerves.

neuralgia Pain in the distribution of a nerve, *e.g. trigeminal n.* Severe pain in the distribution of the trigeminal nerve (*see* CRANIAL NERVES (5)). *Sciatica* is neuralgia of the sciatic nerve distribution. The cause may be irritation of the nerve by some bony structure or a tumour but frequently the cause cannot be ascertained. For intractable pain interruption of the sensory fibres of the nerve is often helpful.

neurapraxia A temporary block to nerve conduction as after giving a local anaesthetic.

neurasthenia Nervous exhaustion.

neurectomy Excision of part of a nerve.

neurilemma The sheath of a nerve fibre.

neurinoma Tumour of neurilemma.

neuritis Inflammation of a nerve.

neuroblast Embryonic nerve cell.

neuroblastoma Malignant growth of sympathetic nerve ganglia, especially adrenal medulla. Strictly a tumour of neuroblasts.

neurodermatitis *See* LICHENIFICATION.

neuroepithelium Specialized nerve epithelium, *e.g.* the retina, which consists of nerve endings, rod and cone-shaped cells of the optic nerve.

neurofibroma Tumour arising from connective tissue surrounding peripheral nerves.

neurofibromatosis Von Recklinghausen's disease. Generalized distribution within the body of neurofibromas.

neuroglia Connective tissue cells of the central nervous system are collectively known as glia. Neuroglia are cells with long fibrous processes which are derived from embryonic nervous tissue and are closely related to Schwann cells. Their exact supportive function is not known. Microglia are similar to lymphocytes.

neuroleptic Drug affecting nervous system.

neurologist Physician who specializes in neurology.

neurology Study of diseases of the nervous system.

neuroma A tumour composed of nerve tissue.

neuromuscular junction The

junction between a motor
nerve and the effector
muscle. *See* MOTOR END-
PLATE.

neuron Nerve cell which conducts the nerve impulses. It
consists of a cell body from
which extend collecting
branches (dendrites) and a
long process (axon) along
which the impulse passes to
the effector organ or to other
nerves. Upper motor neurone
arises in the cerebral cortex,
passes down and liaises with
lower motor neurone which
supplies skeletal muscles.
Connections between nerves,
and between nerves and effector organs are through
synapses.

neuropathic Relating to
neuropathy.

neuropathy A disorder
affecting the structure and
function of the nervous system, especially applied to the
peripheral nervous system.

neuroplasty Operative repair
of a nerve.

neurorrhaphy Operation to
suture a severed nerve.

neurosis A disorder of
mental function whereby
patients are abnormally emotionally vulnerable but retain
appreciation of external
reality; *cf*. psychosis. Neuroses include behaviour disorders such as hysterical and
obsessive compulsive reactions and disturbances of

'affect', as, for example, in
anxiety states.

neurosurgery Surgery of
peripheral and central nervous system.

neurosyphilis Involvement of
the central nervous system by
syphilis.

neurotic Relating to a
neurosis.

neurotmesis The nerve trunk
is severed and there can be no
useful recovery without
surgery.

neurotomy Division of a
nerve.

neutral Neither acid nor alkaline.

neutropenia Insufficiency of
neutrophil polymorphonuc-
lear leucocytes in the blood.

neutrophil Predilection for
neutral dyes, *i.e*. not acidophil or basophil. A term used
to described the majority of
polymorphonuclear leu-
cocytes which do not demonstrate any characteristically
staining granules in their
cytoplasm; *cf*. basophil,
eosinophil.

nicotine poisoning Result of
overindulgence in smoking.
Cardinal features are the
paralysis of autonomic ganglia and constriction of the
coronary arteries.

nicotinic acid Pellagra-
preventing factor of vitamin B
complex.

nictitation Involuntary blinking of the eyelids.

nidation Implantation.

Niemann–Pick disease A lip-oid storage disease in which lecithin is deposited. An inherited defect of phospholipid metabolism which leads to widespread deposition of lecithin in the tissues. It is associated with mental retardation.

night blindness Inability to see in the dark, also called *nyctalopia*. Usually the result of vitamin A deficiency.

night sweats Profuse sweating at night characteristic of tuberculosis.

nigrescent Growing black.

nigrites Blackness. *N. linguae*, a condition in which the filiform papillae of the tongue are hypertrophied and darkly pigmented.

nipple Small eminence in the centre of each breast. *N. shields*: coverings of glass or india rubber put on the nipples to protect them when they are sore.

Nissl's granules Stacks of granula endoplasmic reticulum visible in the cell body of neurons.

nit The egg of the louse.

nitrogen A colourless inert gas, forming 78 per cent of the atmosphere and acting as a diluent. Nitrogenous foods, *see* PROTEIN. *N. mustard*: cell-destroying drug, used in the treatment of certain malignant tumours and especially

Hodgkin's disease.

nitrous oxide Laughing gas; an anaesthetic.

NMR *Abbr.* nuclear magnetic resonance.

nocturia Passing urine at night.

nocturnal At night. *N. enuresis*: bedwetting during sleep.

nodding spasm *See* SPASMUS NUTANS.

node A swelling. *Atrioventricular n.*: at the base of the interatrial septum from which impulses pass down the bundle of His. *Heberden's ns.*: deformity of the terminal joints in the fingers in osteoarthritis. *Sinoatrial n.*: the pacemaker of the heart, found at the opening of the superior vena cava into the right atrium. *N. of Ranvier*: the constriction in the neurilemma of a nerve fibre.

nodule A little knob.

non-accidental injury *See* BATTERED BABY SYNDROME.

non-compliance Failure to follow instructions regarding medical treatment.

non compos mentis Not sound of mind.

non-gonococcal urethritis (NGU) *See* NON-SPECIFIC URETHRITIS.

non-specific urethritis (NSU) Urethral infection now known to be predominantly due to chlamydia or mycoplasma.

non-viable Unable to survive,

especially as to a child of less than 28 weeks' gestation.

noradrenaline Hormone of the adrenal medulla. Raises blood pressure by a general vasoconstriction. Given in shock, etc.

normal The average or usual form.

normoblasts Immature nucleated red cells present in bone marrow.

normocyte A normally sized erythrocyte.

nose The organ of smell and used for warming, filtering and moistening the air breathed in.

nosocomial infection Infection originating in, or related to, hospitals.

nosology Classification of disease.

nostalgia Homesickness or yearning for the past.

nostrils The anterior apertures of the nose.

notch Indentation.

noxious Harmful.

NPN *Abbr.* non-protein nitrogen.

NSU *Abbr.* non-specific urethritis.

nucha The nape, or back of the neck.

Nuck *See* CANAL OF.

nuclear magnetic resonance (NMR) *See* MAGNETIC RESONANCE IMAGING.

nucleated With a nucleus.

nucleic acid Long chain of nucleotides. Two major types

are found: deoxyribonucleic acid (DNA) and ribonucleic acid (RNA). DNA is formed from nucleotides the components of which are deoxyribose, phosphoric acid and the four bases adenine, guanine, thymine, cytosine (symbolized A, G, T, C). The chromosomes are composed of a double helix of DNA in which the bases are paired A–T and G–C. The coding of genetic information is considered to occur as triplet combinations of those bases. RNA is composed of ribose, phosphoric acid and the bases adenine, guanine, cytosine and uracil (A, G, C, U). There are several types of RNA: messenger RNA, which is formed as a chain complementary to DNA and which takes the message to the sites of protein synthesis. Transfer RNA transports selected amino acids to the ribosomes. Other types of RNA also exist.

nucleolus A small dense body containing RNA which is situated in the nucleus. *See* CELL. It disappears during mitosis and is thought to represent a condensation of some chromosomal material. Its function continues to remain obscure.

nucleoprotein Compound of nucleic acid and protein, *e.g.* the ribosomes.

nucleotide Compound formed from a pentose sugar, phosphoric acid and a nitrogen-containing base.

nucleus (pl. **nuclei**) (1) Of cell: the spherical body containing the chromosomes. *See also* CELL, *etc.* (2) Of brain: demarcated mass of cell bodies, *e.g.* basal nuclei. *N. pulposus*: a pulpy mass in the centre of the intervertebral disc.

nullipara A woman who has never had a child.

nummulated or **nummular** Coin-shaped.

nutation Involuntary nodding of the head.

nutrient Nourishing. *N. foramen*: opening in a bone for the nourishing vessels.

nutrition Science of feeding.

nyctalopia *See* NIGHT BLINDNESS.

nyctophobia Abnormal fear of darkness.

nymphomania Excessive sexual desire in females.

nystagmus Involuntary oscillations of the eyeball; sometimes congenital; sometimes a symptom of brain disease, ocular affection, or lesion in the internal ear.

O

obesity Excessive body fat.

objective (1) The object glass of a microscope. (2) Pertaining to things lying external to one's self.

oblique diameters of pelvis *See* DIAMETERS.

oblique lie In pregnancy unstable lie intermediate between longitudinal and transverse lies.

oblique muscles (1) Two external muscles of the eyeball, an upper and a lower. (2) Two large muscles of the abdominal wall, an internal and an external.

obsession An idea of which the patient cannot rid himself. Minor obsessions are common in perfectly healthy people; but longstanding ones are especially frequent in the insane.

obsessional neurosis A mental illness in which the patient's mind gets taken up with forbidden thoughts and in which he has to engage in many rituals to try and free himself from these thoughts.

obsolete No longer used.

obstetric Pertaining to the practice of midwifery.

obstetrician Doctor who practises obstetrics.

obturator That which stops up a hole or cavity. The obturator of a sigmoidoscope, for example, is the blunt-ended rod which fills up the end of the instrument when it is introduced into the rectum, and thus prevents any scratching of the mucous membrane. The *o. foramen* is a hole on each side of the pelvis, closed by the powerful *o. ligament*. The *o. muscles* are two muscles on each side in the same region, and there are also *o. vessels* and *o. nerves*.

obtusion A blunting, as of sensitiveness.

occipital Relating to the back of the head.

occipitoanterior, occipitoposterior The two kinds of vertex presentation, according to the back of the head (occiput) being directed forwards or backwards.

occiput The back of the head or skull.

occlusion Closure.

occlusive therapy Application of ointments under impervious dressing.

occult blood Not visible to the naked eye. Term used to describe blood passed in faeces in such small amounts that no dark colour is present. This blood can only be demonstrated by the occult blood test.

occupational disease Illness induced by the patient's occupation.

occupational therapy Any occupation given to a patient to help in his recovery, both mentally and physically.

ocular Relating to the eye.

oculist An eye specialist.

oculogyric Rolling eyes.

oculomotor nerves The third pair of cranial nerves which help to move the eyeball.

Oddi, sphincter of Muscular sphincter at the opening of the common bile duct into the duodenum.

odontalgia Toothache.

odontoid Toothlike. *O. process*: peg-like projection of second cervical vertebra.

odontology Dentistry.

odontoma Tumour arising from a tooth or a developing tooth.

oedema Abnormal amount of fluid in the tissues causing a puffy swelling. The fluid tends to collect in the dependent parts, *e.g. o.* of the ankles.

Oedipus complex A persistence of the normal love of a boy for his mother so that it rivals that of his father. Named after Oedipus who, according to Greek mythology, unknowingly married his mother.

oesophageal Pertaining to the oesophagus. *O. atresia*: a congenital closure of the oesophagus needing urgent operative treatment. *O. varices*; varicose veins in the lower part of the oesophagus resulting from hypertension in the hepatic portal system which occurs in cirrhosis of the liver.

oesophagectasis Dilatation of a stricture in the oesophagus.

oesophagectomy Resection of

the oesophagus.

oesophagitis Inflammation of the oesophagus, especially *reflex o.*, due to hiatus hernia when stomach acid regurgitates into the lower part of the oesophagus causing damage and inflammation of the wall.

oesophagoscope An instrument for viewing the interior of the oesophagus.

oesophagoscopy Study of the oesophagus by means of the oesophagoscope.

oesophagostomy An artificial opening made into the oesophagus.

oesophagotomy Cutting into the oesophagus.

oesophagus The canal which runs from the pharynx into the stomach.

oestrogen or **oestrogenic substance** or **hormone** Any substance, usually a steroid, capable of producing genital tract changes characteristic of the follicular phase of the menstrual cycle: an oestrogen, probably oestradiol, is secreted by the ovaries. Oestrogens are also produced by the placenta during pregnancy and by the adrenal cortex. The female secondary sexual characteristics are under the influence of oestrogens, both natural and synthetic. Oestrogens may be used to control menopausal symptoms and combined with

progestogens are used in the contraceptive pill.

ohm (Ω) Unit of electrical resistance.

ointment A soft application to promote healing, usually consisting of a base impregnated with some drug.

olecranon The bone composing the point of the elbow. The extreme upper end of the ulna, the inner of the two bones of the forearm.

olfactory Relating to the sense of smell.

oligaemia Lack of blood.

oligo- Prefix meaning deficiency (Greek).

oligodendroglia Glial cells, *see* NEUROGLIA, with few dendrites or processes. Probably equivalent to microglia.

oligohydramnios Deficiency of amniotic fluid.

oligomenorrhoea Sparse menstrual flow.

oligospermia Abnormally small numbers of spermatozoa in the semen.

oligotrophia Lack of nourishment.

oliguria A diminution in the amount of urine secreted.

omentocele Hernial sac containing omentum.

omentopexy Fixation of the omentum.

omentum A fold of the peritoneum. The *greater o.* is suspended from the greater curvature of the stomach and hangs in front of the gut. The *lesser o.* passes from the lesser curvature of the stomach to the transverse fissure of the liver.

omphalitis Inflammation of the umbilicus.

omphalocele An umbilical hernia.

onychia Inflammation of the matrix of a nail.

onychocryptosis Ingrowing nail.

onychogryphosis Bizarre overgrowth of the nails, often the nail of the big toe.

onychomycosis Infection of the nails by fungi.

oocyte An ovum before it has left the graafian folllicle.

oogenesis The production of ova in the ovary.

oophorectomy Removal of an ovary. Also called *ovariectomy*.

oophoritis Inflammation of an ovary.

oophoron The portion of the ovary which produces the ova; or the ovary itself.

oophorosalpingectomy Removal of the ovary and its associated fallopian tube.

opacity Want of transparency, cloudiness.

opaque Not transparent.

open fracture *See* FRACTURE.

opening snap Adventitious heart sound which often precedes the mid-diastolic murmur of mitral stenosis.

ophthalmia Inflammation of the eye. The term is applied especially to severe inflammations of the conjunctiva. There is an acute infectious form which occurs in epidemics, especially in schools and military camps. *O. neonatorum*: severe inflammation of the eyes in the newborn, due to gonorrhoeal or septic infection of the conjunctiva during the passage of the head through the vagina.

ophthalmic Pertaining to the eye.

ophthalmitis Inflammation of the eye.

ophthalmologist A surgeon specializing in diseases of the eye.

ophthalmology The study of diseases of the eye.

ophthalmoplegia Paralysis of the muscles of the eye.

ophthalmoscope A small instrument fitted with a lens, used to examine the interior of the eye.

ophthalmotonometer Instrument to measure the intraocular tension of the eye.

opiate An opium preparation. A hypnotic.

opioid A substance having opium-like activity. May occur naturally as in certain neurotransmitters.

opisthotonos Backward retraction of the head and lower limbs with arched back; seen in severe cases of tetanus, meningitis and in strychnine poisoning.

opium A preparation of poppy juice, much used to induce sleep and to allay pain. It contains the alkaloids, morphine, codeine, papaverine and narcotine. Can cause addiction.

opponens Opposing. Applied to muscles, *e.g. o. pollicis* which brings the thumb towards the little finger.

opportunistic infection *See* INFECTION.

opsonins Class of globulins found in the blood serum that are said to prepare the bacteria for phagocytosis.

optic Relating to the sight. *O. atrophy*: degeneration of the optic nerve. *O. chiasma*: the structure in which nerve fibres from the medial surfaces of the retinae cross from one optic nerve to the opposite one. Damage results in loss of the lateral field of vision and tunnel vision. *O. disc*: the point where the optic nerve enters the eye. The point is insensitive to light and is known as the blind spot. *O. neuritis*: inflammation of the optic nerve.

optician One who is trained to test eyes, make and dispense prescriptions for lenses, and fit contact lenses.

optics The study of the properties of light.

optimum The best possible conditions for a particular function.

optometry Measurement of visual powers.

oral Pertaining to the mouth.

orbicularis Name given to a muscle which encircles an orifice, *e.g. o. oris*, around the mouth.

orbit The bony cavity in the skull which holds the eye.

orbital Pertaining to the orbit.

orchidectomy Removal of one or both testicles. Castration.

orchidopexy The bringing down of an imperfectly descended testicle into the scrotum and fixing it there by sutures.

orchiepididymitis Inflammation of the testis and epididymis.

orchis Testicle.

orchitis Inflammation of the testicles.

orf Viral skin infection normally affecting sheep.

organ A part of the body constructed to exercise a special function.

organic Relating to the organs; thus, organic disease of the heart means that the structure itself is affected. *O. chemistry*: chemistry relating to the carbon compounds.

organism A living cell or cells.

orgasm The climax of sexual excitement.

oriental sore Delhi boil.

orientation The location of

one's position and attitude in relation to surrounding objects.

orifice An opening.

ornithosis Respiratory disease of birds, transmissable to man.

orogenital syndrome Syndrome of severe riboflavine deficiency characterized by stomatitis, cheilitis, glossitis and an eczematous eruption round the genitalia.

oropharynx Posterior part of the pharynx below the soft palate and above the hyoid bone.

orphan viruses See AD-ENOVIRUS.

orthodontics The correction of irregular placing of the teeth often undertaken for cosmetic reasons.

orthopaedics The medical specialty concerned with all aspects of the bony skeleton including development, disease and damage.

orthopnoea Breathlessness, the patient gaining relief only in an upright position.

orthoptics Term applied to correcting defective vision in a squint by exercises, etc.

orthosis An external device used to ameliorate physical disabilty.

orthostatic Pertaining to or caused by standing upright.

orthotics The study of design of orthoses.

os (1) Bone. (2) Mouth or opening, *e.g. external o.*, of cervix, etc. *O. calcis*: the bone of the heel.

oscheal Pertaining to the scrotum.

oscillation A swinging movement.

Osgood–Schlatter disease Osteochondritis of unknown cause affecting the tibial tuberosity.

Osler's disease Polycythgaemia.

Oster's nodes Small tender inflamed areas in the skin due to small emboli; occurs in subacute bacterial endocarditis.

osmole Unit for measuring ability of dissolved substances to cause osmosis and osmotic pressure; is equal to one gram molecule (or mole) of nondiffusible and non-ionizable dissolved substance.

osmolality Degree of osmotic activity shown by solution or mixture, expressed in osmoles or milliosmoles (mosmols).

osmosis When a solution of a substance is separated from the solvent by a semipermeable membrane impermeable to the solute, solvent passes through the membrane. If aqueous solutions are separated by such a membrane, the water will move in such a way as to equilibrate the strength of the solutions. This process is known as osmosis.

osmotic fragility test Method of determining the fragility of red blood cells.

osmotic pressure Pressure required to prevent the passage of water by osmosis. The osmotic pressure depends on the number of solute molecules in solution.

osseous Like bone, bony.

ossicle Literally, a small bone. Name applied to the tiny bones of the middle ear. *See* EAR.

ossification Hardening into bone.

osteitis Inflammation of bone. *O. fibrosa*: a disease of bone caused by an adenoma of the parathyroid glands. As the result of excessive secretion calcium is absorbed from the bones into the blood. *O. deformans*: *see* PAGET'S DISEASE.

osteoarthritis, osteoathrosis Disorder due to excessive wear and tear to joint surfaces. Affecting chiefly weight-bearing joints, late in life, and resulting in pain, especially at night, deficient movement and deformity.

osteoarthropathy Damage or disease affecting the bones and joints.

osteoarthrotomy Excision of joint and neighbouring bone.

osteoblasts Cells producing the intercellular bone matrix in the same way as fibroblasts may be considered to manu-facture connective tissue matrix.

osteochondritis Combined inflammation of bone and cartilage. *O. deformans juvenilis*: *see* PERTHES' DISEASE. *O. dissecans*: separation of loose bodies from the joint surface.

osteochondroma Benign tumour derived from bone and cartilage.

osteoclasis Intentional fracture of bone for therapeutic reasons.

osteoclastoma A benign or malignant tumour of osteoclasts.

osteoclasts Multinucleated cells which break down the calcified bone matrix. Remodelling of bone by the combined activity of osteoclasts and osteoblasts occurs continuously during bone growth.

osteocyte Osteoblasts which have become incorporated into bone.

osteodystrophy Abnormal growth of bone.

osteogenesis Formation of a bone. *O. imperfecta*: abnormally fragile bones.

osteogenic sarcoma Sarcoma derived from osteoblasts.

osteolytic Bone destroying.

osteoma A bony tumour.

osteomalacia Softening of bones in adults.

osteomyelitis Inflammation of bone including the marrow, the bone around it and the cartilage covering the end of the bone.

osteopath One who practises osteopathy.

osteopathy The study and treatment of disease based on the belief of maladjustments in the joints of the body as a cause of disease. The majority of osteopaths are not medically qualified.

osteopetrosis *See* ALBERS–SCHONBERG'S DISEASE.

osteophony Conduction of sound by bone.

osteophyte A bony outgrowth or nodosity; occurs in osteoarthritis.

osteoplastic Pertaining to the repair of bones.

osteoporosis Fragility of bones due to reabsorption of calcium.

osteosarcoma A malignant tumour growing from a bone.

osteosclerosis Increase in bone density.

osteotome A surgical instrument resembling a chisel and used for cutting through bones. The instrument is bevelled on both sides.

osteotomy Operation of cutting through a bone.

ostium An opening. The orifice of any tubular passage.

otalgia Earache.

otitis externa An inflammation of the outer ear canal. May be allergic (eczematous), due to infection or a combi-

nation of these. In children may be associated with the presence of a foreign body in the ear canal.

otitis interna Inflammation of the inner ear affecting the organs of balance.

otitis media Inflammation of the middle ear.

otolith Calcareous deposits in the internal ear.

otologist Ear specialist.

otology Study of diseases of the ear.

otomycosis *See* OTITIS EXTERNA.

otorhinolaryngology The study of diseases affecting the ear, nose and throat (including the larynx and pharynx).

otosclerosis A chronic, progressive thickening of the structures of the internal ear leading to deafness.

otoscope Auriscope.

ototoxic The term used to describe substances toxic to the inner ear and causing deafness, *e.g.* certain antibiotics including gentamicin.

outlet of pelvis The lower orifice of the bony birth canal bounded by the lower edges of the pubes, ischium, sacrum and coccyx and by the sacrosciatic ligaments.

ova Eggs usually of worms and other gut parasites.

ovarian cyst Cyst of the ovary; may be developmental or associated with ovarian tumour.

ovarian follicle *See*
FOLLICLE.

ovarian tumour A growth in
the ovary which can be benign
or malignant.

ovariectomy Oophorectomy.
Surgical removal of ovary.

ovaries (sing. **ovary**) Two
small oval bodies situated on
either side of the uterus; the
female organs in which the
ova are formed. They are also
endocrine glands.

ovariotomy The operation of
cutting into an ovary.

ovaritis *See* OOPHORITIS.

overcompensation (1)
Homeostasis is achieved by
the body compensating for
changes brought about in
various circumstances. When
the compensatory mechanism
too far outweighs the change
which it opposes, overcompensation is said to have
taken place. (2) In psychiatry
applies to exaggerated compensatory behaviour, *e.g.* extreme aggressiveness in
response to a feeling of in-
adequacy.

overdosage Excessive concentration of a drug in the
blood. This may be an ac-
cumulation from repeated
doses or from too high a dose
(sometimes deliberate). May
also be caused by the body's
inability to excrete or break
down the drug.

overextension Extension beyond the normal, *e.g.* of a

joint or muscle.

oviduct The fallopian tube
between the ovary and the
womb, conveying the ova. *See*
OVARIES.

ovulation The development
and discharge of ova from the
ovary.

ovum The egg cell produced
in the female ovary.

oxaluria Presence of oxalic
acid crystals in the urine.

oxidation Process involving
the loss of electrons from the
oxidized substance.

oximeter An instrument for
transcutaneous measurement
of blood or tissue oxygen
levels.

oxycephaly Abnormal
development of the skull with
resultant egg-shaped ap-
pearance.

oxygen Gas forming 20 per
cent of the atmosphere.
Essential for human life. *O.
administration*: by (1) nasal
catheters at approximately 2
litres per minute. This will
raise the alveolar oxygen to
approximately 30 per cent.
(2) *O. tent*: rate of flow depends upon amount of disturbance for nursing care. With
average care, the alveolar
oxygen can be kept at 45 per
cent. (3) *O. masks*: there are
various types available: some
allow different concentrations
of oxygen dependent upon
the oxygen flow to the mask;
some allow humidification to

be provided. Oxygen may be used in high concentrations following open heart surgery. *O. debt*: if the metabolic requirement for oxygen exceeds the supply, the metabolic processes are carried out under partially anaerobic conditions until at a later time the 'oxygen debt' is repaid.

oxygenation To saturate with oxygen.

oxyhaemoglobin Oxygenated haemoglobin.

oxyntic Term applied to cells secreting hydrochloric acid in the stomach.

oxytocic Having an effect like oxytocin in stimulating uterine contractions.

oxytocin Polypeptide hormone secreted by the posterior lobe of the pituitary which produces a strong contraction of uterine muscle.

oxyuriasis Infection with Oxyuris vermicularis.

Oxyuris vermicularis Threadworm found in the rectum and large intestine, especially in children.

ozaena Atrophic rhinitis.

ozone O_3. An oxidizing agent sometimes used as a disinfectant.

P

Paccini's corpuscles Specialized sensory receptors which register pressure and to some extent vibration. They are situated in the deeper connective tissues of the skin and consist of nerve-endings surrounded by concentric lamellae of fibrous tissue.

pacemaker *See* ATRIOVENTRICULAR BUNDLE. *Artificial p.*: electrical appliance which can be fitted surgically to act as the initiator of the cardiac impulse if the sinoatrial node does not function normally.

pachy- A prefix denoting thickness.

pachydermia Thickening of the skin.

pachymeningitis Inflammation of the dura mater, with thickening of the membrane.

pack Moistened material applied to the patient.

paediatrician Specialist in diseases of children.

paediatrics Study of diseases of children.

Paget's disease (1) Of bone, Osteitis deformans, is a disorder of unknown cause which usually affects a number of bones to greater or lesser extent. Clinically the features are pain, tendency to pathological fractures and hyperdynamic circulation. (2) Of nipple. Eczema of the nipple associated with underlying duct carcinoma of the breast.

pain Specific form of unpleasant, sensory experience, usually aroused by incipient or actual damage to cells or tissue.

palate   The roof of the mouth.

palatoplegia   Paralysis of soft palate.

palliative   A medicine which relieves but does not cure.

pallidectomy   Operation used in Parkinson's disease to decrease the activity part of the lentiform nucleus in the base of the brain.

pallidotomy   Operation performed to relieve tremor in Parkinson's disease. Fibres from the cerebral cortex are severed.

pallor   Paleness.

palm   The hollow or flexor surface of the hand.

palmar   Pertaining to the palm of the hand.

palpation   Examination by the hand.

palpebra   The eyelid.

palpitation   Rapid beating of the heart, producing consciousness of the heart's action.

palsy   Paralysis. *See* ERB'S PARALYSIS.

pan   A prefix signifying all, total.

panacea   A medicine which is claimed or advertised to cure all diseases.

panarthritis   Generalized inflammation of joints.

pancarditis   Generalized inflammation of the heart.

Pancoast's tumour   Tumour occurring at the apex of the lung, involving the lower part of the brachial plexus and producing Horner's syndrome and pain, weakness and wasting down the arm.

pancreas   Sweetbread. A gland situated in the mesentery in relation to the duodenum and crossing the midline of the body. It secretes an alkaline mixture of digestive enzymes through the pancreatic duct into the duodenum when stimulated by the hormone secretin. Contains groups of cells which secrete insulin into the blood. *See* ISLETS OF LANGERHANS.

pancreatectomy   Excision of the pancreas.

pancreatin   Extract of pancreatic glands used in the treatment of mucoviscidosis.

pancreatitis   Inflammation of the pancreas.

pancreozymin   Hormone of duodenal origin which stimulates secretion of pancreatic enzymes.

pandemic   A widely spread epidemic.

panhypopituitarism Simmond's disease. Deficient secretion of all the anterior pituitary hormones with secondary reduction in production of hormones by the thyroid and adrenal cortex.

pannus   Vascularization of the cornea; in joints the replacement of cartilage by granulation tissue.

panophthalmia or **panophthalmitis** Generalized inflammation of the eyeball.

panotitis Inflammation of the middle and internal ear.

Papanicolaou stain Stain frequently employed for the examination of vaginal and cervical smears. *See* CERVICAL SMEAR.

papilla (pl. **papillae**) (1) A small nipple-shaped eminence. (2) The optic disc. *Circumvallate p.*: these are found at the root of the tongue. *Filiform p.*: the common *p.* of the tongue and found at its tip. *Fungiform p.*: the broad *p.* of the tongue.

papillitis Inflammation of the optic disc.

papilloedema Oedema of the optic nerve.

papilloma Benign neoplasm of epithelial cells.

papovaviruses Group of viruses associated with induction of papillomata and polyoma in rabbits and in warts in man.

papule A small solid pimple.

para-aminobenzoic acid (PABA) A bacterial growth factor antagonized by the sulphanilamides.

para-aortic Near the aorta.

paracentesis Withdrawing fluid from body cavity. *See* ASPIRATION.

paracusis Disordered hearing.

paraesthesia Disordered sensation, such as tingling and pins and needles.

parainfluenza Used of viruses suspected of causing common cold. They included Sendai, haemadsorption 1 and 2, and croup-associated viruses.

paralysis Loss of nervous function, usually motor, but may be applied to *sensory p.* In *motor p.* the loss of nerve function results in the inability to stimulate contraction of muscles. This does not necessarily mean that the muscles become flaccid since this follows only the *p.* of lower motor neurones. *Upper motor neurone p.* causes *spastic p. P. agitans*: *see* PARKINSON'S DISEASE.

paralytic ileus Intestinal obstruction due to paralysis of muscles of peristalsis.

paramedian Close to the middle.

paramedical Associated with and supporters to the medical services, *e.g.* physiotherapy, radiotherapy and occupational therapy.

paramenstruum The days before and after the menstrual period.

parametritis Inflammation of the parametrium. Also called pelvic cellulitis.

parametrium The connective tissue around the uterus, chiefly found round large vessels and between the layers of the broad ligament.

paramnesia False memory; usually memory of events

which did not occur in the connection related.

paranasal Near the nose. *P. cavities*: the air sinuses.

paranoia Feelings of persecution; may be due to reality or in some psychiatric illness be delusional.

paranoid Relating to paranoia. *P. schizophrenia*: schizophrenia marked by delusions and hallucinations.

paraphimosis Retraction of the prepuce behind the glans penis with inability to restore it to the natural position.

paraplegia Paralysis of both lower limbs.

pararectal Around the rectum.

parasite Any living thing which lives on or in another organism.

parasiticide Substance lethal to parasites.

parasympathetic system Part of the autonomic nervous system.

parathormone The hormone of the parathyroid glands. Shortened form of parathyroid hormone.

parathyroid Small endocrine glands which control calcium and phosphate metabolism. They are usually four in number and they are situated in the vicinity of the thyroid gland.

paratyphoid An infectious disease resembling typhoid fever and caused by an organism not identical with but closely allied to the bacillus of typhoid. *See* ENTERIC.

paravertebral To one side of the spinal column.

parenchyma The functional part of an organ.

parenteral treatment Therapy by drugs given by routes other than the alimentary tract.

paresis A partial paralysis.

parietal The two bones which form the crown and sides of the cranium. *See* FONTANELLE.

parietes The walls of any cavity of the body.

parity The number of children a woman has borne.

Parkinson's disease Degeneration affecting the basal ganglia of the brain especially affecting the substantia nigra and the surrounding tissues. It is characterized by a combination in varying degrees of muscular rigidity and a tremor which is temporarily abolished by the voluntary movement of the part affected.

paronychia Whitlow; inflammation and abscess at the end of a finger near the nail.

parosmia Perverted sense of smell.

parotid Near the ear; applied to a salivary gland under the ear.

parotitis Inflammation of the parotid gland. (1) Mumps.

(2) Spread of infection from a septic mouth.

paroxysm A sudden temporary attack.

paroxysmal nocturnal dyspnoea Attacks of breathlessness occurring at night due to accumulation of fluid in the lungs resulting from left ventricular failure.

paroxysmal tachycardia This is due to the regular and rapid discharge of impulses from an ectopic focus in the atrial walls of the heart. The focus thus replaces the sinoatrial node as the cardiac pacemaker and drives the heart at a rate of about 180 beats per minute (normal about 80). Attacks may last anything from a minute to several days.

parrot disease Psittacosis.

parthenogenesis Development of an ovum into a new individual without being fertilized.

parturition The act of giving birth to a child.

passive Submissive. Not active or spontaneous. *P. immunity*: *see* IMMUNITY. *P. movements*: these are performed on a patient's joints by a physiotherapist to increase the mobility, prevent contractures and to improve the circulation.

Pasteurella Plague bacteria.

pasteurization Method of sterilization of fluids intro-duced by Pasteur which involves heating for 30 minutes at 70°C

patch test Local application of possible antigen to the skin to test for sensitivity.

patella The kneecap. A sesamoid bone in front of the knee joint.

patella bursae The bursae around the patella. Inflammation of the prepatellar bursa used to be called housemaid's knee, as it occurs after much kneeling.

patellectomy Operation to excise the patella.

patent Open. *P. ductus arteriosus*: failure of the ductus arteriosus to close at birth. *P. foramen ovale*: failure of closure of the foramen ovale.

pathogenesis The origin and progress of disease.

pathogenic Capable of causing disease.

pathognomonic Characteristic of, or peculiar to, a particular disease.

pathological Relating to pathology. Morbid, abnormal. *P. fracture*: *see* FRACTURE.

pathology The study of disease, particularly regarding the changes in the tissues resulting from disease.

pathophobia Neurotic fear of disease.

patient compliance The act of following instructions with regard to taking prescribed drugs.

patulous Open wide.

Paul's tube Transparent drainage tube.

Paul–Bunnell test A serological test for glandular fever (infectious mononucleosis).

PCOD *Abbr.* polycystic ovarian disease.

peau d'orange Orange-skin appearance of skin overlying carcinoma of the breast which is caused by obstruction to superficial lymphatics.

pectin A polysaccharide found in fruit.

pectoral Relating to the chest. *P. muscles* are on the anterior surface of chest.

pectus The thorax, chest.

pediatrics *See* PAEDIATRICS.

pedicle The stalk of a collection of tissue which contains the supply of vessels and nerves.

pediculosis Infestation with lice.

pediculus The louse, a parasite infesting the hair and skin. *P. capitis* infests the head; *p. corporis*, the body and clothing; *p. pubis*, the pubic hair. These three varieties are different in shape and size.

pendunculated Possessing a pedicle.

Pel–Ebstein fever A regularly remitting fever which sometimes occurs in Hodgkin's disease.

pellagra Syndrome caused by deficiency of nicotinic acid

characterized by dementia, diarrhoea and dermatitis.

pellet Small pill.

pellicle A thin skin or membrane.

pelvic Relating to the pelvis. *P. inflammatory disease*: *see* PYOSALPINX. *P. extenteration*: operative removal of organ from pelvis.

pelvimetry Measurement of internal diameters of pelvis.

pelvis The bony cavity composed of the hips and the lower bones of the spine and holding the bowels, bladder and organs of generation. *Renal p.*: the cavity of the kidney draining into the ureter.

pemphigus Disease characterized by the formation of large blisters on the skin and mucous membranes. *P. neonatorum* is a misnomer, it is an acute staphylococcal impetigo occurring in newborn infants.

pendulous Hanging down.

penetration Entering into.

penicillin First of the antibiotic agents to be used in therapy. It is a substance synthesized by the *Penicillium* mould.

penis The male sexual organ containing the urethra.

pentagastrin test meal Test of responsiveness of gastric mucosa to stimulation by the hormone pentagastrin.

pentose Monosaccharide sugar with five carbon atoms, *e.g.* ribose, deoxyribose.

pentosuria   Renal defect in which there is failure to reabsorb pentoses from the urine with the result that the urine contains sugar.

pepsin   An enzyme which breaks down proteins in acid solution to form peptides (a peptidase). It is secreted in the stomach with hydrochloric acid.

peptic   Pertaining to digestion. *P. ulcer*: a gastric, duodenal or gastrojejunal ulcer. *P. ulcer diet*: diet used in the treatment of peptic ulcer. Formerly a bland one but now more varied.

peptide   Compound of two or more amino acids. The peptide link, which is split by peptidases (*see* PEPSIN), is formed between the amino group of one amino acid and the carboxyl group of the next. When many are joined together they form so-called polypeptides, which join together to form protein.

perception   An awareness. Receiving impressions through the senses.

percussion   Striking upon the body, the sound heard being helpful in diagnosis. The note emitted is resonant or dull according to the condition of the organ underneath.

perforation   A hole in an organ caused by disease or injury. The act of perforating.

peri-   Prefix signifying around, near, about (Greek).

perianal   Around the anus.

periarteritis   Inflammation of the outer coat of an artery. *P. nodosa*: a disease of unknown cause which is characterized by the production of multiple nodules in the connective tissues surrounding the smaller arteries. The symptoms and signs associated with this disorder depend on the distribution of the lesions.

periarthritis   Inflammation of the tissues round a joint.

pericardial   Pertaining to the pericardium. *P. adhesions*: fibrosis of the pericardium which may follow pericarditis in which the two layers of the pericardium become stuck together.

pericardiotomy   An opening made into the pericardium.

pericarditis   Inflammation of the pericardium.

pericardium   Membranes which surround the heart leaving a potential space and thus enabling changes in shape and volume of the heart to take place.

perichondritis   Inflammation of perichondrium.

perichondrium   The membranous covering of a cartilage.

pericolitis   Inflammation round the colon.

pericranium   The membrane covering the bones of the skull.

perilymph Clear fluid in the osseous labyrinth of the ear.

perimeter The outside or circumference, often applied to the width of visual fields.

perimetritis Inflammation of the peritoneum covering the uterus.

perinatal The period of time before, during and after childbirth.

perineal Pertaining to the perineum. *P. body*: wedge-shaped muscular body which forms the focus of the pelvic floor.

perineorrhaphy Operative repair of perineal tear.

perinephric Round about the kidney. *P. abscess*: a collection of pus in the tissues round the kidney.

perineum The region of the pelvic floor anterior to the anus.

perineurium A sheath investing a bundle of nerve fibres.

periodic syndrome Cyclical vomiting attacks of unknown cause which may occur in children. Often associated with headache, fever and abdominal pain.

periodontal disease Inflammation of the gums and roots of the teeth. Leads to gum retraction, bone erosion and loosening of attachment of the teeth.

periosteal Pertaining to periosteum. *P. sarcoma*: sarcoma growing from periosteum.

periosteum The membrane covering a bone.

periostitis Inflammation of the periosteum.

peripheral Relating to the circumference or outer surface. *P. neuritis*: inflammation of the peripheral nerves.

periproctitis Inflammation of tissue around rectum or anus.

perisalpingitis Inflammation of peritoneum covering the uterine tube.

perisplenitis Inflammation of the connective tissues surrounding the spleen.

peristalsis The contractions and movements of the alimentary tract forcing on the contents.

peritomy Incision of the conjunctiva near the margin of the cornea for the cure of pannus.

peritoneal Pertaining to peritoneum. *P. dialysis*: see DIALYSIS.

peritoneum The membrane or sac which surrounds the intestines and most other abdominal viscera, and which also lines the abdominal cavity. It secretes a serous fluid which reduces friction.

peritonitis Inflammation of the peritoneum.

peritonsillar abscess Abscess in the pharynx near the tonsils. *See also* QUINSY.

periurethral Around the urethra.

permanent teeth Teeth of the second dentition.

permeable Capable of being penetrated.

pernicious Tending to a fatal issue. *P. anaemia*: anaemia resulting from cyanocobalamin (vitamin B_{12}) deficiency. *P. vomiting*: see VOMITING OF PREGNANCY.

pernio, perniosis Chilblains.

peroneal Pertaining to the fibula. *P. muscular atrophy*: a familiar condition of muscular wasting.

peroral Through the mouth.

perseveration A recurring idea, feeling or way of action from which the patient finds it difficult to escape.

persistent ductus arteriosus *See* PATENT DUCTUS ARTERIOSUS.

personality Individual characteristics of behaviour.

perspiration Sweat.

Perthe's disease Pseudocoxalgia. Osteochondritis affecting the head of the femur. Usually occurs in boys before their teens.

pertussis Whooping cough. A disease of childhood characterized by a cough with a typical 'whoop' on inspiration. Caused by haemophilus pertussis.

pes Foot. *P. cavus*: exaggerated longitudinal arch of foot. *P. planus*: flat foot; loss of longitudinal arch.

pessary (1) A device placed in vagina to remedy malpositions of uterus or vaginal prolapse. (2) A medicated vaginal suppository. (3) A contraceptive device worn in the vagina.

pestilence Epidemic disease.

petechiae Small red spots on the skin formed by effusion of blood.

petit mal *See* EPILEPSY.

Petri dish A small flat glass dish used in bacteriological laboratories.

pétrissage A type of kneading massage.

petrous Stony; a term given to a hard part of the temporal bone.

Peyer's patches Collections of lymphoid tissue associated with the small intestine.

pH Expression of the hydrogen ion concentration of a solution. $pH = -$ logarithm (H^+) where (H^+) represents the hydrogen ion concentration. The scale ranges from 0 to 14. Between 0 and 7 is *acid* and between 7 and 14 is *alkaline*; 7 is neutral.

phaeochromocyte One of two cell types present in the adrenal medulla and in the sympathetic ganglion.

phaeochromocytoma Adrenal medullary tumour which secretes adrenaline and noradrenaline, causing episodes of raised blood pressure.

phage typing Method of

identifying bacteria which depends on their sensitivity to lysis by bacteriophage viruses.

phagocytes The polymorphonuclear white cells of the blood, so called from their property of being able to ingest and destroy microorganisms which may be circulating in the blood or attacking the tissues.

phagocytosis Process of ingestion of material by cells such as phagocytes and macrophages. Most cells are considered to be capable of phagocytosis at least to some extent. In an attempt to distinguish this type of ingestion from the defensive, *e.g.* antibacterial, ingestion of the phagocytes and macrophages, the term pinocytosis has been introduced. The mechanism is similar but the average size of ingested particles is smaller.

phalanges The small bones of the fingers and toes.

phallus The penis.

phantom limb Sensation often experienced by patient, after an amputation, that the limb is still there.

pharmaceutical Pertaining to drugs.

pharmacogenetics Study of genetically determined variations in response to, and metabolism of, drugs.

pharmacokinetics The study of drug transport, metabolism

and excretion.

pharmacology The study of drug action.

pharmacy The science of preparing and mixing medicines or drugs. The place where drugs are dispensed.

pharyngeal Pertaining to the pharynx. *P. pouch*: an outpouching of the mucosal lining of the pharynx through a weakness in the muscular wall. Associated with regurgitation of food, difficulty in swallowing and the presence of a lump in the neck.

pharyngectomy Excision of part of the pharynx.

pharyngismus Spasm of the pharynx.

pharyngitis Inflammation of the pharynx.

pharyngolaryngectomy Surgical removal of part of the larynx and the pharynx usually combined with reanastomosis of the pharyngeal stump with the oesophagus.

pharyngoplasty An operation to reconstruct the pharynx.

pharyngotomy Surgical removal of the pharynx.

pharyngotympanic tube Eustachian tube.

pharynx The musculomembranous sac at the back of the mouth leading to the oesophagus and to the larynx.

phase-contrast microscopy Microscopic examination of living unstained biological material using two light-beams.

phenol Substance consisting of benzene nucleus to which hydroxyl groups are attached. In pharmacology applies especially to carbolic acid, C_6H_5OH, used in liquid form as dental analgesic, in aqueous form as antiseptic, in other solutions as a sclerosing agent for haemorrhoids, intrathecal injection for intractable pain. It is poisonous, and sufficient can be absorbed through intact skin to be fatal.

phenotype Property shown by an individual, due to the expression of characters of his genotype.

phenylalanine Essential amino acid.

phenylketonuria (PKU) Genetically determined error of metabolism in which there is an inability of the liver to convert phenylalanine to tyrosine. Instead phenylalanine is broken down to phenylpyruvic acid which is excreted in the urine. There is associated mental deficiency. Screening is done for this and other inborn errors of metabolism by the Guthrie test soon after birth.

phimosis Contraction of the orifice of the prepuce; usually treated by the operation of circumcision.

phlebectomy Excision of a vein.

phlebitis Inflammation of the veins.

phlebolith Calcified venous thrombus.

phlebothrombosis Thrombosis in veins, particularly the veins of the legs, due to prolonged haemostasis.

phlebotomist Person employed to take blood samples.

Phlebotomus Genus of disease-carrying flies.

phlebotomy Bleeding a patient by opening a vein. Venesection.

phlegm Thick mucoid expectoration.

phlegmasia Inflammation. *P. alba dolens*: white leg; a form of phlebitis occurring sometimes after labour. The leg becomes swollen, white and tense, and is very painful.

phlyctenule Red pimples on surface of eye. *Phlyctenular conjunctivitis*, a form of disease when phlyctenules appear on the conjunctiva, each becoming the centre of a small inflamed patch. They then rupture, forming a small ulcer which readily heals. *Phlyctenular keratitis*, when the cornea is similarly affected.

phobia Fear of sufficient intensity to affect the life of the patient, *e.g.* cancerophobia, claustrophobia.

phonation The utterance of vocal sounds.

phonetic Relating to the voice.

phonocardiogram Instrument recording heart sounds.

phonocardiograph Instrument recording heart sounds.

phosphate Salt of phosphoric acid.

phosphaturia Excess of phosphates in the urine.

phospholipid A lipid containing phosphates, *e.g.* lecithin. Phospholipids are particularly useful in living systems for forming membranes.

phosphonecrosis Necrosis of the jaw, caused by inhaling phosphorus; occurs in certain trades, such as matchmaking, but is rare.

photobiology The study of the effect of light on life.

photochemistry The study of the effect of light on chemical reactions.

photophobia Intolerance of light.

photosensitization Tendency of tissues to react abnormally to light, usually as the result of the presence in tissues of certain chemicals which magnify the damaging effect of the incident radiation.

phrenic Relating to the diaphragm.

phrenicotomy Division of the phrenic nerve.

phrenoplegia Paralysis of the diaphragm.

physic (1) The art of medicine. (2) Any medicinal preparation.

physical abuse *See* BATTERED BABY SYNDROME.

physician Qualified medical practitioner.

physicist An expert in the science of physics.

physics The science which deals with the forces and forms of nature.

physiological saline A solution, 0.9 per cent of sodium chloride in water.

physiology The study of processes occurring in living systems.

physiotherapy Therapy by physical means, *i.e.* heat, light, electricity, massage, etc.

physique The form and constitution of the body.

phytic acid Substance which prevents absorption of calcium from the gut. Found in wholemeal flour but partially destroyed if yeast is used in preparation of bread.

pia mater The fine membrane surrounding the brain and spinal cord.

pica A desire to eat substances unsuitable for food. Occurs most commonly in small children who are emotionally upset.

Pick's disease (1) Disorder affecting serous membranes resulting in effusions in the peritoneum, pericardium and pleura. The cause is unknown. (2) Presenile dementia due to cerebral atrophy.

picornavirus A group of

RNA virus including polio, coxsackie and rhinovirus.

PID *Abbr*. (1) Pelvic inflammatory disease. (2) Prolapsed intervertebral disc.

pigeon chest A narrow chest with prominent sternum.

pigment Coloured material, *e.g.* haemoglobin, melanin.

piles Enlarged veins about the anus; haemorrhoids.

pilonidal Containing hair as in some cysts. *P. sinus*: sinus leading from encysted hairs usually in the sacral region.

pilosis Abnormal growth of hair.

pimple A papule.

pineal body The so-called 'third eye'. Develops from outgrowths of the forebrain, part of which forms an eye-like structure in the lamprey. In man it is a gland-like structure whose function is entirely unknown.

pinguecula Small yellow patch of connective tissue on conjunctiva occurring in old age.

pink eye Infectious conjunctivitis.

pinna The outspread part of the ear.

pinocytosis Particles are surrounded by cell membrane and are included in the cytoplasm. *See* PHAGOCYTOSIS.

pint Twenty fluid ounces (568ml).

pipette A small graduated glass tube for taking up liquids.

pisiform Pea-shaped; applied to a bone of the wrist.

pitting (1) Pits are formed in the skin on pressure, as in oedema. (2) Pits occurring in the nails as in psoriasis.

pituitary gland Endocrine gland in the base of the skull. There are two lobes separated by a cleft. The anterior lobe secretes thyrotrophic hormone (TSH), corticotrophic hormone (ACTH), gonadotrophic hormones (FSH, LH), growth hormone (GH) and prolactin. The posterior lobe secretes antidiuretic hormone (ADH) and oxytocin.

pityriasis rosea Skin disease characterized by scaly, erythematous macular eruption. Thought to be caused by a virus related to the measles virus.

placebo Medicine made of inert material and flavouring which may be used as a control during trials on an active drug or as a token to satisfy a patient's need for help.

placenta The afterbirth; a circular flesh-like tissue through which the mother's blood nourishes the fetus; it is expelled from the womb after the birth of the child. *P. praevia*: the placenta attached partially or totally to the lower uterine segment thus impairing the normal delivery of a baby by obstruction and by inevitable haemorrhage.

placental barrier Layer of placental epithelium separating maternal from fetal blood.

plagiocephaly Type of craniostenosis in which there is unilateral involvement of a coronal or lambdoid suture thus producing an asymmetrical head.

plague An acute epidemic infectious disease caused by *Pasteurella pestis* derived from infected rats and transmitted to man by fleas.

plantar Relating to the sole of the foot. *P. response*: reflex movement of toes when the sole of the foot is stroked.

plasma The liquid in which the cells of the blood are suspended. *P. proteins*: these are fibrinogen, albumin and globulins.

plasmapheresis Therapeutic process where the patient's blood is removed, separated and the plasma substituted from another source. New plasma/red cell mixture is then returned to patient.

Plasmodium *See* MALARIA.

plaster (1) Adhesive tape used to secure dressings, etc. (2) Plaster of Paris. Material used to immobilize part of the body.

plastic surgery Restoration of tissue to its normal shape and appearance by operative means.

platelets Blood cells concerned with the clotting of blood.

Platyhelminthes Flat worms.

play therapist A person who guides constructive play activity in hospitalized children.

pleomorphism Having several different forms.

plethora Fullness; an excess of blood.

plethysmograph A device to record changes in volume of an organ of the body under various conditions.

pleura A thin membrane which covers each lung and lines the inner surface of the thoracic cavity.

pleural rub A grating feeling and sound produced by friction between the layers of the pleura.

pleurisy Inflammation of the pleura.

pleurodynia Pain in the side, usually intercostal myalgia. *See* BORNHOLM DISEASE.

plexus A network of vessels or nerves.

plica A fold.

plicate Folded.

plication An operation which involves folding of a structure.

plombage Filling a cavity with an inert substance.

plumbism Lead poisoning.

Plummer–Vinson syndrome Also known as Kelly–Patterson syndrome. Glossitis and dysphagia due to iron deficiency.

PMB *Abbr*. postmenopausal bleeding.

PMS *Abbr*. premenstrual syndrome.

pneumatocele A swelling containing air or gas.

pneumaturia Diagnostic feature of vesicointestinal fistula. Air is passed per urethra.

pneumococcal Pertaining to the pneumococcus.

pneumococcus A microbe which causes pneumonia. *See* BACTERIA.

pneumoconiosis Fibrosis of the lungs caused by working in an atmosphere contaminated with irritant dusts. *See* SILICOSIS, BAGASSOSIS and BYSSINOSIS.

pneumocystis carinii An organism causing pneumonia, usually in debilitated or immunosuppressed individuals. *See* ARC.

pneumomycosis Fungus disease of the lungs.

pneumonectomy Surgical removal of a lung.

pneumonia An infective disease characterized by inflammation of the lungs. In double pneumonia, both lungs are diseased. *Hypostatic p*. is caused by lack of movement in a debilitated patient. May occur after operation or in the aged. *Lobar p*., affecting one or more lobes of the lung. *Lobular p*., *see* BRONCHOPNEUMONIA.

pneumonitis Inflammation of the lung.

pneumoperitoneum Air in the peritoneal cavity.

pneumothorax Air in the pleural space. *Spontaneous p*. due to rupture of one of the air passages which may lead to a rise in pressure inside the chest (*tension p*.) and difficulty in breathing. *Artificial p*.: air is introduced into the chest through a needle or incision.

pock A pustule or the scar left by it.

podalic version A turning round of the fetus in utero so that the breech presents in delivery.

poikilocytosis Variation in the form of the red blood cells.

poison A substance deleterious to the body if absorbed in toxic concentrations. The term is usually reserved for substances which are toxic in low concentrations, *e.g.* cyanide.

polar body Two small cells formed after mitotic division of the primary oocyte.

polio Prefix denoting grey. Journalese abbreviation of poliomyelitis.

polioencephalitis Inflammation of the grey matter of the brain.

poliomyelitis Acute virus-mediated infection causing degeneration of the anterior horn cells of the spinal cord and consequent paralysis of the appropriate muscles.

Politzer's bag An india rubber bag with long tube and nozzle. Used for inflating the middle ear through the nose and eustachian tube.

pollution The act of rendering impure.

poly- A prefix denoting much or many (Greek).

polyarteritis nodosa *See* PERI-ARTERITIS NODOSA.

polyarthralgia Pain in many joints.

polyarthritis Inflammation of many joints.

Polya's operation Operation for duodenal ulcer in which the stump of the stomach is anastomosed to the side of the jejunum.

polychondritis Inflammation of cartilaginous tissues at several sites in the body.

polychromasia Term given to staining characteristics of young red blood cells.

polycystic Composed of many cysts. *P. ovarian disease. See* STEIN–LEVENTHAL SYNDROME.

polycythaemia (1) *Primary p.*: an increased number of red cells. (2) *Secondary p.*: increase in the number of red blood cells in the blood due to stimulation of the bone marrow, *e.g.* by anoxia at high altitudes or due to respiratory disease.

polydactyly The presence of supernumerary fingers or toes.

polydipsia Abnormal thirst.

polyglandular Pertaining to several glands.

polyhedral Having many surfaces.

polymazia Accessory breasts.

polymenorrhoea Frequent menstruation.

polymorphonuclear Having nuclei of various shapes. Name given to the most numerous form of white blood cell, of which there are normally about 70 per cent of total. These are the chief phagocytes, and therefore they are increased in number in the presence of most bacteria.

polymyositis Weakness and wasting of muscles due to inflammation of unknown aetiology.

polyneuritis Multiple neuritis. *Syn.* peripheral neuritis.

polyopia Seeing multiple images of the same object.

polypeptide *See* PEPTIDE.

polypoid Like a polypus.

polyposis intestini Familial adenomatous polyposis of the colon. An inherited disorder. Distinguish from *Peutz-Jegher's intestinal polyposis* in which there is characteristic circumoral pigmentation.

polyp A tumour, usually benign, raised above or pedunculated from the surface of the body or of a hollow organ, *e.g.* ear, nose, uterus or rectum.

polypus A small tumour occurring in the ear, nose, uterus or rectum.

polysaccharides A group of carbohydrates which contain more than two molecules of simple carbohydrates combined with each other, *e.g.* starch, glycogen.

polyuria Excessive production of urine.

polyvalent As applied to sera, meaning those which are active against many different strains of the same microorganisms.

pompholyx A vesicular eruption occurring on the palms and soles. Probably a form of eczema.

pons Part of the brain stem between the medulla oblongata and the thalamus.

pontine Pertaining to the pons.

POP *Abbr.* (1) Persistent occipitoposterior presentation of the fetus. (2) Plaster of Paris. (3) Progestogen-only pill.

popliteal Pertaining to the popliteal space, the area behind the knee.

pore A small space.

porphyria General term used to describe a variety of syndromes due to an excess of porphyrins in the blood and tissues.

porphyrins Pyrrole derivatives produced in the metabolism of haemoglobin.

portal hypertension Hypertension in the hepatic portal system usually resulting from cirrhosis of the liver.

portal vein A vein carrying blood between capillary networks, usually *hepatic p.v.*

position Attitude or posture.

positive pressure ventilation (PPV) Artificial respiration by blowing air into the lungs.

posological Pertaining to dosage.

posset In infant feeding, to regurgitate a feed.

possum *Abbr.* Patient-operated Selector Mechanism. An electronic device which can be operated with minimal muscle effort and can be used by a severely disabled patient for opening and shutting doors, controlling lighting, typing, etc.

post Behind or after.

postclimacteric After the menopause.

postdiphtheritic paralysis Paralysis as a result of the diphtheria toxin acting on the nervous system. These may be palatal, ocular, cardiac, pharyngeal, laryngeal and respiratory paralysis.

postencephalitis Condition which may remain after encephalitis.

posterior chamber of eye Small space lying behind the

iris and containing aqueous humour.

posterior nerve root Dorsal nerve root. *See* NERVE ROOT.

postganglionic Behind or after a ganglion.

postgastrectomy syndrome A number of syndromes may follow gastrectomy including dumping syndrome hypoglycaemic attacks and malnutrition.

posthumous After death.

postmaturity Birth of an infant considered to have matured beyond the normal fetal stage. More than one of the following criteria should be satisfied: pregnancy exceeding 290 days; fetal length exceeding 54 cm; fetal weight exceeding 4 kg. The skin is often dry and scaling, the nails may have grown beyond the ends of the fingers and toes and the liquor may be stained with meconium.

postmortem After death. Usually *p. examination. See* NECROPSY.

postnatal Following birth.

postoperative After operation.

postpartum After labour. *P. haemorrhage* is excessive vaginal bleeding occurring either immediately after the birth of the baby (primary), or within a few days (secondary).

postprandial After meals.

postural Pertaining to post-

ure, *e.g. p. drainage*, position adopted to facilitate expectoration of material in lung diseases.

postvaccinial Occurring after vaccination.

potassium deficiency Blood electrolyte disturbance usually resulting from diarrhoea and vomiting. Causes muscle weakness and eventually cardiac failure.

potential (1) Capability; *e.g. p. space*, a space which is capable to forming. (2) *Electrical p.*, the tendency of electrons to flow in a specified direction, measured in volts.

Pott's disease Tuberculosis of the spine.

Pott's fracture Fracture dislocation of the ankle in which the fibula and the medial malleolus are fractured with lateral displacement of the foot.

pouch of Douglas *See* DOUGLAS'S POUCH.

pouch, pharyngeal *See* PHARYNGEAL POUCH.

pouch, postprostatic Diverticulum of the bladder which sometimes develops behind a hypertrophied middle lobe of the prostate.

pouch, urethral Diverticulum of the male urethra.

poultices Hot moist material applied as an external counterirritant.

Poupart's ligament The ligament of the groin, stretching between the anterior superior spine of the ilium and the os pubis.

poxviruses Group of large DNA viruses associated with vaccinia, variola and allied animal diseases.

PR *Abbr.* per rectum. Examination made with one finger in the rectum, by which information can be obtained of the condition of the rectum and adjacent structures.

preauricular sinus Opening at the root of the tragus of the ear due to imperfect fusion of the processes which form the ear.

precancerous A state before a cancer has arisen but which may become cancerous.

precipitate labour Labour which is concluded in a time very much shorter than the average.

precipitin An antibody forming an insoluble complex with an antigen. Basis of much serological testing.

precocious puberty Two groups are recognized. (1) Those in which true sexual maturity is reached at an early age and in which ovulation or spermatogenesis commences. (2) Those in which there are advanced secondary sex changes but no spermatogenesis or ovulation occur.

precordium The area of the chest over the heart.

precursor Forerunner.

predigestion Breakdown of foodstuffs before ingestion.

predisposed Susceptible.

pre-eclampsia State before eclampsia develops and when it can still be prevented. There is proteinuria, raised blood pressure and swelling of the ankles.

prefrontal Lying in the anterior part of the frontal lobe of the brain. *P. leucotomy*: SEE LEUCOTOMY.

pregnancy The state of being with child. Usual period 280 days. *See also* ECTOPIC GESTATION.

premature labour Labour at or before 36 weeks of gestation and resulting in a low birth weight baby, *i.e.* one weighing 2.5 kg or less.

premedication Drug given as a narcotic before a general anaesthetic.

premenstrual Before menstruation. *P. syndrome*: syndrome consisting of tension, anxiety, aches, depression and often accident-proneness which occurs for a few days before menstrual period in some women. It is thought to be hormonal in origin.

premolar The two bicuspid teeth in each jaw which lie between the canine and the molars. *See* TEETH.

premonitory Giving warning beforehand.

prenatal Prior to birth, during the period of pregnancy.

prepuce Loose skin covering the glans penis: foreskin.

presbyopia Longsightedness due to inability to make the lens of the eye convex by contraction of the ciliary muscles, *i.e.* failure of adaptation of the lens.

prescription A formula written by the physician to the dispenser. Consists of the heading, usually the symbol R/ meaning 'take', the names and quantities of the ingredients, the directions to the dispenser, the directions to the patients, the date and the signature.

presentation The part of the fetus which first engages or tends to engage in the pelvis is said *to present*, and the description of this part is the presentation.

presenting symptom The symptom of a disease which causes the patient to seek medical advice.

pressor Substance causing rise in blood pressure, *e.g. P. amines* are substances such as noradrenaline and adrenaline which constrict the blood vessels and cause an elevation of the blood pressure.

pressure areas Parts of the body where the bone is near the skin surface and where a pressure sore is likely to occur if there is prolonged pressure owing to diminished blood supply to these parts.

pressure points Points at which pressure may be applied to check haemorrhage.

pressure sore Ulceration of skin over pressure areas.

presytole Period in the cardiac cycle before systole.

priapism Painful erection of the penis.

prickle cells Epidermal cells, so-called because they have specialized areas of attachment to each other (called desmosomes) which allow extracellular fluid to circulate between them.

prickly heat Miliaria papillosa.

primary complex *Syn.* Ghon focus. First site of infection in tuberculosis. Healing usually takes place uneventfully.

primary health care The first contact between patient and medical practice, usually with general practitioner.

primary lesion Original lesion from which others may arise.

primary sore Initial site of infection in syphilis.

primigravida A woman pregnant for the first time.

primipara A woman who has borne one child.

primordial Pertaining to the beginning.

probe A slender rod, sometimes of silver, used for exploring wounds.

process A prolongation or eminence of a part.

procidentia　A falling down, especially of the uterus. Complete prolapse of the uterus outside the vagina.

proctalgia　Pain about the rectum.

proctectomy　Excision of rectum.

proctitis　Inflammation of the rectum.

proctocele　Prolapsed rectum.

proctoclysis　Introduction into the rectum of saline solution for absorption.

proctorrhaphy　Suturing of the rectum.

proctoscope　An instrument for viewing the interior of the rectum.

prodromal period　The period that elapses in an infectious disease between the appearance of the first symptoms and the development of the rash, *e.g.* in smallpox, three days.

progeria　A condition in which premature senility is combined with infantilism.

progestogen　Synthetic drug with progesterone-like activity used in contraceptive and similar drugs.

progesterone　A steroid hormone secreted by the corpus luteum responsible for preparing the reproductive organs for pregnancy and for maintaining these changes if pregnancy occurs. A synthetic form used with oestrogen in the contraceptive pill.

proglottis　Segment of tapeworm.

prognosis　The considered opinion as to the course of a disease.

progressive muscular atrophy　Loss of power and wasting of muscles. Degenerative changes are found in the motor cells of the brain and anterior horns of the spinal cord. *See also* MOTOR NEURONE DISEASE.

projection　Painful thoughts, feelings and motives are relieved by transferring them on to someone else, *e.g.* blaming one's own mistake on to another person.

prolactin　Milk production stimulating hormone of the anterior lobe of the pituitary.

prolapse　Falling forwards or downwards. *Genital p.*: weakness of the ligaments of the uterus and walls of the vagina; 'dropped womb'. *See also* CYSTOCELE, RECTOCELE, PROCIDENTIA: *p. intervertebral disc*: slipped disc.

proliferation　Reproduction. Cell genesis.

promontory　A projecting part. An eminence.

pronation　Downward turning of the palm of the hand.

prone　Lying with the face downward.

propensity　Inclination or tendency.

prophylactic　Tending to prevent disease.

proprietary name The name under which a drug is marketed as compared to the generic name which describes the chemical compound.

proprioceptor Sensory end organ which detects changes in tension of muscles.

proptosis oculi Protrusion of eyeballs.

prostacyclin A substance produced by the vascular endothelium which inhibits platelet aggregation.

prostaglandins A group of substances present in most tissue which locally mediate many physiological activities, *e.g.* uterine contractions. Also involved in inflammatory reaction.

prostate A gland associated with the male reproductive system. Its size and secretion are under the influence of androgens. Its function is not clear but it appears to supply supportive substances to the spermatozoa in the seminal vesicles.

prostatectomy Operation of removing the prostate gland. The operation may be suprapubic when the bladder is first incised, or retropubic through an abdominal incision.

prostatic Pertaining to the prostate. *P. bar*: form of benign prostatic enlargement.

prostatitis Inflammation of the prostate gland.

prosthesis The replacement of an absent limb or organ by an artificial apparatus.

prostration Extreme exhaustion.

protein Very complex organic compound, made up of a large number of amino acids, which are synthesized by living systems, *see* NUCLEIC ACIDS. There are 20 different amino acids commonly found in proteins and these are arranged in different sequences which give the specific characteristics to the proteins.

proteinuria Protein in the urine.

proteolysis The breakdown of proteins to form polypeptides, peptides and amino acids.

proteolytic enzymes Enzymes capable of proteolysis. Several different such enzymes are usually required to digest protein.

prothrombin The precursor of thrombin. *See* BLOOD COAGULATION.

protoplasm The substance of a cell, thus excluding material which has been ingested or is to be secreted.

prototype The original form from which others are copied.

protozoa A class of unicellular organisms forming the lowest division of the animal kingdom, *e.g.* an amoeba.

proud flesh Excessive granulation tissue in a wound.

provitamin A precursor of a vitamin.

proximal Nearest to the centre or origin.

prurigo A skin disease marked by irritating papules.

pruritus Itching.

pseudarthrosis A false joint arising from failed union of a fracture.

pseudo- A prefix meaning false or spurious (Greek).

pseudoangina A neurotic disease resembling angina pectoris.

pseudobulbar palsy A form of motor neurone disease affecting the nerves arising from the brain stem.

pseudocholinesterase An enzyme having cholinesterase-like activity but present in plasma rather than nerve endings.

pseudocoxalgia *See* PERTHE'S DISEASE.

pseudocyesis Changes mimicking pregnancy but without a fetus.

pseudohermaphrodite Individual in whom the secondary sexual characteristics do not correspond to the generative organs. In females this may be due to hypersecretion of androgens by the adrenal cortex. In males the condition is genetically determined and presumably due to a metabolic abnormality whereby oestrogens are produced by the adrenal cortex or by the

testes. In true hermaphroditism there is ambivalence in the development of the organs of generation.

pseudomyxoma peritonei Condition in which rupture of a mucinous ovarian cyst or mucocele of the appendix gives rise to huge jelly-like deposits throughout the peritoneal cavity and causes intestinal obstruction.

pseudopodium Temporary protrusion of cell serving as method of locomotion and phagocytosis.

psittacosis A virus disease found in parrots and other birds which is communicable to man. It manifests itself as an atypical pneumonia.

psoas An important muscle attached above to the lumbar vertebrae and below to the femur. It flexes the femur on the trunk. *P. abscess. See* ABSCESS.

psoriasis Abnormality of keratinization producing skin lesions consisting of raised, red, scaly areas.

psyche The mind.

psychiatric social worker One who works under a psychiatrist to rehabilitate mentally ill people.

psychiatrist A physician who specializes in psychiatry.

psychiatry The study and treatment of mental disorders.

psychoanalysis A method of

treatment for psychiatric conditions based on Freudian theories whereby relief is allegedly obtained by tracing neuroses to their genesis.

psychogenic Originating in the mind.

psychologist One who studies psychology.

psychology The study of behaviour patterns.

psychoneurosis *See* NEUROSIS.

psychopath Somebody suffering from a severe personality disorder.

psychopathology The pathology of mental diseases.

psychosis An organic disorder of the mind.

psychosomatic Relating to mind and body. A physical symptom or illness may have a psychological aetiological component, *e.g.* ulcerative colitis, peptic ulcer, asthma.

psychotherapeutics, psychotherapy Treatment of the mind. A term which includes any treatment for functional nervous disorders, *e.g.* by hypnotism, suggestion, psychoanalysis, etc.

psychotic Relating to a psychosis.

pterygium Mucous membrane growing on the conjunctiva and tending to grow on to the cornea.

pterygoid Literally, wing-shaped.

pterion The point of junction of the frontal, parietal, temporal and sphenoidal bones.

ptosis Drooping of the upper eyelid.

ptyalin An enzyme found in saliva which can digest starch (amylase).

ptyalism Excessive salivation.

ptyalolith Stone in a duct of a salivary gland.

puberty The period of sexual development.

pubes The pubic bones.

pubiotomy Cutting the pubis; an operation sometimes performed to enlarge a contracted pelvis and so facilitate delivery. *Syn.* symphisiotomy.

pudenda The external female genital organs.

pudendal block Method of anaesthesia in second stage of labour by injecting pudendal nerves transvaginally.

puerperal Relating to the six weeks following childbirth. *P. fever*: fever associated with sepsis of the genital tract following delivery. Elevation of temperature on about the tenth day of the puerperium may be a sign of phlebothrombosis. *P. psychosis*: psychosis occasionally occurring after delivery probably due to hormonal alterations occurring at that time.

puerperium The period after a confinement until the uterus is involuted.

Pulex irritans Common flea. *See* FLEA.

pulmonary Relating to the lungs. *P. embolism*: *see* EMBOLISM. *P. hypertension*: increase of the pressure in the pulmonary circulation. *P. oedema*: exudation of fluid into the lungs. *P. stenosis*: narrowing of the pulmonary valve of the heart. *P. valve*: the valve at the exit of the right ventricle into the pulmonary artery.

pulp The interior, fleshy part of vegetable or animal tissue.

pulsation Beating of the heart, or of the blood in the arteries.

pulse *See* ANACROTIC.

pulsus alternans Alternate weak and strong pulse waves.

pulsus bisferiens Double pulse wave which occurs in patients with combined aortic stenosis and regurgitation.

pulsus paradoxus The pulse decreases on inspiration and may disappear. It is the result of pericardial constriction.

pulvis A powder.

punctate Dotted.

puncture To make a hole with a sharp instrument.

PUO *Abbr*. Pyrexia of unknown origin.

pupa Second stage of insect development following the larval stage.

pupil The orifice in the centre of the iris.

pupillary Pertaining to the pupil.

purgative A medicine for causing evacuation of the bowels.

purpura Purple-coloured spots due to haemorrhage into the tissues. There are many causes of purpura which may be roughly categorized as due to: (1) deficiency of clotting mechanism, *e.g.* essential thrombocytopaenia; (2) capillary damage; (3) both.

purpura, Henoch–Schönlein This is a syndrome also known as anaphylactoid purpura characterized by urticaria, pain, and effusions into the joints, intestinal bleeding and colic and purpura. Usually occurs in children and often follows a streptococcal throat infection.

purulent Pus-like.

pus Matter. Consists of dead leucocytes in an albuminous fluid.

pustula maligna Anthrax.

pustulation The formation of pustules.

pustule A pimple containing pus.

putrefaction The rotting away of animal matter. Decomposition advanced to an offensive stage.

PV *Abbr*. per vaginam. Examination of the pelvic organs by inspection or palpation through the vagina.

pyaemia The circulation of septic emboli in the bloodstream causing multiple abscesses.

pyarthrosis Suppuration in a joint.

pyelitis Inflammation of the kidney.

pyelography To demonstrate kidneys, ureters and bladder following intravenous injection of contrast medium opaque to x-rays. *Intravenous p.*: to demonstrate renal tract following intravenous injection of radio-opaque dye concentrated in the urine. *Retrograde p.*: to demonstrate kidneys and ureters following introduction of ureteric catheter into which contrast medium is injected.

pyelolithotomy Operation to remove a stone from the renal pelvis.

pyelonephritis Inflammation of the kidney and its pelvis.

pyknic A body type which tends to be thickset.

pyknosis Contraction of nuclear material to form a dense mass. Often seen preceding cellular death.

pyloric stenosis Narrowing of the pylorus. (1) A condition found in infants, more commonly male than female. It is not apparently present at birth and is usually noted after the age of ten days. Projectile vomiting after all feeds, constipation, wasting, are the chief symptoms, while on examination visible peristalsis may be present and a

hard tumour to the right of the umbilicus may be felt. Condition is supposed to be due to muscular spasm and consequent hypertrophy of muscle surrounding the pylorus, so preventing the passage of food. The stomach is always dilated. The condition can be treated in its early stages by gastric lavage, and small and frequent feeds; but once a tumour is felt, it is best to open the abdomen and divide hypertrophied muscle (Ramstedt's operation). (2) In adults when it is usually due to a gastric ulcer, or to a neoplasm.

pyloroplasty Operation for widening a contracted pylorus.

pylorus Region of the junction between the stomach and the duodenum. There is a thickening of the circular muscle at this point which acts as a sphincter allowing the passage of food out of the stomach.

pyoderma Any septic skin lesion.

pyogenic Pus-producing, forming pus.

pyometra Pus retained in the uterus.

pyonephrosis Pus in the kidney.

pyorrhoea A flow of pus. Generally used as meaning the same as *p. alveolaris*, a condition in which pus oozes out from the gums around the roots of the teeth. This is also known as Rigg's disease.

pyosalpinx   (1)Abscess in one of the fallopian tubes.

pyramid   Elevation on the medulla oblongata caused by the pyramidal tract. (2) The eminence of renal cortical tissue on which the collecting tubes open into the renal pelvis.

pyramidal   Shaped like a pyramid. *P. cells*: cells in the cerebral cortex giving out impulses to voluntary muscles. *P. system*: tracts in the brain and spinal cord transmitting impulses from the pyramidal cells.

pyrexia   Fever. Elevation of the body temperature. *Intermittent p.*: temperature is high at night but below normal in the morning. *Remittent p.*: temperature high at night, less in the morning, but never reaching normal.

pyridoxin   Formerly called vitamin B_6. Required as coenzyme in cell metabolism.

pyrosis   *See* HEARTBURN.

pyuria   Pus in the urine.

Q

'Q' fever   Also called Queensland fever. An acute disease resembling pneumonia and caused by Rickettsia burnetii.

quack   One who pretends to knowledge or skill, usually medical, which he does not possess.

quadriceps   Four-headed: name given to four separate muscles, covering the front of the thigh, which are all inserted into the tubercle of the tibia, and extend the knee.

quadriplegia   Paralysis of both legs and arms. Also known as tetraplegia.

quadruple vaccine   A vaccine for immunization against poliomyelitis, diphtheria, tetanus and pertussis.

quarantine   A period of separation of infected persons or contacts from others, and which is necessary to prevent the spread of disease.

quartan   *See* MALARIA.

Queckenstedt's test   To elicit the presence of spinal block, *e.g.* tumour. A lumbar puncture is performed. If the manometer shows no increase of intraspinal pressure when the jugular veins are pressed, there is spinal block.

quickening   The first perception of movement of the fetus in the womb, usually felt by the mother at the end of the fourth month.

quiescent   Not active. Dormant.

quinsy   A peritonsillar abscess, situated immediately outside the capsule of the tonsil. *See* TONSILLITIS.

R

rabies A specific and fatal infective disease which chiefly
affects rodents and canines;
transmissible to man through
the saliva by means of a bite
from an infected dog. *Syn.*
hydrophobia.

racemose Resembling a
bunch of grapes. *R. glands*:
having the cells arranged in
saccules with numerous ducts
leading to a main duct, *e.g.*
salivary glands.

radial Relating to radius.

radiation Emanation of
energy from a source. The
energy may be in a number of
different forms. The usual
form is that of photons which
according to their frequency
of emission are known as
radiowaves, light, x-rays,
gamma rays, etc. Subatomic
particles such as electrons,
neutrons, protons, and posi-
trons, mesons and many sub-
nuclear particles may also be
radiated. High-energy neutrons may be produced by
atomic explosions and certain
special equipment. Electrons
are also a natural product of
radioactivity and are known
as beta rays. Radiation dam-
ages living tissue. *R. sickness*:
illness resulting from overex-
posure to radiation.

radical That which goes to
the root; thus radical treatment aims at an absolute
cure, not palliation.

radiculitis Neuritis affecting
the nerve root.

radioactive fallout Radioactive isotopes distributed in
the atmosphere as a result of
atomic explosions. It constitutes a biological hazard
since isotopes may be ingested in food.

radioactive isotopes Radio-
isotopes. Variants of elements which exhibit the same
chemical properties as those
elements but which have a
greater number of neutrons in
their nucleus, *i.e.* have a
higher atomic number. For
example radioactive carbon
C^{14} (usually written ^{14}C) has
an excess of 2 neutrons over
carbon ^{12}C. There is tendency
for ^{14}C to decompose giving
rise to ^{12}C. As a result of this
decomposition energy is emitted, which in the case of
radioactive carbon is in the
form of electrons. *See* BETA
RAYS.

radioactivity Spontaneous
decomposition of an element
with emission of energy.

radiobiology The study of the
effects of radiation on living
tissue.

radiographer Person trained
to take x-rays.

radiography Science of examination by means of x-rays.

radiologist A doctor who has
made a special study of
radiology.

radiology Study of diagnosis by means of x-rays.

radiosensitive Term applied to a structure, especially a tumour, responsive to radiotherapy.

radiotherapy Treatment of disease, particularly cancer, by radiation.

radium Natural radioactive element.

radius The outer bone of the forearm.

radon Radioactive gas derived from radium. *R. seeds*: sealed containers of radon.

râle Slight rattling sound heard in the air passages upon auscultation.

Ramstedt's operation *See* PYLORIC STENOSIS.

ramus A branch, thus ramification of vessels.

ranula Cyst of sublingual gland.

raphe Fibrous junction between muscles.

rarefaction The process of becoming less dense.

rash Skin eruption.

rat-bite fever Disease which occurs in China and Japan. It is conveyed by the bite of an infected rat. The organism is known as Spirillum minus.

Rathke's pouch Diverticulum in the roof of the developing mouth which becomes part of the pituitary gland.

rationalization A justification to oneself of one's action or behaviour. The rationalization is based on unconscious or instinctive motives.

raucous Hoarse.

Raynaud's disease Inherited idiopathic hypersensitivity of the digital vessels to cold. Affects women.

Raynaud's phenomenon Syndrome characterized by intense spasm of the digital arteries producing cold, white, pulseless fingers often associated with impairment of sensation and fine movement. There are many possible causes, *e.g.* vibration syndrome.

reaction Response to stimulus.

reagent An agent taking part in a reaction.

recalcitrant Resistant, especially of a disease to its treatment.

recall Bring back a memory.

receptaculum chyli The lower expanded portion of the thoracic duct.

receptor A sense organ which receives stimuli, *e.g.* light, sound, vibration, movement, pressure, etc. and converts this information into nerve impulses which are transmitted via the sensory nerves.

recessive Tending to disappear. In genetics: a gene which tends not to be expressed unless it is present in a homozygous state; *cf.* dominant.

recipient One who receives,

e.g. a recipient of blood transfusion.

Recklinghausen's (von) disease
See NEUROFIBROMATOSIS.

recrudescence Return of symptoms.

rectal Relating to the rectum.

rectocele Prolapse of posterior vaginal wall. Strictly the term applies to any herniation of the rectum.

rectoscope Proctoscope.

rectosigmoidectomy Operation to excise the rectum and the sigmoid colon.

rectovesical Of the rectum and the bladder. *R. space*: the space between the rectum and bladder in men.

rectum The lower part of the large intestine from the colon to the anal canal. *See* BOWEL.

rectus Straight; applied to certain muscles. *R. abdominis*: two external abdominal muscles, one each side of the midline, running from pubic bone to ensiform cartilage and the fifth, sixth and seventh ribs. It is enclosed in a strong sheath. There are also four short muscles of the eye, external, internal, superior and inferior rectus. *R. femoris*: muscle on the front of the thigh, one of the four forming the quadriceps extensor.

recumbent Lying down.

recuperate To get better.

recurrent Returning. *R. laryngeal nerve* is so-called because this branch of the vagus (*see* CRANIAL NERVES) comes back from below the thyroid to supply the larynx.

red blood cell or **corpuscle**
These are the blood cells which contain haemoglobin (*erythrocytes*). There are about 5,000,000/ml of blood and they carry nearly all the oxygen required by the body cells. Red blood cells are formed in the bone marrow, normally at a rate of about a million a second and are notable for the absence of a nucleus in the mature state. They do not divide and have a lifetime of about 120 days when they are destroyed in the spleen.

reduction (1) Replacing to a normal position, *e.g.* after fracture, dislocation or hernia. (2) In chemistry: the addition of electrons to the reduced substance.

referred pain Pain felt in the distribution of a sensory nerve supplied from the same segment as the nerve stimulated, *e.g.* pain felt in the shoulder due to irritation of the diaphragm, for both are supplied by nerves from the same spinal segments.

reflex An immediate response to a stimulus without voluntary control. In its simplest form involves nerve fibres of a single spinal segment. More complex reflexes

229

include those responsible for accommodation of eyes to light and distance. Autonomic reflexes are mediated via the parasympathetic nerves and smooth muscle, *e.g.* the *gastrocolic r.* Reflex activity may be taught, *i.e.* *conditioned r.*

reflux Flowing back, *e.g.* *oesophageal r.* is the flow of stomach acid into the oesophagus.

refraction The bending of light rays as they pass from one medium to another. This bending is an essential part of the process by which the image of an object is focused on the retina of the eye. Errors of refraction are caused when the eyeball is too short or too long or when the muscles which make the lens focus are weakened through disease or age; the rays of light are prevented from converging accurately on the retina. Spectacles will correct the error in most cases.

refractory Stubborn; not amenable to treatment.

refrigeration The cooling of part of the body to reduce its metabolic requirements or to anaesthetize a part.

regeneration Renewal of damaged tissue such as regenerating nerve fibres.

regimen A rule of diet or of hygiene, or of life.

regional ileitis *See* CROHN'S DISEASE.

regression Reverting to a more primitive stage. In psychology reverting to childlike behaviour as may be seen in severe physical illness or emotional upset.

regurgitation Backward flow as occurs with defective valves, *e.g.* in the heart and veins. Also applied to the reverse flow of gastric contents.

rehabilitation Fitting a patient to take his place in the world again, *e.g.* rehabilitation of an amputee.

Reiter's syndrome Syndrome consisting of arthritis, conjunctivitis and urethritis and occasionally other manifestations, *e.g.* fever, rash, malaise, etc. The cause is not known.

rejection Refusal to accept; used especially of grafted tissues and organs.

relapse A return of disease after convalescence has once begun.

relapsing fever Famine fever. A tropical disease caused by spirochaetes of the genus Borrelia.

relaxation Reduction of muscle tone.

relaxin An ovarian peptide hormone involved in cervical softening.

remission Period when a disease subsides and shows no symptoms.

remittent Returning at

regular intervals; applied to certain fevers. *R. pyrexia*: *see* PYREXIA.

renal   Relating to the kidney. *R. calculus*: stone in the kidney. *R. colic*: colic of the ureter due to stone in the ureter or renal pelvis. *R. dwarfism*: dwarfism due to malfunction of the kidneys, usually due to stunting of skeletal growth due to *renal rickets*. See FANCONI SYNDROME. *R. failure*: *Acute* presents as a sudden inability of the kidneys to produce urine. Chronic: *see* NEPHRITIS. *R. threshold*: concentration of substance in the blood at which it appears in the urine. *R. tubular acidosis*: defective renal tubular function in which there is a failure to secrete hydrogen ions into the urine with consequent inability to reduce the acidity of the blood in the normal way. Consequently there is excessive loss of compensatory ions with generalized metabolic disturbance.

renin   Renal enzyme produced in response to sodium loss. Involved in the angiotensin system.

rennin   Enzyme secreted in the stomach of infants which clots milk by converting caseinogen to casein which precipitates as a calcium salt.

repetitive strain injuries   *See* TENOSYNOVITIS.

replantation   Used especially of replacing tooth in socket.

repression   (1) In psychiatry: the shutting away of undesirable information from consciousness. (2) In genetics: the ability to prevent certain types of protein synthesis from taking place within a cell.

resection   A complete removal.

resectoscope   Instrument to view and remove pieces of tissue in transurethral prostatectomy.

reservoirs of infection   Parts of the body with high population of potential pathogenic organisms, *e.g.* skin, gut.

residual air   That remaining in the lungs after forced expiration.

residual urine   That left in the bladder after the organ has apparently been emptied naturally, measured by catheterization.

resistance   The degree of opposition to an action.

resolution   (1) A resolve. (2) Stage in an inflammation, in particular, term used in pathological description of lobar pneumonia.

resonance   Increase of sound by reverberation, applied to voice sounds in auscultation.

resorption   Absorption of secreted matter.

respiration   Breathing. Rate should be: in infants 50 to the minute, in children 36, in adults 16. *Inverted r.*: the pause is after inspiration instead of after expiration; noticed in babies with bronchopneumonia.

respirator (1) Appliance worn over the mouth and nose to prevent the inhalation of poisonous gas. (2) Apparatus used to assist the muscles of respiration when paralysed, *e.g.* in poliomyelitis. A variety of types of these respirators exists.

respiratory Pertaining to breathing. *R. acidosis*: acidosis caused by inability to excrete CO_2 (carbon dioxide), usually the result of chronic lung disease. *R. alkalosis*: alkalosis due to hyperventilation with excessive loss of CO_2. *R. distress syndrome*: also known as the pulmonary syndrome of the newborn. Very much more common in premature babies. Rapid heart beat, grunting respiration and intercostal inspiratory recession are followed by respiratory failure. *See also* HYALINE MEMBRANE, SURFACTANT. *R. quotient (RQ)*: this is the ratio of the volumes of carbon dioxide expired and the oxygen consumed during the same time.

restitution An obstetric term meaning the rotation of the fetal head towards the right or left side immediately after it has completely passed the vulva; the occiput is thus turned (in a vertex presentation) towards the same side of the mother as that on which it originally entered the pelvis.

resuscitation Reviving those who are apparently dead.

retardation A slowing down of activity; backwardness.

retching Ineffectual efforts to vomit.

retention A holding back. Inability to void urine.

reticular Resembling a network. Applied to tissue.

reticulocyte Immature red blood cell in which nuclear remnants persist as basophilic threads in the cytoplasm.

reticulocytosis Excessive reticulocytes found in the bloodstream.

reticuloendothelial system A system of phagocytic macrophages in the blood and tissues which free the body fluids of foreign particles. They can be recognized by injecting particles of indian ink or certain other dyes into the body. The particles are selectively taken up by cells of the reticuloendothelial system. *See also* MACROPHAGE, PHAGOCYTE, KUPFFER CELLS, etc.

reticulosis A group of neoplasms arising from lymphoid tissue, *e.g.* Hodgkin's disease, lymphosarcoma.

reticulum cell sarcoma A reticulosis similar to Hodgkin's disease. It is alleged to arise from a more primitive cell than other reticuloses, a so-called stem cell known as a reticulum cell.

retina Layer lining the interior of the eye which contains the light-sensitive receptors, the rods and the cones.

retinal Pertaining to the retina

retinitis Inflammation of the retina.

retinoblastoma Tumour arising from germ cells in the retina.

retinopathy Pathological lesion affecting the retina, *e.g. diabetic r., hypertensive r.*

retraction Withdrawal or shortening. Retraction of the lower segment of the first stage of labour. There is a progressive increase in the tone of the longitudinal muscle fibres with consequent shortening of the muscles.

retractor Instrument used to withdraw structures obscuring the field of operation.

retro- Prefix denoting backwards, behind (Latin).

retrobulbar Behind the globe of the eye.

retrocaecal Behind the caecum.

retroflexion A bending back, as of the body of the uterus on the cervix.

retrograde pyelography *See* PYELOGRAPHY.

retrogression Retreating.

retrolental fibroplasia The posterior part of the capsule of the lens of the eye becomes fibrosed and blindness may result. It occurred in babies, usually premature, who were given too high a concentration of oxygen after birth, but this condition is seldom seen since this danger was recognized.

retroperitoneal Behind the posterior layer of the peritoneum.

retropharyngeal Behind the pharynx. *R. abscess:* a collection of pus behind the wall of the pharynx and anterior to the cervical vertebrae. An acute abscess may develop from inflammation of two glands near the midline, a chronic one from cervical caries.

retropubic Behind the pubis. *R. prostatectomy: see* PROSTATECTOMY.

retrospection Looking back into the past.

retrosternal Behind the sternum.

retroversion A turning backwards. The uterus is normally turned considerably forwards, that is, the cervix is directed towards the lower end of the sacrum and the fundus towards the suprapubic region. Any deviation from this in the backward direction is termed retroversion. *R. of the gravid uterus* may prevent the enlarging uterus from rising out of the pelvis.

rhachitis Technical misnomer for rickets.

rhagades A crack or fissure of skin causing pain; a term especially used of radiating scars at angle of mouth due to congenital syphilis. Now most commonly due to ill-fitting dentures or vitamin deficiencies.

rhesus (Rh) factor *See* BLOOD GROUPING.

rheumatic Pertaining to rheumatism. *R. fever*: acute rheumatic fever is a disorder affecting connective tissue, particularly that of the heart and the joints. The cause is considered to be an allergic reaction to toxins from haemolytic streptococcus (Lancefield group A). *R. heart disease*: chronic rheumatic heart disease is the result of severe damage and deformation of the valves of the heart due to rheumatic fever.

rheumatism General nontechnical term covering diverse conditions which have in common rather ill-defined pains in the muscles or joints.

rheumatoid Similar to rheumatism. *R. arthritis*: a subacute or chronic form of arthritis. Gross changes occur in the joints leading to

deformity and ankylosis.

rhinitis Inflammation of the nose.

rhinolith A calculus formed in the nose.

rhinoplasty Surgical reconstruction of the nose, *e.g.* following severe fracture of the nasal bones with resulting deformity.

rhinorrhoea Discharge from the nose.

rhinoscope Nasal speculum.

rhinovirus A large group of viruses causing the common cold.

rhizotomy Division of spinal nerve roots.

rhodopsin Visual purple contained in the retina.

rhonchus A dry wheezing sound heard in the chest on auscultation. May be high pitched or sibilant, low pitched or sonorous.

rhythm A patterned sound or movement.

riboflavine Vitamin B_2. It forms part of a number of enzymes required for oxidative metabolism in cells.

ribonuclease Enzyme which degrades RNA.

ribonucleic acid (RNA) *See* NUCLEIC ACID.

ribosomes Minute intracytoplasmic bodies composed of ribonucleic acid (RNA) and protein, present in most animal cells and plentifully in those actively growing or synthesizing secretory proteins.

ribs Long lateral bones enclosing the chest. The upper seven ribs on each side join the sternum by separate cartilages, and are called true ribs. The lower five ribs being termed false ribs. Of the latter, the upper three pairs are attached to the sternum by a common cartilage on each side, while the lower two ribs on each side are not attached to the sternum at all, and are therefore called floating ribs.

ricewater stools Characteristic stools of cholera.

rickets Deficiency of calcification of the skeleton and bowing of the long bones. The cause is vitamin D deficiency occurring in infancy. If blood calcium drops there may be tetany. *Renal r.*: due to excessive urinary calcium loss osteoporesis develops and simulates true rickets.

Rickettsia Group of organisms which fall between bacteria and viruses in a classification based on size and properties. Typhus fever is a rickettsial disease.

Riedel's thyroiditis A fibrosing inflammation of the thyroid.

Rigg's disease *See* PYORRHOEA.

rigor Sudden feeling of cold accompanied by shivering which raises the body temperature above normal. Due to disorder of the thermo-regulatory system of the brain caused by toxins, etc. Common in malaria. *R. mortis*: the stiffening of the body after death.

rima A fissure; thus *r. glottidis*, slit between vocal cords.

ring pessary Pessary in circular form.

Ringer's solution Physiological saline which includes sodium, potassium, calcium, magnesium and some other ions normally present in extracellular fluid.

ringworm Fungus infection of keratinized structures such as hair, nails and skin. There are several species of fungus which are parasitic to man.

Rinne's test A vibrating tuning-fork is placed on the mastoid process until no longer heard, then quickly put in front of the meatus; normally the vibration is still heard. The test is negative when obstruction exists in the external or middle ear.

risus sardonicus A convulsive grin, symptomatic of tetanus.

RNA *Abbr.* ribonucleic acid. *RNA viruses*: viruses in which genetic material is RNA.

ROA *Abbr.* right occipito-anterior presentation of fetus.

rodent ulcer Basal cell carcinoma of the skin. More common on parts of the skin exposed to the sun. Only spreads locally.

rods Sensitive light receptors in the retina.

Roentgen rays X-rays.

Romberg's sign Inability to stand erect when the eyes are closed and the feet placed together; seen in tabes dorsalis.

ROP *Abbr.* right occipito-posterior presentation of fetus.

rosacea Vasculomotor disturbance affecting the face with associated hyperplasia of the sebaceous glands.

roseola A rose-coloured rash.

rotation Twisting. Applied to the twisting of the head upon the shoulders of the fetus as it passes down the birth canal and follows the curves.

rotators Muscles which cause circular movement.

roughage Cellulose part of food which gives bulk and aids peristalsis.

round ligaments Ovarian ligaments. *R.l. of the uterus*: the continuation of the ovarian ligaments. Run from corner of uterus to the inguinal region. No function known.

roundworm *See* ASCARIS LUMBRICOIDES.

RQ *Abbr.* respiratory quotient.

rubefacients Mild irritants which cause redness of the skin.

rubella Also called German measles. A mild infectious disease caused by a virus. Incubation period 14–20 days, infectivity less than measles. There may be slight catarrh and fever and swelling of sub-occipital glands. The rash begins on the face and spreads to the body and fades quickly. Complications are few but if a woman has the disease during the first four months of pregnancy, she may have a deformed child with eyes, ears and heart commonly affected. All girls and women should now be immunized against rubella at least three months before becoming pregnant.

rugae Wrinkles or creases.

rugose Wrinkled.

rumination Regurgitation of feeds by infants. Analogous to chewing the cud. Can cause failure to thrive. Infant may be seen inducing a vomit with fingers at the back of the mouth.

rupture A bursting or breaking. Popular term for a hernia.

Ryle's tube A form of naso-gastric tube.

S

Sabin's vaccine A vaccine against poliomyelitis which consists of an attenuated strain of virus which is taken orally; *cf.* Salk vaccine.

sac A small pouch, such as a hernial sac.

saccharin A glucoside used as a sugar substitute, having no food value.

Saccharomyces A group of fungi including yeasts. One is the cause of thrush.

sacculated Bagged or pursed out.

sacral Pertaining to the sacrum. Sacral analgesia, *see* CAUDAL ANALGESIA.

sacroiliac synchondrosis or **joint** The articulation between the sacrum and the hipbone. Normally there is no movement at this joint. During pregnancy the joint becomes more movable and this, to a slight extent, facilitates the birth of the child.

sacrum The division of the backbone, forming part of the pelvis.

saddlenose A flattened bridge of the nose.

sadism A sexual perversion in which pleasure is derived from inflicting cruelty upon another.

sagittal Arrowlike. *S. section*: section made by cutting through a specimen from top to bottom so that there are equal right and left halves. *S. suture*: the suture between the parietal bones.

St Vitus' dance Chorea.

sal A salt.

saline A solution of salt (NaCl). In medical practice this normally refers to 'physiological' saline.

saliva The secretion of the salivary glands.

salivary glands Three pairs of glands. The sublingual and submaxillary are situated in the floor of the mouth, the parotid above the angle of the lower jaw. *See* PAROTID.

salivation The act of secretion of saliva.

Salk's vaccine A vaccine against poliomyelitis made from dead virus and given by injection. Seldom used.

Salmonella Group of Gram-negative bacteria which include the typhoid bacteria and a number of others causing food poisoning.

salpingectomy Removal of one or both fallopian tubes.

salpingitis Inflammation of a tube, usually applied to the fallopian tubes.

salpingocyesis Tubal pregnancy.

salpingography Technique of examination of the fallopian tubes by x-rays.

salpingo-oophorectomy Removal of fallopian tubes and ovaries.

salpingostomy Artificially opening a fallopian tube whose aperture has been closed by inflammation.

salpinx A tube, either eustachian or fallopian.

salt A substance resulting from the combination of an acid and a base.

salve An ointment.

Samaritans Voluntary organization offering help initially by telephone to people in distress and possibly suicidal.

sanatorium Any institution for convalescent patients can technically be called a sanatorium. Formerly used for the open-air treatment of tuberculosis.

sandfly fever Tropical disease due to infection by organism transmitted by sandfly bites.

sanguine (1) Full-blooded. (2) Hopeful.

sanguinous Bloodstained. Containing blood.

sanitary Pertaining to health.

sanitation The use of methods conducive to public health.

sanity Being of sound mind.

saphena varix Saccular enlargement of the termination of the long saphenous vein often without obvious varicose veins.

saphenous Applied to certain structures in the leg. *S. nerve*: large branch of the femoral nerve. *S. opening*: just below groin near inner side of thigh where superficial saphenous vein passes deep to enter femoral vein. *S. veins*: superficial leg veins. *Long s.v.*: begins on the foot and extends to the groin. *Short s.v.*: joins the popliteal vein at the knee.

sapo Soap. *S. mollis*: soft soap.

saponify To make into a soap. Deposits of calcium soaps occur in acute peritonitis by saponification of peritoneal fat.

saprophytes Organisms that exist only in dead matter.

Sarcina A genus of Schizomycetes which form rectangular bundles as they divide; usually non-pathogenic.

sarcoid Resembling flesh.

sarcoidosis A syndrome resulting from what appears to be a disturbance of the immunological mechanism. It is characterized by widespread lesions of a characteristic histological appearance resembling tuberculosis. Symptoms depend on the situation of these lesions. In a proportion of cases there is an associated disturbance of calcium metabolism.

sarcolemma The membrane which covers each fibril of muscle.

sarcoma Malignant tumour of mesodermal origin.

Sarcoptes scabiei The itch mite or insect causing scabies. It burrows into the skin where it lays its eggs which hatch out. The 'burrows' often terminate in a papule on the skin. The disease is treated with benzyl benzoate.

sartorius The long ribbon-shaped muscle of the front of the thigh.

saturation The condition of holding in solution the full amount of a solid capable of being dissolved.

scab An incrustation formed over a wound.

scabies *See* SARCOPTES.

scald Burn caused by hot fluids.

scale Aggregation of keratinized cells.

scalenus anterior syndrome Is characterized by pain in the arm and tingling of the fingers with loss of power and muscle wasting due to compression of the lower fibres of the brachial plexus by the scalenus anterior muscle.

scalp The skin covering the cranium.

scalpel Knife used in surgery and dissection.

scanning speech Speech in which syllables tend to be separated. Usually a sign of a lesion affecting the cerebellum.

scaphocephaly Deformity of skull due to premature fusion of sutures producing a long narrow head.

scaphoid Boat-shaped. The name of a bone of the carpus and of the tarsus.

scapula The shoulder blade.

scar The connective fibrous tissue found after any wound has healed.

scarification Shallow incisions just penetrating the epidermis.

scarlatina Scarlet fever. The cardinal sign is a widespread erythematous rash produced by a toxin released by haemolytic streptococci which are commonly found in the throat where they give rise to an infection.

Scarpa's triangle The femoral triangle bounded by Poupart's ligament, the adductor longus and sartorius.

SCBU *Abbr.* special care baby unit.

Scheuermann's disease Vertebral osteochondritis found in adolescents. It affects the two rings of cartilage and bone around the margin of both superior and inferior surfaces of the vertebral body. The condition does not cause general ill health.

Schick test Skin test to detect whether an individual has immunity against diphtheria. Small amounts of diphtheria toxin are used.

schistosomiasis *See* BILHARZIA.

Schizomycetes Yeasts.

schizophrenia The generic term used for a group of disorders characterized by a progressive loss of emotional stability, judgement and contact with reality. The cause is not yet known but there are probably genetic and biochemical components.

Schlatter's disease *See* OSGOOD SCHLATTER DISEASE.

Schlemmin's canal Lymphatic channel leading to a venous plexus at the root of the ciliary body of the eye. It allows the intraocular fluid (aqueous humour) to drain.

Failure of the canal to drain results in raised hydrostatic pressure in the anterior chamber of the eye (glaucoma).

Schwann cell Supporting cell of the peripheral nervous system, *See* NEUROGLIA. The Schwann cells invest the nerves and form the myelin sheath which surrounds many of the larger fibres.

sciatica Neuralgia of the sciatic nerve the large nerve of the thigh. It may be caused by pressure on the nerves in the spinal canal or the pelvis.

scintillography Imaging technique based on visual recording of radioactive emission from an organ after administration of a radioisotope selectively concentrated in that organ.

scirrhous Hard and fibrous in nature.

scissor leg deformity Deformity due to exaggerated tone in the adductor muscles usually resulting from cerebral damage.

sclera The opaque outer coat of the eyeball, forming five-sixths of the globe of the eye, the remaining one-sixth being formed by the cornea. *See* EYE.

scleritis An inflamed sclera.

sclerodactylia *See* ACRO-SCLEROSIS.

scleroderma Disorder of connective tissue in which there is probably increased amounts

of elastic fibres laid down resulting in loss of elasticity of the connective tissues and atrophic changes in the structures which they support.

sclerosis Hardening. *See also* MULTIPLE SCLEROSIS.

sclerotic Pertaining to the sclera.

sclerotomy An operation on the sclerotic coat of the eye, for the relief of glaucoma.

scolex Head of a tapeworm.

scoliosis Lateral curvature of the spine.

scotoma A blind spot in the field of vision.

screening Radiological examination by means of a fluorescent screen. Term used more generally for ways of detecting early disease in clinically healthy people.

scrofuloderma Tuberculosis of the skin.

scrotocele Hernia in the scrotum.

scrotum The bag which holds the testicles.

scruple A weight equal to 20 grains apothecaries' weight, or 1.295 grams.

scurf Dandruff. Large aggregates of exfoliating epidermal cells.

scurvy Syndrome of extreme vitamin C deficiency. *See* VITAMINS. Principal features are haemorrhage into the tissues and swelling of mucous membranes.

scybala Faeces passed as

hard dry masses.

sebaceous Fatty, secreting oily matter. *S. glands*: of skin, secrete fatty material called sebum. *S. cysts*: dilatation of one of these glands, due to blocking of its opening on to the skin. A cyst is filled with sebum.

seborrhoea Excessive secretion of the sebaceous glands.

sebum The oil of the skin, secreted by the sebaceous glands.

second intention The healing of a wound by means of granulation, and the growing of new skin.

second stage of labour Childbirth between the completion of cervical dilation and the delivery of the infant. It normally lasts up to two hours and is marked by strong contractions of the uterus and the instinctive desire to push of the mother to push in a way to expel the baby.

secondary disease A disease consequent on another disease already active.

secondary haemorrhage *See* HAEMORRHAGE.

secretin A hormone formed in the mucous membrane of the duodenum. It is carried by the blood to the pancreas, exciting it to activity. It also stimulates the secretion of bile.

secretion The active produc-tion, filtering or extrusion of material from cells. Certain cells have specialized secretory activity (gland cells).

section Usually applied to thin slices of tissue cut for microscopical examination.

sedative Allaying excitement or pain.

sedimentation rate *See* ESR.

segment A small piece; a section; a subdivision.

segregation A setting apart. Isolation.

sella turcica Pituitary fossa of the sphenoid bone.

semen The fluid emission which contains the spermatozoa.

semicircular canals Three canals of the internal ear, the sense organs of equilibrium or balance. *See* EAR.

semilunar cartilages Two crescentic cartilages, an internal and an external, lying in the knee joint between the femur and tibia. These may be torn and displaced, giving rise to pain and deformity and fluid in the knee joint. Usually removed by operation.

seminal Relating to the semen. *S. vesicles*: sac-like storage organs for semen.

seminoma Malignant neoplasm of the testicular cells.

senescence The process of growing old.

Sengstaken tube Oesophageal tube used to compress bleeding varices.

senility Degenerative
changes due to advanced
age.

sensible Perceptible.

sensitive Able to react to a
stimulus.

sensitization Act of producing an immunological
state in which there is a dis-
proportionately adverse reaction to a substance (antigen or
hapten).

sensory nerves Afferent
nerves carrying sensory information to the central nervous
system; *cf.* motor nerve.

sepsis The condition of being
infected by pyogenic bacteria.

septate uterus and vagina
Developmental abnormality
of the uterus and/or vagina in
which a longitudinal septum
divides the organ into two
parts.

septic Pertaining to sepsis.

septicaemia The circulation
and multiplication of microorganisms in the blood. It is a
very serious condition if a
suitable antibiotic is not
readily available.

septum The division between
two cavities; such as *s. ven-
triculorum*, which separates
the right ventricle of the heart
from the left.

sequelae Morbid conditions
remaining after, and consequent on, some former
illness.

sequestrectomy Operation to
remove sequestrum.

sequestrum A fragment of
dead bone.

serosa A serous membrane.
Serous membranes line the
large lymph spaces, *e.g.*
pleural, pericardial, peritoneal cavities.

serositis An inflamed serous
membrane.

serotonin 5-hydroxy-
tryptamine (5-HT), an amine
found in blood platelets, the
intestines and brain sub-
stance, inactivated by monoamine oxidase.

serpiginous Serpent-like in
shape.

serrated With a saw-like
edge.

serum That part of the blood
which remains after the cells,
platelets and fibrinogen have
been removed, usually by allowing the blood to clot. It
consists of a saline solution
containing a number of proteins and lipids. Of particular
interest are serum albumin
and globulin.

sesamoid bones Small foci of
bone formation in the tendons of muscles. The patella
is the largest.

sessile Having no stem, applied to tumours.

sex chromosomes These are
defined as chromosomes of
which there is a homologous
pair in the nuclei of one sex
and a heterologous pair in the
nuclei of the other. In humans
the homogametic sex (XX) is

female and the heterogametic sex (XY) is male.

sex-linkage This refers to genes whose locus is on one of the sex chromosomes.

sexually transmitted diseases (STDs) The venereal diseases. Infectious diseases transmitted during sexual intercourse, *e.g.* gonorrhoea, syphilis, etc.

Sheehan's syndrome Panhypopituitarism resulting from thrombosis of the pituitary blood supply occurring in association with postpartum haemorrhage.

Shiga's bacillus Shigella dysenteriae.

shingles *See* HERPES ZOSTER.

shock Severe circulatory disturbance characterized by fall in blood pressure, weak rapid pulse, thirst, and pallor. The usual cause is rapid diminution in the blood volume.

short circuit Anastomosis between gut or blood vessels which allows the contents to bypass a section of the normal pathway.

shortsighted Myopic.

shoulder presentation A form of transverse lie which must be converted into breech or vertex before delivery is possible.

show Popular term for the discharge of slightly blood-stained mucus common at the beginning of labour.

sialectasis Dilatation of salivary gland due to obstruction to the flow of saliva.

sialogogue Substance which stimulates salivation.

sialolith A salivary calculus.

sibling One of two or more children of the same parent.

sickle-cell anaemia Hereditary anaemia found sometimes in Negroes or those of Mediterranean origin. The red blood cells become sickle-shaped or crescentic in deoxygenated state due to content of abnormal haemoglobins.

side effect An effect of a drug other than the desired therapeutic effect.

siderosis (1) Inhalation of iron particles causing pneumoconiosis. (2) Excess of iron in the blood.

SIDS *Abbr.* sudden infant death syndrome. *See* COT DEATH.

sight The power of seeing.

sigmoid Like the Greek letter sigma, applied especially to a bend in the pelvic colon just before it becomes the rectum.

sigmoidoscope An instrument for viewing the interior of the rectum and sigmoid flexure of the colon.

sigmoidostomy Opening into sigmoid colon.

sign An indication of the presence of disease.

signatura A label.

silicones Polymers consisting

of alternate silicon and oxygen atoms, with organic groups sometimes attached to the silicon atoms.

silicosis Lung disease due to the inhalation of very fine particles of silica which irritate the lungs causing fibrotic changes. *See* PNEUMOCONIOSIS.

Simmond's disease *See* PANHYPOPITUITARISM.

simple fracture *See* FRACTURE.

Sim's position The patient lies in the semiprone position across the bed. The buttocks are brought to the edge of the bed. The right knee is flexed more than the left. Used for vaginal examination.

sinciput The upper fore part of the head.

sinew A tendon uniting a muscle to a bone.

sinistral Pertaining to the left side.

sinoatrial node Cells found in the heart at the junction of the superior vena cava and the right atrium. The node is the pacemaker of the heart.

sinus (1) A passage leading from an abscess, or some inner part, to an external opening. (2) A dilated channel for venous blood, *e.g. lateral s.*: a large venous channel on the inner side of the skull. It passes near the mastoid antrum and empties itself into the jugular vein. (3) Air

sinuses, hollow cavities in the skull bones which communicate with the nose. They are the frontal, maxillary, ethmoidal and sphenoidal sinuses. *S. arrythmia*: irregular cardiac rhythm due to the controlling effect of the vagus on the sinoatrial node. The heart rate increases in inspiration and slows during expiration.

sinusitis Inflammation of an air sinus.

sinusoid Like a sinus. Channels for small blood vessels as found in the liver, suprarenal glands, etc.

situs inversus viscerum A developmental anomaly in which there is complete transposition of the organs from right to left and vice versa.

Sjögren's syndrome Syndrome characterized by dry mouth, defective lacrimation and rheumatoid arthritis.

skeleton The bony framework of the body.

Skene's glands These open into the posterior wall of the female urethra, just within the orifice; almost always infected in acute gonorrhoea.

skin Outer covering of the body consisting of epidermis and its appendages (hair, sweat glands) supported by specialized dermal connective tissue.

skull The bony framework of the head.

sleeping sickness (1) Tropical disease due to a trypanosome. The tsetse fly carries the organisms which are transferred to healthy individuals by the bite of the fly. (2) *See* ENCEPHALITIS LETHARGICA.

slough Dead matter thrown off by gangrene or ulcers.

smallpox Variola. A highly infectious disease caused by a virus. Incubation period 12–14 days. Smallpox has been almost eradicated on a world scale by vaccination and enforcement of quarantine regulations.

smegma Thick white secretion forming under the prepuce.

Smith-Petersen nail Inserted to fix the two fragments of bone in a fracture of the neck of the femur.

snare A looped wire instrument for encircling and strangling some piece of tissue which it is desired to remove, *e.g.* a nasal polypus.

Snellen's test types A chart showing letters of different size and used for testing vision. The patient sits at a distance of 6 metres from it. If only the large top letter can be seen the patient's vision is termed 6/60, *i.e.* he can see at 6 metres what the normal eye can see at a distance of 60 metres.

snow blindness Ophthalmia with photophobia caused by the glare from snow.

sodium chloride *See* SALINE.

soft sore A venereal sore not due to syphilis. Also known as chancroid, and non-infecting sore. The causative organism is Ducrey's bacillus.

solar plexus A plexus of nerves and ganglia in the upper region of the abdomen.

soleus A muscle in the calf of the leg.

solution A liquid containing a solid which has been dissolved in it.

solvent A liquid able to dissolve another substance. *S. abuse*: addiction, often at a young age, to substances used in solvents. Includes 'glue sniffing'.

somatic Pertaining to the body.

somnambulism Walking and carrying out other activities while asleep. *Syn.* sleepwalking.

Sonne dysentery Dysentery caused by Shigella sonnei bacteria.

soporific Agent causing sleep.

souffle A soft blowing sound. During late pregnancy the *funic s.* can sometimes be heard by auscultation of the maternal abdomen, a sound synchronous with the fetal heart and supposed to be produced in the umbilical cord. The *uterine s.* is a blowing murmur heard over the uterus due to pulsations in the maternal arteries.

sound A probe-like instrument used for exploring cavities, such as the uterus, bladder, etc.

Southey's tubes Small perforated metal tubes, used to drain oedematous tissue.

spasm (1) Sudden convulsive involuntary movement. (2) Sudden contraction of a muscle or muscles, especially of the unstriped muscle coats of arteries, intestines, heart, bronchi, etc. The effect of such spasm depends on the part affected: thus asthma is believed to be due to spasm of the muscular coats of the smaller bronchi; and renal colic is due to spasm of the muscle coat of the ureter.

spasmolytic Substance which relieves spasm.

spasmus nutans A condition known as nodding spasm in babies, in which the head is continually nodding or turning from side to side.

spastic (1) In a state of spasm. (2) Popular term for cerebral palsy. In patients with this disease the muscles are often spastic, *i.e.* hypertonic, and there is excessive neuromuscular excitability.

spasticity The condition of being spastic. Occurs in upper motor neurone lesions.

spatula (1) A flat, flexible, blunt knife, used for spreading ointments and

poultices. (2) A tongue depressor.

species A group of organisms having many of the same characteristics. In natural history various species form a genus or class of animals.

specific Applied to a medicine or treatment, it means the particular remedy for a certain disease; applied to a disease, it means due to a distinct specific microorganism which causes that disease alone. *S. gravity*: the ratio between the weight of a substance and the weight of an equal volume of water, the latter being taken, as a matter of convenience, to be 1.000. The specific gravity of a liquid depends on the amount of solid in solution.

spectroscope An instrument for the production and examination of spectra in luminous bodies.

spectrum The band of colours formed when rays of white light are passed through a prism.

speculum A polished instrument for examining the interior cavities of the body, especially the vagina, the rectum, the ear, and the nose.

speech The power of speaking; conveying a meaning by vocal sounds. *S. centre*: the part of the brain controlling speech. *S. therapist*: one trained to treat defects and disorders of language, voice and speech.

Spencer–Wells forceps The usual forceps for haemostasis during operations.

sperm *See* SPERMATOZOA.

spermatic cord Composed of arteries, veins, lymphatics and nerves, and the vas deferens, the duct of the testicle; it suspends the testicle from the abdomen.

spermatocele A unilocular retention cyst from some portion of the epididymis.

supermatogenesis The process of formation of sperm. *See* MEIOSIS.

spermatozoa The male generative cells; minute animated cells found in the semen, which are possessed of the power of self-propulsion by means of a flagellum, and which can fertilize the ovum, or female germ cell.

spermicide Substance destroying spermatozoa.

sphenoid Wedge-shaped. The name of one of the bones forming the base of the skull.

sphenoidal Pertaining to the sphenoid bone.

spherocyte A spherical rather than biconcave red blood cell.

spherocytosis Familial disorder of red cell production leading to spherocyte production. Haemolytic anaemia and jaundice result.

sphincter A circular muscle which contracts the orifice of an organ.

sphincterotomy Division of sphincter muscles.

sphygmocardiograph Apparatus recording both pulse and heart beats.

sphygmograph An instrument affixed to the wrist, which moves with the beat of the pulse and registers the rate and character of the beats.

sphygmomanometer An instrument for measuring the arterial tension (blood pressure) of the circulation.

spica A spiral bandage done with a roller in a series of figure eights. Most used for the shoulder, groin, thumb, and great toe.

spicule Fragment of bone.

'spider' naevus (pl. **naevi**) Dilatation of small blood vessels arising from a central arteriole. These may occur in the skin during pregnancy or under oestrogen stimulation. The distribution of the vessels gives the spots the appearance of a spider.

spigot Wooden or plastic peg closing a tube.

spina bifida Malformation due to failure of the neural arch of one or more of the vertebrae to fuse in the midline. As a result the vertebral canals is exposed at this site and may herniate through the opening. *See* MENINGOCELE. The defect most commonly occurs in the lumbosacral region. *S. b occulta*: incomplete closure of the neural arch which may be indicated by a pigmented or hairy patch over the affected part of the spine.

spinal Relating to the spine. *s. analgesia* or *anaesthesia*: infiltration of local anaesthetic agents into the cerebrospinal fluid by means of a lumbar puncture. This procedure results in a block to the nerves below the level of the injection. *S. column*: the backbone. It is composed of seven cervical, twelve thoracic and five lumbar vertebrae and the sacrum with its five fused vertebrae and the coccyx or tailbone. *S. cord*: the portion of the central nervous system within the spine. It contains many nerve cells and bundles of nerve fibres connecting the various levels of the spinal cord with the brain; 31 pairs of nerves form the connections with the peripheral nervous system of the trunk and limbs. *See* also NERVE ROOT. *S. curvature*: the normal curvature of the spine is divided into primary curvature (giving an ape-like stooping posture) and secondary curvatures (cervical and lumbar). For abnormal spinal curvature *See* SCOLIOSIS, KYPHOSIS, LORDOSIS.

spine The backbone or spinal column.

Spirillum Corkscrew-shaped bacteria.

spirochaetaemia The presence of spirochaetes in the blood.

spirochaete Elongated spiral bacteria which move by flexions of the body. Pathogenic spirochaetes cause diseases such as syphilis and Weil's disease.

spirograph Instrument for recording respirations.

spirometer An instrument for measuring the capacity of the lungs.

splanchnic Pertaining to the viscera. *S. nerves*: group of sympathetic nerve fibres which supply the viscera.

splanchnicectomy Surgical removal of the splanchnic ganglia and transection of the splanchnic nerves.

splanchnology The study of the viscera.

splay foot Flatfoot. Pes planus.

spleen A mass of lymphoid tissue situated in the mesentery of the abdomen. Unlike the lymph nodes the spleen acts as a filtration organ for blood. The spleen forms an important part of the reticuloendothelial system and is the generative centre for the formation of many lymphocytes. The spleen is largely responsible for the removal of red blood cells at the end of their lifespan.

splenectomy Removal of the spleen.

splenic anaemia Banti's syndrome. It is characterized by anaemia and splenomegaly associated with portal hypertension due to hepatic cirrhosis.

splenic flexure Bend of the colon on the left side, near the spleen.

spleniculus Name given to accessory spleen, several of which may be present.

splenitis Inflammation of the spleen.

splenomegaly An enlarged spleen.

'splinter' haemorrhages Haemorrhage from longitudinal capillaries in the nail bed giving the appearance of splinters under the nail. Characteristically occur in subacute bacterial endocarditis.

splints Used to immobilize a limb in the case of a fracture, disease or deformity.

spondyle A vertebra.

spondylitis Inflammation of a vertebra or vertebrae. *Ankylosing s.*: condition of unknown origin occurring characteristically in young men and comprising the ossification of spinal ligaments with ankylosis of the cervical and sacroiliac joints.

spondylolisthesis The vertebral arch of the fifth lumbar vertebra gives way so that the body of the affected vertebra becomes displaced.

spondylosis Term used to describe non-specific degenerative changes in the intervertebral discs with peripheral ossification. Known as osteoarthritis of the spine.

spongioblastoma A rapidly growing locally malignant brain tumour.

spontaneous fracture Fracture due to disease affecting the bone, either abnormality of development or rarefaction of the bone from other causes.

sporadic A disease which is not epidemic, but occurs in one or two isolated cases in a district.

spore Reproductive body which gives rise to new individual organism. Produced by protozoa, fungi and bacteria, spores constitute a method of wide dispersal of population and a means of survival through unfavourable conditions. Important spore-forming bacteria are Clostridium welchii and Clostridium botulinum.

sporotrichosis Fungus infection giving rise to intradermal garnulomas.

spotted fever (1) Meningococcal bacteraemia giving rise to meningitis and foci of infection in dermal blood vessels. (2) Rocky Mountain spotted fever is a rickettsial disease transmitted by the dog tick.

sprain Severe strain of a joint without fracture or dislocation, but with swelling and often with effusion into joint; may be associated damage to ligaments.

Sprengel's deformity Congenital upward displacement of the scapula.

sprue A disease of tropical climates which causes inflammation of the mucous membrane of the alimentary canal, characterized by soreness of tongue and mouth, chronic diarrhoea, wasting and anaemia.

spurious pains False labour pains, leading to no result, and sometimes occurring several days before confinement.

sputum Expectorated matter. Different types are: *mucoid s.*, which occurs in the early stage of irritation; *mucopurulent s.*, develops at a later stage, pus is mixed with mucus; *rusty s.*, tenacious sputum, occurs in lobar pneumonia — copious foul-smelling sputum occurs in bronchiectasis; *foaming s.*, occurs in oedema of the lung. Separate pellets or nummular sputum occurs in pulmonary tuberculosis. It may be streaked with blood.

squamous Scaly.

squint *See* STRABISMUS.

staccato or **scanning speech** Hesitation between syllables, and when the sound comes it comes explosively. It is a type of incoordination, and occurs in cerebellar lesions.

stages of labour *See* LABOUR.

stain Coloured compound used to dye tissues for microscopical examination, *e.g.* eosin, haematoxylin.

stamina Vigour. Staying power.

Stanford–Binet test A test of intelligence.

stapedectomy Removal of the stapes.

stapedius A muscle of the middle ear.

stapes One of the three ossicles of the middle ear; stirrup-shaped. *See* EAR.

Staphylococcus Genus of Gram-positive bacteria which grow in clusters in culture (Greek staphyle = bunch of grapes). Many staphs are commensals on the skin. Some are serious pathogens and several strains have evolved which are insensitive to penicillin and other antibiotics.

staphyloma Any protrusion of the sclerotic or corneal coats of the eyeball due to inflammation.

staphylorrhaphy Operation to suture cleft soft palate.

starch Carbohydrate made up of a chain of monosaccharide sugars, *i.e.* a poly-saccharide.

stasis Standing still. Most commonly used for arrest of the circulation of either blood or lymph, but also for intestinal stasis, a holding up of the contents of the bowel.

status asthmaticus Severe asthmatic attack lasting for more than 24 hours.

status epilepticus When a series of major epileptic fits occur without intervening recovery of consciousness the patient is said to be in status epilepticus.

status lymphaticus Sudden death from apparently trivial cause associated with hyperplastic lymphatic tissue. The existence of this syndrome has been disputed.

STD *Abbr.* sexually transmitted disease.

steapsin Lipase.

steatoma Tumour composed of fatty tissue.

steatorrhoea The passage of pale, bulky, offensive stools with a high fat content and which tend to float on water. Often the first symptom of any malabsorption syndrome.

steatosis Fatty degeneration.

Stegomyia Variety of mosquito.

Stein–Leventhal syndrome Syndrome characterized by obesity and hirsutism in women. The ovaries are enlarged with multiple follicular cysts. Amenorrhoea, oligomenorrhoea or anovulatory menstrual cycles may be present. *Syn.* PCOD, polycystic ovarian disease.

Steinmann's pin A fixation pin inserted through a bone in order to apply extension in the case of fractures. *See* EXTENSION.

stellate ganglion Star-shaped sympathetic ganglion situated in the neck. *See* SYMPATHETIC NERVOUS SYSTEM.

stenosis Contraction of a canal or an orifice.

Stensen's duct The duct of the parotid salivary gland, the opening of which is opposite the upper first molar tooth.

stercobilin The colouring matter of the faeces. It is derived from bile pigment.

stercolith Faecolith. Compacted mass of faeces.

stereognosis Recognition of the form of objects by handling them.

sterile Barren; unable to have children. In surgical practice, sterile means entirely free from germs of all kinds, a result brought about by heat or by antiseptic chemicals or by ionizing radiation.

sterility The condition of being sterile.

sterilization (1) Made incapable of progeny, *e.g.* by removal of ovaries, tying the fallopian tubes, hysterectomy or, in the male, vasectomy or tying the vas deferens. (2) Rendering germ-free.

sternal puncture Technique employed to obtain sample of red bone marrow for investigation. A needle is inserted into the sternum under local anaesthesia, and a small amount of the marrow aspirated.

sternomastoid muscle Muscle of neck, running from the inner end of the clavicle and upper border of the sternum to behind the ear. *See* TORTICOLLIS.

sternomastoid tumour Swelling in sternomastoid muscle found in neonates and associated with torticollis.

sternum The breastbone.

steroids A group of substances with a common basic structure. Slight differences in the chemical configuration produce greatly divergent biological effects, *e.g. see* ADRENAL CORTEX.

sterols Steroids with an alcohol (−OH) side group, *e.g.* cortisol (= hydrocortisone).

stertor Snoring type of respiration.

stethoscope Instrument for listening to sounds, *e.g.* heart sounds, respiratory sounds.

Stevens–Johnson syndrome Severe form of erythema multiforme in which mucous membranes may be extensively involved.

sthenic Strong, active.

stigma (pl. **stigmata**) Mark on the skin. Also any permanent condition indicative of some constitutional peculiarity.

stilette A sharp probe.

stillborn Any baby born dead after more than 28 weeks gestation.

Still's disease A form of rheumatoid arthritis occurring in children. The syndrome is characterized by polyarthritis, lymphadenopathy and splenomegaly.

stimulant Substance causing an increase in the activity of living material.

stimulus An agent provoking activity.

stitch (1) Suture. (2) Pain in the side due to spasm of the diaphragm.

Stokes–Adams syndrome Syncope due to cerebral hypoxia resulting from heartblock.

stoma (1) Normal body opening *e.g.* mouth. (2) Artificial opening *e.g.* colostomy.

stomach The dilated portion of the intestinal canal into which the food passes from the oesophagus, and where it undergoes partial digestion. *S. pump*: apparatus used to aspirate the contents of the stomach.

stomatitis Inflammation of the mouth.

stone (1) A measure of

weight, 14 lb (6.3 kg). (2) A concretion.

stools Discharge of faeces from the bowels.

strabismus Squint; divergent when the eye turns out, convergent when it turns in.

strain (1) To filter. (2) Condition resulting from unsuitable use of a part.

strangulated Constricted, so that the blood supply is cut off. *See* HERNIA.

strangury Painful micturition.

strapping Material used to bind up injuries.

stratified In layers.

stratum A layer.

Streptococcus Genus of Gram-positive bacteria which grow in chains. Pathogenic cocci produce toxins responsible for scarlet fever, rheumatic fever and acute glomerulonephritis.

stress incontinence Incontinence of urine or faeces when the intra-abdominal pressure is raised as in coughing or sneezing, etc.

striae gravidarum Lineae albicantes. Scars on the abdomen and thighs due to stretching of the dermis during rapid expansion of the abdomen. Frequently this is seen in association with pregnancy (stretch marks).

striated muscle Striped voluntary muscle; *cf.* smooth muscle.

stricture Contraction. Usually applied to the urethra, with consequent inability to pass urine.

stridor A harsh sound during breathing, caused by obstruction to the passage of air.

stroke Cerebrovascular accident. *See also* HEATSTROKE.

stroma The connective tissue.

Stryker bed Bed designed to allow rotation of patient without painful or dangerous handling, *e.g.* for spinal injuries or burns.

stupor State of unconsciousness.

Sturge–Weber syndrome Syndrome characterized by capillary naevus on the face in the distribution of the fifth cranial nerve associated with angiomas of the cerebral cortex which may cause focal epilepsy, hemiparesis and mental deficiency.

stye Suppuration around an eyelash follicle.

styptic Agent which arrests bleeding.

sub A prefix denoting beneath or under (Latin).

subacute Less than acute, *i.e.* fairly gradual onset; *cf.* chronic, long in duration. *S. bacterial endocarditis.* Bacterial colonization of defective heart valves with consequent bacteraemia and distribution of septic emboli throughout the body. *S. combined* *degeneration of the cord*: degeneration of the posterior and lateral columns of the spinal cord due to vitamin B_{12} deficiency.

subarachnoid haemorrhage Haemorrhage into the subarachnoid space.

subarachnoid space The space between the arachnoid membrane and the pia mater. It contains cerebrospinal fluid.

subclavian Under the clavicle: thus the subclavian artery and vein are vessels passing under the clavicle.

subclinical Without any obvious signs of the disease.

subconscious Thought processes which occur without the awareness of the individual, *i.e.* he is unconscious of these processes (equals unconscious 'mind'). It must be assumed that most of the neuronal activity in the central nervous system is subconscious. Only some of the products of nerve activity reach awareness. This consciousness of thought is probably a quantitative measure of the number of neurons conducting complementary impulses. The mechanism of 'awareness' is, however, a philosophical problem.

subcutaneous Under the skin.

subinvolution Failure of involution of the uterus after delivery.

subjacent Lying below.

subjective Internal: pertaining to one's self.

subliminal Below the threshold.

sublingual Under the tongue.

subluxation Less than dislocated, *i.e.* partial dislocation.

submandibular Beneath the mandible.

submaxillary Beneath the maxilla.

submucous Beneath a mucous membrane.

subnormal Below normal.

subphrenic Under the diaphragm. *S. abscess*: a collection of pus beneath the diaphragm.

substrate Compound on which an enzyme acts.

subtotal hysterectomy The removal of the uterus, excluding the cervix. Now rarely performed.

succenturiate lobe An extra lobe of the placenta.

succus entericus The digestive juice secreted by the glands in the small intestine.

succussion Sound made on shaking a patient if fluid is present in a hollow cavity.

sudamina Sweat rash.

sudden infant death syndrome (SIDS) *See* COT DEATH.

sudorific An agent causing perspiration.

suffused Congested. Bloodshot.

suggestibility A state when the patient readily accepts

other people's ideas and influences.

suicide To kill oneself.

sulcus A furrow.

sulphonamides A group of drugs which have bacteriostatic properties used in the treatment of certain infections.

sunstroke *See* HEATSTROKE.

superciliary Having to do with the eyebrows.

supercilium The eyebrow.

superego A Freudian term. Control from within of instinctive acts such as aggression. Possibly the adoption of parental attitudes taught in childhood.

superfecundation The fertilization of two ova discharged at the same ovulation by two distinct acts of insemination effected at a short interval.

superfetation Condition of doubtful authenticity in which twins are derived from separate ovulations and separate acts of coitus during different intermenstrual periods.

superior Above. The upper of two organs.

superovulation Use of gonadotrophin in high dose to intentionally stimulate ripening of large numbers of ovarian follicles to maximize oocyte numbers available for IVF or GIFT.

supination Turning the palm of the hand upwards.

supine Lying face upwards; in the case of the forearm, having the palm uppermost.

suppository Rectally administered cones containing a medicament in a base which is soluble at body temperature.

suppression To prevent some activity, *e.g.* glandular secretion, cough, etc.

suppuration The formation of pus.

supraorbital Above the orbit.

suprapubic Above the pubes.

suprarenal Above the kidney. *S. glands*: *see* ADRENAL GLANDS.

sural Relating to the calf of the leg.

surface The outer part. *S. markings*: lines drawn on the skin to show the position of structures beneath it.

surfactant The phospholipids, mainly lecithin, that reduce the surface tension exerted by fluid in the neonatal bronchial tree and allow expansion at the first breath. Deficiency is associated with respiratory distress syndrome.

surgery (1) The part of medicine concerned with diseases needing treatment by operation. (2) A physician or surgeon's consulting room.

surgical Pertaining to surgery. *S. emphysema*: air or gas in connective tissue introduced via a break in a viscus or by a surgical manoeuvre.

susceptible Liable to, *e.g.* infection.

suspension (1) Hanging. (2) Undissolved particles dispersed in a liquid.

suspensory bandage A bandage to support the testicles.

sutures (1) Silk, thread, catgut, nylon, etc., used to sew a wound. (2) The union of flat bones by their margins, *e.g.* bones of the skull.

swabs Small pieces of wool, gauze over wool, or gauze only, used for cleansing wounds and for removing blood at operations.

sweat Perspiration. The fluid secreted on to the skin by the sweat glands.

sycosis barbae Inflammation of the hair follicles especially of the beard and whiskers.

symbiosis The living together of two organisms, whose mutual association is necessary to each, although neither is parasitic on the other.

symblepharon Adhesion of the eyelids to the eyeball.

Syme's amputation Amputation through the ankle joint.

sympathectomy Surgical transection of sympathetic nerves usually with excision of part of the sympathetic chain.

sympathetic nervous system Part of the autonomic nervous system. The preganglionic fibres leave the spinal cord between segments T_1–T_2 and synapse in the various ganglia. The postganglionic fibres are unmyelinated. Some sympathetic fibres leave the CNS in the cranial nerves.

symphysiotomy The operation of dividing the symphysis pubis (of the mother) so as to facilitate delivery in certain cases of contracted pelvis.

symphysis Growing of bones together. The *s. pubis* is the bony mass bounding the front of the pelvis, at the lower end of the abdomen. *See* PELVIS.

symptom A noticeable change in the body and its functions, evidence of disease. Usually meaning the change complained of by the patient.

symptomatology A study of the symptoms of disease.

synapse Region where nerve cells communicate. There is no continuity between the neurons and impulses are transmitted from one nerve cell to another by the passage of chemical messengers which stimulate the postsynaptic nerve cell.

synarthrosis Immovable union of bones, *e.g.* the cranial bones.

synchondrosis A joint whose surfaces are united by cartilage.

syncope Transient loss of consciousness.

syndactyly   Webbed fingers.

syndrome   Collection of symptoms and/or signs which comprise a recognizable pattern of disease.

synechia   Adhesion of the iris to the cornea, or to the crystalline lens.

synergy   The working together of two or more agents.

synonyms   Different words having the same meaning.

synovectomy   Operation to remove synovial membrane.

synovial fluid   The liquid which lubricates the joints.

synovial membrane   That lining a joint cavity but not covering the articular surfaces.

synovitis   Inflammation of the synovial membrane of a joint.

synthesis   The building up of complex substances by the union and interaction of simpler materials.

synthetic   Pertaining to synthesis. Artificial.

syphilide   Lesion of the skin due to syphilis. May be papular, macular, squamous, etc.

syphilis   One of the sexually transmitted diseases. Now rarely seen. Caused by a specific spirochaete. *Treponema pallidum. S.* may be congenital or acquired. *Congenital s.* may be inherited from the mother. The chief symptoms in young babies: wasting, snuffles, rashes, enlargement of liver and spleen. If the child survives, he/she may later show pallor, malnutrition, depressed bridge of nose, rhagades, square skull, thickening of tibiae, corneal opacities, Hutchinson's teeth. *See* RHAGADES, HUTCHINSON'S TEETH. *Acquired s.* is divided into three stages. (1) First stage or *primary s.* with local symptoms, 2–3 weeks after infection. Hard chancre on penis, vulva, or cervix. Inflamed glands in groin. Lesions infective, *see* CHANCRE, (2) Second stage or *secondary s.*, 1–2 months after infection, with rashes, sore throat, mucous patches, condylomata, general enlargement of glands, anaemia and fever. Infective, *see* CONDYLOMA. (3) Third stage or *tertiary s.*, 2–10 years, or even longer after infection. Non-infective. Manifestations, include gummata, tabes, GPI. *See* GENERAL PARALYSIS OF THE INSANE.

syringe   An instrument for injecting fluids, or for exploring and aspirating cavities.

syringomyelia   Progressive degenerative disease affecting the brain stem and spinal cord in which the tracts of fibres subserving pain and temperature are mainly affected.

syringomyelocele   Form of myelocele in which there is a communication between the mass and the canal of the spinal cord.

system An organized scheme. A series of parts concerned in a basis function such as nutrition by the alimentary system.

systemic Affecting the whole body. *S. lupus erythematosus*: one of the so-called 'collagen diseases'. *See* LUPUS ERYTHEMATOSUS.

systole The period when the heart contracts. *See* DIASTOLE.

systolic blood pressure Upper limit of arterial blood pressure, *cf.* diastolic pressure.

systolic murmur Adventitious sound heard during systole.

T

TAB *Abbr.* triple vaccine to prevent typhoid, paratyphoid A and paratyphoid B.

T bandage A special bandage used for keeping dressing on the perineum.

tabes Wasting. *T. dorsalis* (locomotor ataxia): syphilis affecting the posterior columns of the spinal cord which carry the sensory fibres from the trunk and limb. Sometimes it is associated with general paralysis of the insane (GPI) when the syndrome is known as taboparesis. *T. mesenterica*: tuberculosis of peritoneal glands.

tachycardia Increased heart rate.

tactile Relating to touch.

Taenia Tapeworm. *T. solium, t. saginata* and *t. echinococcus* are parasitic to man.

talc French chalk. Used as dusting powder.

talipes Clubfoot. Term used to cover a group of foot deformities in which the sole of the foot is no longer plantigrade. The term talipes is qualified by four adjectives which describe the elements of the deformity: equinus, valgus, varus and calcaneus. The commonest deformities are *t. equinovarus* and *t. calcaneovalgus*.

talus The ankle.

tampon A plug of wool or gauze introduced into the vagina, used by women during menstruation.

tamponade Compression. Usually *cardiac t.* in which the action of the heart is impeded by the presence of fluid in the pericardium.

tantalum A resistant metal sometimes used in bone surgery for plates or wire.

tapeworm *See* TAENIA.

tapping *See* ASPIRATION.

tar Dark liquid obtained from pinewood. It has antipyretic and antiseptic properties. *Coal t.*: black liquid distilled from coal. It contains benzene, phenol, cresols, naphthalene, etc.

target cell Erythrocyte with dark central area and dark peripheral ring, seen in forms of anaemia.

tarsal Bones of the ankle. There are seven in man forming a group which articulate with the tibia and fibula and the metatarsal bones.

tarsalgia Pain in the foot.

tarsectomy Excision of part of the tarsal group of bones.

tarsoplasty Plastic surgery of the eyelid.

tarsorrhaphy Stitching the eyelids together.

tarsus (1) The seven small bones of the foot. (2) The cartilaginous framework of the eyelid.

tartar Deposit on the teeth of calcium salts derived from saliva.

taste bud Specialized sensory end organ, situated on the tongue and oral mucosa, which is sensitive to taste.

taurocholic acid One of the bile acids.

taxis Locomotion of an organism or a cell in response to a directional stimulus, *cf.* kinesis.

Tay–Sachs' disease Amaurotic familial idiocy. Degenerative disease of infancy affecting the brain and optic nerves. Most commonly found in Ashkenazi Jews and may be inherited by a recessive gene.

TBI *Abbr.* total body irradiation.

tears Secretion of the lacrimal gland.

tease To divide a tissue into shreds.

teat Nipple.

technique Method.

teeth Teeth are derived from ectodermal buds. There are two dentitions in man: primary dentition (milk teeth, temporary teeth, deciduous teeth) which erupt in the first two years of life; and secondary dentition (permanent teeth) which erupt from about the sixth year onwards with corresponding shedding of the primary teeth. Each tooth is composed of dentine which is surrounded by a material known as 'cement' except the erupted portion which is covered by a hard material called 'enamel'. The blood supply and nerve supply of the tooth is contained in the central pulp cavity.

tegument The skin.

tela Tissue formed like a web.

telangiectasis, talangioma Lesion consisting of a number of tortuous dilated capillaries which have a web-like appearance.

telemetry Physiological monitoring at a distance using radio transmission of signals to a recording display unit.

Used to monitor fetal or adult heart rate in ambulant patients.

telepathy The transference of thought from one person to another. There is considerable doubt as to whether this is possible and the question is under investigation.

teletherapy Radiotherapy using cobalt or caesium, the application of which can be controlled at a distance.

temper tantrums Behaviour disorder in children. Particularly common around the age of two years.

temperament A person's mental outlook.

temperature A measurement of the degree of heat. The average normal temperature of the human body is 37°C (98.4°F). The average temperature of a sick-room should be about 16°C (65°F).

temples The part of the forehead between the outer corner of the eye and the hair.

temporal Relating to the temple. Thus *t. artery, t. bone, t. lobe* of the brain.

temporal arteritis Giant cell arteritis. A disease of unknown aetiology characterized by general malaise, aches and muscle pains and acute inflammation of the arteries, particularly those of the scalp. A cause of unilateral blindness.

temporomandibular joint syndrome Pain on jaw movement resulting from poor dental occlusion.

tendinitis Inflammation of a tendon.

tendo Achilles The stout tendon of the calf muscles at the back of the heel.

tendon A sinew, a cord of fibrous white tissue by which a muscle is attached to a bone or other structure.

tenesmus Painful straining to empty the bowel. May be a symptom of a neoplasm in the rectum.

tennis elbow Painful disorder affecting the fibres by which the extensor muscles of the forearm are attached to the external epicondyle. The precise nature of the disorder is not known.

tenoplasty Plastic surgery to a tendon.

tenorrhaphy Operation to suture a tendon.

tenosynovitis Inflammation in the sheath of a tendon. *Syn.* repetitive strain injury.

tenotomy Cutting a tendon.

tension The act of stretching.

tensor A muscle which stretches.

tent *Intracervical t.*: a device used to induce dilatation by gradual expansion and/or chemical means. *Oxygen t.*: enclosure in which the patient is surrounded by an atmosphere of high oxygen content.

Steam t.: tent erected around a bed to provide a moist atmosphere. Screens and an old sheet or blanket are used. Steam is directed inside from a kettle. Temperature of tent, 21°C (70°F).

tentorium cerebelli The part of the dura mater which separates the cerebral spheres from the cerebellum.

tepid Just warm.

teratogen Agent inducing fetal malformation.

teratoma A neoplasm arising from totipotent cells, *i.e.* cells which like the cells of an early embryo possess the ability to differentiate into all the components of the body. The origin of these cells is disputed. An example of a teratoma is a 'dermoid' tumour which may contain hair, muscle, teeth, glandular structures, etc.

teres Round and smooth. *Ligamentum t.*: ligament of the head of the femur.

terminology Nomenclature.

tertian *See* MALARIA.

tertiary syphilis *See* SYPHILIS.

test (1) Trial. (2) A reaction distinguishing one substance from another.

test tube baby Popular term for infant conceived with in vitro fertilization (IVF).

testicles The testes.

testis (pl. testes) Organ whch produces spermatozoa.

testosterone A steroid hormone with androgenic properties. *See* ANDROGEN. Probably the principal sex hormone secreted by the testes.

tetanus Lockjaw. Disease caused by Clostridium tetani characterized by rigidity and spasm of the muscles. The causative organism is anaerobic and thrives in wounds contaminated by soil or road dust containing the spores. A powerful toxin is produced by the Clostridium which reaches the spinal cord by retrograde spread up the motor nerves, and is responsible for the clinical features. Infants usually have a course of immunization against tetanus and a booster dose can be given after an accident.

tetany A condition marked by spasm of the extremities, particularly of hands and feet (carpedal spasm) due to faulty calcium metabolism. It may be due to dysfunction of the parathyroid glands, alkalosis, rickets.

tetracyclines Group of chemically related antibiotics which include Aureomycin (chlortetracycline), Terramycin (oxytetracycline) and Achromycin (tetracycline hydrochloride), etc.

tetradactylous Having only four digits on each limb.

tetralogy of Fallot *See* FALLOT'S TETRALOGY.

tetraplegia Paralysis of all four limbs.

thalamus Collection of neurons in the forebrain which serves as a major coordinating region for sensory information.

thalassaemia Genetically determined abnormality in which there is continued production of fetal haemoglobin. The clinical features are those of haemolytic anaemia. Two forms are recognized; one in which the condition is homozygous (*t. major*), and the other heterozygous (*t. minor*). The latter is generally symptomless.

thalidomide Non-barbiturate sedative found to induce fetal malformations if taken by pregnant women.

theca A sheath. Examples are the meninges of the spinal cord, and the synovial sheaths of the flexor tendons of the fingers.

thecoma Benign tumour of ovarian theca mainly fibromatous, but includes fatty and sometimes epithelial elements.

thenar Relating to the palm of the hand at the base of the thumb.

theory Logical principles relating to a subject.

therapeutics Branch of medicine which deals with treatment.

thermography Study of temperature variations in parts of the body by scanning infraradiations emitted by skin. Used to detect vascular disorders and tumours of soft tissues such as the breast.

thermolabile Describing a substance which undergoes change with temperature.

thermometer An instrument used to record variations of temperature. *Clinical t.*: a small thermometer used for taking the temperature of the body. It is graduated from 35°C (95°F) to 43.5°C (110°F). It is made so that the mercury does not fall when the thermometer is taken from the patient. After the temperature has been recorded the mercury is shaken down. *Low reading t.*; necessary for detecting hypothermia. *See* TEMPERATURE.

thermophilic Describing an organism which flourishes at high temperatures.

thermostat Apparatus which is made to regulate heat automatically.

thesaurosis A sarcoidosis-like condition with inflammation resulting from hairspray aspiration.

thiamine Aneurine, vitamin B_1, thiamine diphosphate (cocarboxylase) is an important coenzyme concerned in carbohydrate metabolism. Thiamine deficiency causes beriberi.

Thiersch Type of skin graft in which the epidermis and upper part of the dermis are employed.

thigh Part of the lower limb above the knee.

Thomas splint (1) Knee splint for immobilizing a fractured femur or tibia and fibula. It consists of two sidepieces of metal with a crosspiece at foot, and an oblique ring for fixation in groin. Leg is kept in position by pieces of material slung between sidepieces and adjusted to the fracture. (2) Hip splint used for immobilization of the hip.

thoracic Pertaining to the thorax. *T. duct*: the largest lymphatic vessel. It receives the fat absorbed from the intestine and the lymph from the greater part of the body. It ascends from the abdomen through the thorax to the left side of the neck, where it empties itself into the angle of union between the left internal jugular vein and the subclavian vein.

thoracocentesis Puncture of the thorax, *e.g.* aspiration of pleural effusion.

thoracolysis The severing of adhesions between the two layers of the pleura.

thoracoplasty Operation in which part of the chest wall is resected in order to collapse the underlying lung. Formerly used in the treatment of tuberculosis.

thoracoscopy Endoscopy of the pleural cavity.

thoracotomy Operation of opening the thorax.

thorax The chest; the cavity which holds the heart and lungs.

threadworm Oxyuris vermicularis. Small worm parasitic in the rectum; common in children.

threonine An amino acid.

thrill A vibratory impulse perceived by palpation.

thrombectomy Removal of a blood clot.

thrombin Essential factor required in the blood clotting mechanism. *See* BLOOD COAGULATION.

thromboangiitis Inflamed blood vessel with formation of a blood clot. *T. obliterans*: inflammatory, obliterative disease of the blood vessels, especially in the limbs.

thromboarteritis Arteritis with thrombosis.

thrombocytes Blood platelets.

thrombocytopenia Deficiency of platelets in the blood. *See* IMMUNE THROMBOCYTOPENIC PURPURA.

thromboendarterectomy Operation to remove a clot from a blood vessel.

thrombokinase *See* THROMBOPLASTIN.

thrombolytic An agency which breaks down clots.

thrombophlebitis Inflammation of a vein with thrombosis. *T. migrans*: recurrent thrombophlebitis affecting superficial veins in different sites. There is sometimes an association with carcinoma of the pancreas or stomach.

thromboplastin An enzyme converting prothrombin to thrombin in the clotting mechanism. May be derived from many tissues and from platelets.

thrombosis Coagulation of blood in the vessels. The clot thus formed is termed a *thrombus*.

thrombus (pl. thrombi) A clot of blood found in the heart or in a blood vessel.

thrush Infection of mucous membrane, *e.g.* mouth or vagina, by Candida albicans. This fungus infection gives rise to white patches on the membrane.

thymectomy Operation to remove the thymus gland. Sometimes performed for myasthenia gravis.

thymocytes Lymphocytes in the cortex of the thymus gland.

thymoma Malignant neoplasm of the thymus.

thymus A gland at the root of the neck; it is situated in the anterior mediastinum, is largest in children, reaches its maximum size in puberty and thereafter slowly atrophies.

The function of the thymus is not clear. It appears to be concerned with the immunological mechanisms of the body. It has been suggested that it acts as a 'priming station' for lymphocytes where they are selected for release into the general circulation. At the present time its function is uncertain.

thyroglossal cyst Cyst in the thyroglossal duct which is the embryonic canal formed by the migration of the presumptive thyroid cells from the surface of the tongue.

thyroid cartilage The large cartilage of the larynx forming the 'Adam's apple'.

thyroid crisis Acute severe thyrotoxicosis which may follow subtotal thyroidectomy in the absence of preoperative antithyroid treatment.

thyroid gland A bilobed ductless gland lying in front of the trachea. Its secretion, thyroxine, controls metabolism, growth and development. Congenital lack causes cretinism. Undersecretion in later life causes myxoedema. Excessive secretion causes thyrotoxicosis.

thyroidectomy Operative removal of the thyroid gland.

thyrotoxicosis Hyperthyroidism, syndrome due to an excessive production of thyroid hormone which has the effect of uncoupling oxidative phosphorylation, *i.e.* reducing the production of ATP by oxidative metabolism, in the cells. As a result the metabolic rate is speeded up in an attempt to maintain the yield of ATP. Clinically, hyperthyroidism is characterized by tachycardia, sweating, tremor, weight loss and increased appetite. Hyperthyroidism may be primary when the thyroid is at fault, or secondary when there is excessive stimulation of the thyroid by TSH from the pituitary. Recently a gammaglobulin with thyroid stimulatory properties has been identified and is known as long-acting thyroid stimulant (LATS) which is considered to be the cause of the exophthalmos often associated with hyperthyroidism.

thyrotrophic Stimulating the thyroid. *T. hormone* is produced by the pituitary.

thyroxine The active principle of the secretion of the thyroid gland. A substance rich in iodine.

TIA *Abbr.* transient ischaemic attacks.

tibia The shin bone; the larger bone of the leg below the knee. *See* SKELETON.

tic Spasmodic twitching of muscles, usually of face and neck. *T. douloureux*: trigeminal neuralgia.

tick A bloodsucking parasite.

T. fever: (1) Relapsing fever. (2) Rocky Mountain fever, a rickettsial fever.

tidal air That which is inspired and expired during normal breathing.

Tietze syndrome A self-limiting costochondritis of unknown origin.

tincture An alcoholic solution of a drug.

tinea Ringworm.

tinnitus aureum A ringing in the ears.

tissue An aggregate of similar cells performing a similar function. *T. culture*: method by which cells and tissues are grown under artificial conditions after their removal from the parent organism.

titration Quantitative analysis by volume by means of standard solutions.

titre A standard of purity or strength.

TMJ *Abbr.* temporomandibular joint syndrome.

tocography Method of recording alterations in the intrauterine pressure.

tocopherol Vitamin E. Its precise function is unknown but it is widely used as an antioxidant in medical preparations.

tolerance Ability to tolerate a substance. Usually applied to (1) *immunological t.*, in which there is no immunological reaction to a potential antigen; or (2) *t. to drugs, e.g.* barbiturates, morphine, etc. when the dose requires to be increased to achieve the same effect. The mechanism of this is not clear but it has been suggested that there is an increased synthesis of the enzymes responsible for the breakdown of the drug.

tomography Technique in radiography which brings into focus only those objects lying in the plane of interest, while blurring structures on either side of the object's plane; also known as body section radiography.

tone (1) State of tension as found in muscles. (2) Quality of sound.

tongue The muscular organ which lies in the floor of the mouth, and whose chief functions are to assist in the mastication and tasting of food and vocalization. *T. tie*: extremely rare condition in which the tongue is rendered immobile by adhesions to the floor of the mouth. Minor degrees of tongue tie are common and not a cause for delayed speech.

tonic (1) A traditional medicine which was thought to increase general physical wellbeing after an illness. (2) Term applied to continuous spasms; *cf.* clonic.

tonometer Instrument for measuring tension, *e.g.* intraocular.

tonsillectomy Operative removal of the tonsils.

tonsillitis Inflammation of tonsils.

tonsillotome Instrument for cutting off a tonsil.

tonsils Two oval bodies of lymphoid tissue on either side of the throat at the opening of the pharynx.

toothed Dentate. Possessing teeth.

tophus (pl. **tophi**) Concretion of uric acid salts found on the ear lobes or interpharyngeal joints characteristic of gout.

topical Pertaining to a particular locality. Local.

topography A study of the various areas of the body.

torpor Lethargy.

torsion Twisting.

torso The trunk.

torticollis Wryneck. The head is flexed and drawn to one side as the result of contraction of the sternomastoid muscles either due to spasm or fibrosis in the body of the muscle.

total body irradiation (TBI) Radiotherapy applied to the whole body, *e.g.* to treat marrow malignancy.

tourniquet An instrument used to exert pressure on an artery and so arrest bleeding.

toxaemia Toxins in the circulation. *See also* PRE-ECLAMPSIA, PRE-ECLAMPTIC TOXAEMIA.

toxic Poisonous. *T. shock*

syndrome: fever, malaise and diarrhoea thought to be due to absorption of toxins from the vagina in women using tampons.

toxicology The study of poisons.

toxicosis Any disease due to poisoning.

toxin A poison, usually of bacterial origin.

toxoid A non-poisonous modification of a toxin. Sometimes used to immunize against disease. *T. antitoxin*: a mixture of toxoid and its antitoxin.

toxoplasmosis Infection by Toxoplasma gondii. The clinical manifestations vary in severity. In infants severe encephalitis may occur. Other results of infection include nephritis, pneumonia, rashes and lymphadenopathy.

trabecula A septum extending into an organ from its capsule or wall.

trabeculotomy An operation for glaucoma.

trace elements Mineral substances whose presence in minute amounts in the diet is necessary for the maintenance of health, *e.g.* cobalt, copper, manganese, etc.

tracer Radioactive isotope or substance containing a radioactive isotope which enables the substance to be traced in metabolic systems.

trachea The windpipe; the air passage from the larynx to the bronchi. *See* BRONCHI.

tracheitis Inflammation of the trachea.

trachelorrhaphy The operation of suturing a torn cervix uteri.

tracheobronchitis Inflammation of trachea and bronchi.

tracheostomy Incision into the trachea to provide an accessory airway.

tracheotomy Incision of the trachea.

trachoma Conjunctivitis due to Chlamydia trachomatis which untreated results in blindness.

traction Pulling, as for example in traction of a limb to facilitate correct apposition.

tragus The small eminence just inside the ear.

trait A special characteristic of the individual.

trance State of unnatural sleep; catalepsy.

tranquillizer Drug with sedative and tranquillizing action, such as chlorpromazine. Used to relieve anxiety, tension and agitation in mental illness. May be useful in the control of pain during a terminal illness. While the patient is taking this drug, the action of a hypnotic or analgesic is made more powerful.

transabdominal Through the abdomen.

transaminase Enzyme which

transfers amino(–NH$_2$) groups from one substance to another. Enzymes of this type are liberated into the bloodstream from damaged cells, particularly muscle cells, and the estimation of the *serum ts* (glutamic-oxaloacetic transaminase or GOT and glutamic-pyruvic transaminase or GPT) is sometimes helpful in the diagnosis of conditions in which there is muscle damage, *e.g.* myocardial infarction, dermatomyositis, etc.

transference A psychoanalytical term. The patient transfers his own emotions on to the analyst, *e.g.* he may develop an intense love or hatred of him. Also used if the patient transfers his own emotions on to someone else as when he blames someone else for what he has done himself.

transfusion *See* BLOOD TRANSFUSION.

transillumination The method whereby suppuration in the maxillary or frontal sinus is detected. The patient is placed in a completely darkened room, and a bright light placed in the mouth. The affected side is not so highly illuminated as the sound side.

transmigration The passage of cells through a membrane.

transperitoneal Through the peritoneum.

transplant Term generally

used for surgery to replace a diseased organ such as a kidney, lung or heart with a healthy one from a dead person, living relative or possibly an animal.

transplantation Operation to remove a portion of tissue from one part of the body to another.

transposition of vessels Defect of development in which the pulmonary artery arises from the left ventricle and the aorta from the right ventricle.

transudation Oozing of fluid through a membrane or from a tissue.

transurethral Via the urethra.

transverse Across. A transverse incision is from side to side. *T. process*: lateral projection of the neural arch of a vertebra with which the head of a rib articulates.

transvestism Psychiatric condition in which there exists an anomaly of instinct. The patient wears the clothes characteristic of the opposite sex. Transvestites may identify themselves completely with the opposite sex and develop delusional convictions of this kind.

trapezium First bone in the second row of the carpal bones.

trapezius A large muscle, running from the nape of the neck and the upper part of the spine, to the clavicle and scapula.

trapezoid Second bone in second row of the carpal bones.

trauma Injury.

Trematoda Parasites which affect man, causing bilharzia.

tremor Involuntary trembling.

Trendelenburg's operation Used to treat varicose veins. The long saphenous vein is ligated in the groin.

Trendelenburg's position Operation position with patient supine tilted with the head down.

Trendelenburg's sign Test of the ability of the abductor muscles of the hip to steady the pelvis when one leg is raised from the ground.

trephining Removing a circular piece of tissue to gain access to the enclosed structure, *e.g.* trephining the bone of the skull.

Treponema pallidum The infecting agent of syphilis.

trial of labour Attempt to achieve spontaneous delivery in any case where there is doubt about a normal delivery; always done in hospital where there may be speedy intervention if necessary.

triangular bandage Made by cutting a 90 cm square of linen diagonally across. It is very useful in emergencies and for minor casualties.

triceps Certain muscles with three heads, especially the one at the back of the arm which extends to the elbow.

trichiasis Inversion of the eyelashes towards the eye.

trichinosis Infection with a parasitic worm, Trichina spiralis, which is parasitic in pigs and sometimes in man.

Trichocephalus dispar The whipworm. A parasite of the human large intestine.

Trichomonas vaginalis A protozoon, motile by means of flagellae. It is a common cause of vaginitis.

trichonosis Abnormality of hair.

trichophytosis fungal infection of the hair.

Trichuris Type of threadworm.

tricuspid valve Valve with three cusps, particularly the heart valve between the right atrium and right ventricle.

trigeminal Triple. *T. nerves*: fifth pair of cranial nerves. They are motor and sensory and each has three branches supplying the skin and structures of the face, tongue and teeth. *T. neuralgia*: pain in the face of unknown cause. The distribution is confined to branches of the trigeminal nerve. The pain is paroxysmal and precipitated by mild stimuli such as washing the face or eating. *See also* TIC DOULOUREUX.

trigger finger A thickening of

the tendon sheath at the metacarpophalangeal joint often of the first finger of the right hand. The finger can be bent but not straightened without help.

trigone A triangle. *T. vesicae*: triangular space in the bladder, immediately behind the opening to the urethra.

trimester A three-month period.

triplegia Paralysis of three limbs.

triplets Three children resulting from one pregnancy.

triploid Having three times the haploid number of chromosomes in a nucleus.

trismus Lockjaw. Occurs as a reflex in dental caries. Is also a symptom of tetanus.

trisomy Presence of additional somatic chromosomes.

trocar The perforating instrument used with a cannula to draw off fluids from the body.

trochanter Two processes at the junction of the neck and shaft of femur.

trochlear (1) Relating to a pulley. (2) Relating to the trochlear nerve. *T. nerves*: the fourth pair of cranial nerves. Motor nerves to the eyes.

trophic Relating to nutrition. *T. ulcers* occur where nutrition is poor, particularly if there is paralysis.

trophoblast The outer ecto-

dermal layer of the embedding ovum.

trophoblastic disease Placental neoplasia. *See* MOLE, HYDATIDIFORM.

Trousseau's sign Sign of increased nervous excitability due to hypocalcaemia. A sphygmomanometer cuff is inflated above the patient's systolic blood pressure for three minutes. Spasm in the flexor muscles produces the classical main d'accoucheur.

trunk The torso.

truss An apparatus for retaining a hernia in place.

trypanosoma A genus of microscopic parasites which cause sleeping sickness and other diseases.

trypanosomiasis Infection with trypanosomes.

trypsin A peptidase, which breaks down proteins and peptides at certain peptide links.

trypsinogen A precursor of trypsin.

tryptophan An essential amino acid.

tsetse fly Genus of dipteran insects which are carriers of trypanosome diseases such as sleeping sickness.

tubal Relating to a tube, and especially to an oviduct. *T. gestation* or *pregnancy*: pregnancy in a fallopian tube. *See* ECTOPIC PREGNANCY.

tubercle (1) A small eminence. (2) The small greyish

nodule which is the specific lesion of the tubercle bacillus.

tuberculide Any skin rash due to tuberculous infection.

tuberculin A preparation from cultures of the tubercle bacillus used in diagnosis of tuberculosis.

tuberculoma Walled-off region of caseating tuberculosis.

tuberculosis Infection by Mycobacterium tuberculosis.

tuberculous Connected with tuberculosis.

tuberosity Bony eminence.

tuberous sclerosis *See* EPILOIA.

tubo-ovarian Connected with both the fallopian tube and the ovary (*e.g.* abscess, cyst).

tubular necrosis Acute renal failure with reduced renal flow.

tubule Small tube.

tularaemia Deer fly fever caused by pasteurella tularensis.

tumefaction Becoming swollen.

tumour A lump. Frequently used synonymously with neoplasm.

tunica A term applied to several membranes, *e.g. T. vaginalis*: the serous coat of the testicle.

turbinate bones Three thin convoluted bones situated on the lateral wall of the nasal fossa.

turbinectomy Operation of excise a turbinate bone.

turgid Swollen, distended.

Turner's syndrome Gonadal dysgenesis is caused by an abnormality of the sex chromosomes (XO). There are multiple abnormalities comprising the syndrome, webbing of the neck, cubitus valgus, failure of gonad development and often coarction of the aorta.

tussis A cough.

twins Two children from a single pregnancy. *Identical t.*: twins developing from the same egg.

tylosis Thickening of the skin of the soles and palms.

tympanic membrane The membrane separating the middle from the external ear, commonly called the eardrum.

tympanites A distended state of the abdomen caused by gas in the intestines.

tympanitis Otitis media.

tympanoplasty Operation to reconstruct sound-conducting mechanism in middle ear.

tympanum Also called tympanic cavity. A part of the middle ear, and comprises a cavity in the temporal bone deep to the tympanic membrane.

typhoid fever An acute infectious disease which flourishes where the standard of hygiene is poor. Caused by ingestion of Salmonella typhi from contaminated food or water supplies. The germs reach the intestines and through the lymph channels produce a bacteraemia. After the first week the germs settle in the spleen. liver and intestines, especially the ileum. Here the lymph follicles known as Peyer's patches are attacked. They become inflamed, raised, and eventually the tissue of the follicle sloughs off. It is at this stage that intestinal haemorrhage or perforation may occur. Incubation period for the disease is 12–14 days and the patient remains infectious until bacteriological tests are negative. The onset is gradual. For 4 or 5 days the temperature is of the stepladder type. If untreated the patient becomes very ill during the second week with high temperature and slow pulse and the stools are often pea soup in character. Rose-coloured spots,in crops, appear on the abdomen, chest and between the shoulder blades. By the third week, if untreated, the patient is delirious. Treatment is with co-trimoxazole, chloramphenicol, usually with dramatic improvement. *See also* ENTERIC FEVER.

typhus fever A highly infectious fever characterized by a petechial rash, high temperature and great prostration. It is caused by Rickettsia bodies from infected lice or rat fleas.

tyrosine An essential amino acid.

U

ulcer Region in which there is a breach in the continuity of an epithelium.

ulcerative Pertaining to ulceration. *U. colitis*: a disease with inflammation and ulceration of the colon. There is diarrhoea, and mucus and blood are passed in the stools. The patient is anaemic. The disease may be mild or severe and pathogenic organisms appear not to cause it, though emotional stress seems to precipitate it.

ulna The inner bone of the forearm.

ulnar artery With ulnar vein and ulnar nerve, runs beside the ulna.

ultrasound Sound of wavelength too high for human hearing (30000 Hz). Used diagnostically and therapeutically. *See* DOPPLER.

ultrasonography Diagnostic imaging from ultrasound reflected from body surfaces between substances of differing acoustic density. Images may be present in different forms in either a static or moving picture.

ultraviolet rays Photons with

higher frequency distribution than the violet end of the visible spectrum. *See* RADIATION.

umbilical cord The funis; the cord connecting the fetus with the placenta.

umbilicated With an appearance like the umbilicus.

umbilicus Region of attachment of the umbilical cord. A small depressed scar on the anterior abdominal wall.

unciform The hook-shaped bone of the wrist.

uncinariasis Infection with hookworm.

unconsciousness A state of being insensible as when anaesthetized.

undulant Wavelike. *U. fever*: *see* BRUCELLOSIS.

unguentum An ointment; abbreviation, *ung*.

unguis A fingernail.

unicellular Composed of one cell.

unilateral Found only on one side.

uniocular Relating to one eye.

union Joining together to form one, especially *u. of fracture*.

uniovular With one ovum. Identical twins come from the same ovum.

uniparous Having borne only one child.

unit An individual thing or group forming a complete whole. A standard of measurement.

upper respiratory tract infection (URTI) The infections include rhinitis, tonsillitis, pharyngitis, laryngitis, otitis media, and are usually of viral origin.

urachus A fibrous cord in the fetus from the bladder to the umbilicus. It becomes the median umbilical ligament.

uraemia Strictly this means an elevation of the urea concentration in the blood above its normal value of about 5 mmol/litre. Generally, however, it is used to describe a syndrome resulting from impaired renal function which may be due to renal or extrarenal causes, *e.g.* dehydration. There are disturbances of salt and water balance and acid–base equilibrium in addition to the elevation of the blood urea.

urate Salt of uric acid.

urea Principal excretory product of protein catabolism. It is water soluble. *U. concentration test*: the normal amount of urea in urine is 2 per cent. If a definite quantity of urea, 15 g in 100 ml water, is given to a fasting subject, the amount of urea eliminated by the kidneys can be estimated by specimens taken one, two and three hours after. The proper excretion of urea shows an adequately functioning kidney. The percentage should rise to 3 or 4. This test is used to estimate renal efficiency.

ureter The canal between the kidney and the bladder, down which the urine passes.

ureteral Pertaining to the ureter.

ureterectomy Excision of a ureter.

ureteric Pertaining to a ureter. *U. reflux*: the flow of urine up the ureters at the same time as voiding to the exterior; can be a contributory cause to recurrent urinary infection in childhood.

ureteritis Inflammation of a ureter.

ureterocele The result of congenital atresia of a ureteric orifice which causes a cystic enlargement of the portion of the ureter situated in the bladder wall.

ureterolith Stone in the ureter.

ureterolithotomy Operation for the removal of a stone impacted in the ureter.

ureterosigmoidostomy Implantation of a ureter into the sigmoid colon.

ureterovaginal Pertaining to a ureter into the vagina.

ureterovesical Pertaining to a ureter and the bladder.

urethra The canal between the bladder and the exterior through which the urine is discharged.

urethral Pertaining to the urethra.

urethritis Inflammation of the urethra.

urethrocele Urethral diverticulum. A small pouch in the wall of the urethra more common in women than in men. The origin is probably the result of a developmental defect.

urethrography X-ray examination of the urethra by means of retrograde injection of a radio-opaque dye.

urethroplasty Plastic repair to the urethra.

urethroscope An instrument for viewing the interior of the urethra.

urethrotomy Incision of the urethra to remedy stricture; the instrument used being a urethrotome.

uric acid Complex nitrogen-containing organic compound only slightly water-soluble. Formed in the breakdown of nucleic acids. It is excreted by primates and Dalmatian dogs but not by other mammals. Patients with gout accumulate uric acid salts in the blood and tissues.

urinalysis Analysis of urine.

urinary Pertaining to the urine. *U. organs*: these include the kidneys, ureters, bladder and urethra.

urination Micturition. The act of dischaging urine.

urine Excretory product of the kidneys.

uriniferous tubules *See* NEPHRON.

urinometer A small glass instrument with a graduated stem, used for measuring the specific gravity of urine.

urobilin Pigmented derivative of urobilinogen.

urobilinogen Derivative of bilirubin which is made in the intestine by the gut bacteria. Some of it is absorbed and there is impaired liver function, may be excreted in the urine.

urochrome Pigment colouring urine.

urogenital sinus Part of the developing genitalia which forms the bladder and urethra. It develops as a ventral diverticulum from the hindgut.

urography X-ray examination of the urinary tract.

urolith A stone found in the urine.

urologist A specialist in urology.

urology The study of diseases of the urinary tract.

uroscopy Examination of the urine.

URTI *Abbr.* upper respiratory tract infection.

urticaria Nettle rash. Allergic reaction affecting the permeability of small blood vessels. Characterized clinically by erythema and the formation of wheals.

uterine Relating to the uterus.

uterovesical Relating to the uterus and the bladder.

uterus Womb. Muscular hollow pelvic organ. In the resting state it measures about 7.50×5.0 cm and is triangular in shape with a cervix about 2.5 cm which projects into the vagina. It is connected bilaterally to the oviducts (fallopian tubes). The uterus has a glandular epithelium lining it and the whole structure is under the control of sex hormones, in particular oestrogens and progesterone. *See* MENSTRUATION. The uterus is the normal site of implantation of the trophoblast. During pregnancy the uterus grows out of the pelvis to occupy much of the abdominal cavity. After delivery, when contraction of the smooth muscle in the wall expels the fetus and placenta, the uterus diminishes in size, returning to its resting state. *See* INVOLUTION.

UTI *Abbr.* urinary tract infection.

utricle (1) The larger sac of membrane in the vestibule of the internal ear. (2) The prostatic vesicle.

uvea, uveal tract The middle coat of the eyeball. The choroid, ciliary body and iris as a whole.

uveitis Inflammation of the uvea.

uvula A small fleshy body hanging down at the back of

the soft palate.

uvulectomy Excision of uvula.

uvulitis Inflammation of the uvula.

V

vaccination (1) Inoculation of cowpox lymph into the arm as a protection from smallpox. No longer done routinely on babies. (2) Protective inoculation with any vaccine.

vaccine An extract or suspension of attenuated or killed organisms. The antigenic properties of the organism are retained and the vaccine is used to immunize the recipient.

vaccinia Cowpox. In man, it gives immunity to smallpox and is therefore used in vaccination against that disease.

vacuole Specialized region within a cell surrounded by plasma membrane. *See also* PHAGOCYTOSIS.

vagal Pertaining to the vagus nerve.

vagina The passage leading from the cervix uteri to the vulva. The lower limit of this canal is formed by the hymen.

vaginal Pertaining to the vagina.

vaginismus Spasmodic contraction of the vagina whenever the vulva or vagina is touched. May be a cause of painful sexual intercourse.

vaginitis Inflammation of the vagina.

vagotomy Surgical division of the vagus nerve sometimes performed on patients with peptic or duodenual ulcers.

vagus *See* CRANIAL NERVES (10).

valgus *See* TALIPES.

valine One of the essential aminoacids.

valsalva manoeuvre Raising the intrathoracic pressure by attempting expiration against the closed glottis. Occurs with lifting and straining at stool.

valve A fold across a channel allowing flow in one direction only.

valvotomy Incision into a valve, especially heart valve. The purpose of the operation is to widen the orifice of a stenosed valve.

valvulitis Inflammation of a valve.

valvulotomy *See* VALVOTOMY.

van den Bergh's test Method by which the amounts of conjugated and unconjugated bilirubin are estimated in the serum. This is sometimes helpful in the differential diagnosis of jaundice.

varicella Chickenpox.

varices (sing. **varix**) Dilated, twisted veins.

varicocele A varicose condition of the veins of the spermatic cord.

varicose ulcer Ulceration of the lower legs due to reduction in the blood supply resulting from the increased venous pressure.

varicose veins Dilated veins in which the valves have become incompetent. As a result the blood flow may become reversed or static. Most common in the legs where the blood pools by gravitation. Other examples are piles and oesophageal varices.

varicotomy Excision of varicose vein.

variola *See* SMALLPOX.

varioloid A mild form of smallpox, sometimes seen in persons who have been previously vaccinated.

varix An enlarged and tortuous vein.

varus *See* TALIPES.

vas A vessels, or duct of the body; as *v. deferens*, the duct of the testis.

vascular (1) Possessing a blood supply. (2) Concerning the blood vessels and the supply of blood. *V. system*: system of the blood vessels.

vasectomy Removal of a part of the vas deferens. Used as a method of male sterilization.

vasoconstriction Contraction of blood vessels.

vasodilatation Dilatation of blood vessels.

vasomotor Concerned with constriction of blood vessels. *V. nerves*: sympathetic nerves

which control the tone of the smooth muscle in the walls of blood vessels.

vasopressin Posterior pituitary extract. *See* PITUITARY GLAND.

vasospasm Spasm of the blood vessels.

vasovagal attack Slowing of the heart rate with a feeling of nausea and grave distress. The attack may last a few minutes or an hour. The cause is unknown.

Vater's ampulla Small dilatation in the terminal portion of the common bile duct where it empties into the duodenum.

VDRL *Abbr.* Venereal Disease Reference Laboratory. *VDRL test*: antigen–antibody test for syphilis. Antibody to syphilis in serum under test is revealed by flocculation of antigen.

vector A carrier. One who conveys the infection to another person.

vegetations Concretion of small clots on the diseased valves of the heart which occur in endocarditis.

vegetative Having the power of growth.

vein A vessel carrying the blood to the heart.

vena cava The superior vena cava and the inferior vena cava are two large veins which return blood from the head and body and empty it into the right atrium of the heart.

venepuncture Inserting a needle into a vein.

venereal Relating to sexual intercourse. *V. diseases*: *see* SEXUALLY TRANSMITTED DISEASES.

venereology The study of venereal disease.

venesection Bloodletting. A vein is opened and blood drained off from it. Frequently performed in the past for almost any ailment. There are very few present-day indications for venesection.

venography X-ray examination of veins following injection of contrast medium opaque to x-rays.

venous Relating to the veins.

ventilation (1) The supply of fresh air. (2) The process of breathing.

ventral Relating to the belly. *V. root*: anterior root, motor root. The nerve root containing the motor fibres.

ventricles The two lower chambers of the heart are known as the right and left ventricles. The cavities in the brain also are known as ventricles.

ventricular septal defect Defect of development in which a passage remains patent between the two ventricles. Usually causes no disability and may close spontaneously during the early years of life. *See also* FALLOT'S TETRALOGY.

ventriculography X-ray examination of the ventricles of the brain. Air or a radio-opaque dye is introduced into the ventricles enabling their size and position to be observed.

ventriculostomy Operation to open a ventricle of the brain usually in order to construct a bypass when the flow of cerebrospinal fluid is obstructed.

ventrosuspension Operation to place a retroverted uterus in anteversion.

venule Small vein.

vermicide Substance able to kill worms in the intestine.

vermiform appendix *See* APPENDIX VERMIFORMIS.

vermifuge Substance used to dispel worms.

verminous Infested with parasites, *e.g.* fleas, lice.

vernix caseosa The sebaceous material which covers the skin of the fetus.

verruca A wart.

version The manoeuvre of altering the presentation of the fetus in the uterus so as to facilitate its delivery. It may be done with or without an anaesthetic or sedative. *Cephalic v.*: turning the fetus, so that the head presents; *podalic v.*: brings about a breech presentation; *bipolar v.*: acting upon both poles of the fetus.

vertebrae The 33 small bones which form the backbone, or spinal column. *See* SKELETON.

vertebrobasilar insufficiency (VBI) Occlusive disease affecting the vertebral and basilar arteries which results in a syndrome characterized by recurrent attacks of blindness, diplopia, vertigo, dysarthria, ataxia, and hemiparesis due to transient cerebral ischaemia.

vertex The crown of the head.

vertigo Giddiness.

vesica The bladder.

vesical Relating to the bladder.

vesicant A blistering agent.

vesicle A small blister. Blisters of greater diameter than 5 mm are termed bullae.

vesicovaginal Relating to the bladder and the vagina.

vesicular breathing The normal sound of inspiration heard on auscultation.

vesiculitis Inflammation of seminal vesicles.

vestibular neuronitis Disorder affecting the vestibular nerve which is characterized by extreme vertigo while the hearing is unaffected. May result from streptomycin toxicity.

vestibule (1) A small cavity of the ear into which the cochlea opens. (2) The space between the labia minora.

vestigial Rudimentary. Bearing a trace of something now vanished or degenerate.

viable Able to live.

vibration syndrome Raynaud's phenomenon and impotence occurring in those working with vibrating machinery.

Vibrio Genus of bacteria with a characteristic curved shape resembling a comma. *V. cholerae* causes cholera.

vicarious Substituted.

villi (sing. **villus**) Fine soft processes of living cells. *Intestinal v.*: in the small intestine, each contains a central vessel or lacteal, surrounded by a plexus of capillaries. *Chorionic v.*: processes arising from the chorion, the outer membrane of the developing ovum. Specialization of a mass of villi ultimately forms the placenta.

villous Resembling villi.

Vincent's angina Infection of the oral mucous epithelium by a symbiotic association of a spirochaete (Borrelia vincenti) and a fusiform Gram-negative bacterium (Fusobacterium planti-vincenti). Many consider these to be a secondary infection following an unrecognized primary lesion of the mucosa, *e.g.* virus infection, vitamin deficiency, etc.

viraemia Presence of viruses in the blood.

virilism The appearance of masculine characteristics in the female.

virology The study of viruses.

virulence Ability of an organism to overcome the resistance of the host.

virus One of a group of disease-produced parasites which require to be inside the host cell in order to replicate. Some of the larger viruses, *e.g.* vaccinia (about 0.2 μm in diameter), have a complex structure. Consists largely of nucleic acid molecules, although divided into *DNA* and *RNA v.* according to nucleic acid contained. *DNA v.* include *pox*, *herpes*, *adeno*, and *papova*. *RNA v.* include *reo*, *toga*, *picorna*, *myxo*, *rhabdo*, *corona* and *arena*.

viscera Plural of viscus.

visceroptosis Prolapse of the abdominal viscera.

viscid, viscous Sticky, thick, adhesive.

viscus An internal organ, *e.g.* the heart, lung, or stomach, etc.

vision The act or faculty of seeing. *Binocular v.*: use of both eyes without seeing double. *Central v.*, *direct v.*: that performed through the centre of the retina. *Double v.*: diplopia, a failure to fuse the images thrown upon the two retinae at the same time: two images are therefore seen and objects appear double. May be due to defect in muscles of the eye or an error of refraction. It is also a symptom of some nervous diseases, *e.g.* encephalitis lethargica. *Peripheral v.*, *indirect v.*: that performed by the peripheral or circumferential portion of the retina. *Stereoscopic v.*: gives perception of distance and solidity.

visual Pertaining to vision. *V. field*: the total area which can be seen at the same time without turning the head.

vital Pertaining to life. *V. capacity*: the amount of air that can be breathed out after a complete inspiration. *V. statistics*: statistics of birth, marriages, deaths and diseases in a population.

vitallium An alloy used in bone surgery for nails, screws, plates, etc.

vitalograph Device for measuring the vital capacity of the lungs.

vitamins Organic substances which an organism requires to ingest from its environment. The reason that vitamins are essential is because the body cannot synthesize these metabolic requirements. At the present time most of the metabolic processes affected by vitamin molecules are unknown. Vitamin deficiencies are recognized by clinical syndromes such as scurvy (vitamin C deficiency). The vitamins presently recognized are as follows:

Fat-soluble vitamins

Vitamin A A carotene derivative. Plays an important role in the regeneration of visual purple in the retina. Effect on cell metabolism unknown. *Deficiency*: xerophthalmia, follicular hyperkeratosis, night blindness.

Vitamin D Group of sterols. Increase absorption of calcium from the gut. Mode of action not known. *Deficiency*: rickets, tetany.

Vitamin E Group of tocopherols. Probably important in metabolism as it is found ubiquitously in the body. Function unknown.

Vitamin K Group of substituted naphthaquinones. Plays an important part in the synthesis of prothrombin by the liver. Mode of action unknown. *Deficiency*: hypoprothrombinaemia, haemorrhage.

Water-soluble vitamins

Vitamin C: ascorbic acid Important factor in production of mucopolysaccharides. Mode of action unknown. *Deficiency*: scurvy.

Vitamin B_1: thiamine Thiamine diphosphate is an important coenzyme in carbohydrate metabolism. *Deficiency*: polyneuritis, beriberi.

Vitamin B_2: riboflavin Essential part of an important respiratory coenzyme. *Deficiency*: non-specific malaise, cerebellar syndromes, glossitis, etc.

Vitamin B_6 Pyridoxine derivative. *Deficiency*: implicated in PMS.

Nicotinic acid Constituent of coenzymes which act as electron transport substances in conjunction with dehydrogenase enzymes. *Deficiency*: pellagra (in association with other deficiencies).

Folic acid group Pteroylglutamic acid and derivatives. Important cofactor in transmethylation. *Deficiency*: megaloblastic anaemia.

Vitamin B_{12}: cyanocobalamin Function unknown. *Deficiency*: megaloblastic anaemia, degeneration of the spinal cord.

The vitamins mentioned are present in adequate quantities in the articles of food in a normal omnivorous diet. Dietary restriction, unless the diet is 'balanced', may lead to vitamin deficiency.

vitelline Pertaining to the vitellus, or yolk.

vitellointestinal duct Embryonic duct between the yolk-sac and the developing gut.

vitiate To corrupt, contaminate.

vitiligo   Disorder of pigment cells in which patches of depigmented skin arise, often in a symmetrical distribution.

vitreous chamber of the eye The region of the eye containing the vitreous humour. *See* EYE.

vivisection   Scientific examination of a living animal.

vocal cords   Two folds of mucous membrane in the larynx attached behind to the arytenoid cartilages, and in front to the back of the thyroid cartilage. Voice is produced by variation in position of these cords when acted on by small muscles of the larynx, and at the same time forcing through them an expiratory blast of air.

volatile   That which evaporates quickly.

volition   The act or power of willing.

Volkmann's ischaemic contracture   Fibrosis in a muscle due to prolonged ischaemia. Most often associated with spasm of the brachial artery following fracture of the humerus which leads to contracture of the forearm flexor muscles.

volt   Unit of electrical potential.

voluntary   Free. Regulated by choice and desire.

volvulus   Twisting of gut about its mesenteric attachment.

vomer   A bone of the septum of the nose.

vomit   To eject the contents of the stomach through the mouth.

vomiting of pregnancy   Early morning vomiting occurring in early pregnancy. Sometimes severe (hyperemesis gravidarum). Probably of hormonal origin.

von Gierke's disease   Glycogen storage disease. Recessively inherited defect in the metabolism of glycogen which prevents utilization of glycogen. As a result the tissues become stuffed with glycogen while hyperglycaemia occurs.

von Recklinghausen's disease *See* NEUROFIBROMATOSIS.

von Willebrand's disease   Autosomal dominant inherited bleeding disorder. Abnormal platelet and endothelium interaction and factor VIII deficiency.

Voss operation   Operation for hip pain due to articular surface damage.

vulvectomy   Excision of the vulva.

vulvitis   Inflammation of the vulva.

vulvovaginal   Pertaining to the vulva and the vagina.

vulvovaginitis   Inflammation of both the vulva and the vagina.

W

Waldeyer's ring Circle of lymphoid tissue in the pharynx formed by the faucial, lingual and pharyngeal tonsils.

Wallerian degeneration Degeneration of a nerve after it has been cut or severed.

wart Hyperplasia of epidermal cells due to a virus infection.

water-borne Spread by water, such as certain diseases, *e.g.* typhoid fever.

water-brash Regurgitation of stomach acid into the oesophagus.

water-hammer pulse Occurs in aortic regurgitation.

Waterhouse–Friderichsen syndrome Syndrome resulting from bilateral adrenal haemorrhage accompanying the purpura of acute septicaemia, usually meningococcal.

weal Raised patch on skin due to intradermal effusion. Sometimes spelt wheal.

wean To cease feeding a baby at the breast.

Weber syndrome Hemianopia caused by posterior cerebral aneurysm.

Weber test Use of a tuning fork placed in mid-forehead to identify deafer ear.

Weil's disease Epidemic spirochaetal jaundice. Disease caused by a *Leptospira* characterized by fever, headache and pains in the limbs. Many patients develop jaundice and purpuric rash.

Weil–Felix reaction An agglutination reaction for typhus.

wen *See* SEBACEOUS CYST.

Werner's syndrome Hereditary syndrome comprising cataract, osteoporosis, subnormal growth and sexual development, early onset of arteriosclerosis and premature greying of hair.

Wernicke's encephalopathy Syndrome occurring in association with alcoholic polyneuritis characterized by vertigo, nystagmus, ataxia and stupor. It is considered to be due to thiamine deficiency.

Wertheim's hysterectomy A radical operation for uterine cancer, whereby the uterus, tubes, ovaries, broad ligaments, pelvic lymph glands and cellular tissue around ureters are removed en masse.

Wharton's duct The duct of the submaxillary gland.

wheal Acute local oedema, *e.g.* as occurs in urticaria. *See* WEAL.

Wheelhouse's operation External (perineal) urethrotomy for stricture of the urethra.

Whipple's disease Intestinal lipodystrophy. Disease of unknown cause in which there is progressive deposition of mucoprotein in the wall of the small intestine.

whipworm *See* TRICHO-CEPHALUS.

white cell   *See* BLOOD CELLS.
white leg   Thrombosis of deep leg veins.
whitlow   *See* PARONYCHIA.
whooping cough   Pertussis.
Widal reaction   Test to identify by an agglutination reaction either typhoid organisms (if serum is known) or typhoid antibodies (in test serum).
Willebrand's disease   *See* VON WILLEBRAND'S DISEASE.
willpower   A voluntary effort which directs our actions and can overcome some primary impulse such as fear.
Wilm tumour   *See* NEPHROBLASTOMA.
Wilson's disease   A rare metabolic disorder, hepatoenticular degeneration, in which copper accumulates in the liver and certain nuclei of the brain.
windpipe   Trachea.
Winslow's foramen   An aperture between the stomach and liver formed by folds of peritoneum. It forms a communication between the greater and lesser peritoneal cavities.
wisdom teeth   The posterior molars. They erupt at about 21 years of age.
withdrawal   In psychology meaning to 'shrink into oneself'. A normal method of adjustment in a frightening situation. *W. symptoms*: symptoms which appear when a drug, to which a person has become addicted, is withheld from him. *W. method*: *see* COITUS INTERRUPTUS.
Wolffian duct   Embryological kidney duct which becomes the epididymis and vas deferens.
womb   The uterus.
Wood's light   Ultraviolet light used to detect fluorescence of ringworm fungus.
woolsorters' disease   *See* ANTHRAX.
word salad   Jumble of incomprehensible phrases. A speech defect occurring in some forms of schizophrenia.
wound   Injury particularly to skin. Usually due to trauma or perforating injury. Maybe iatrogenic as in *surgical w.*
wrist   The joint between the hand and the forearm.
writer's cramp   Spasm of the hand and forearm brought on by efforts to write. Largely due to defective posture when writing.
wryneck   *See* TORTICOLLIS.

X

xanthelasma   Small yellowish nodules located on and near the eyelids.
xanthine   A purine base.
xanthochromia   Term applied to the distinctive yellow colour of cerebrospinal fluid following a subarachnoid haemorrhage. It is due to

haemolysis of the blood in the subarachnoid space.

xanthoderma Yellowness of the skin.

xanthoma A cholesterol-containing tumour.

X chromosome The sex chromosome which is paired in the homogametic sex. Unlike the Y chromosome it carries many major genes.

xenopsylla cheopis A rat flea which can transmit plague and typhus.

xeroderma Excesive dryness of the skin.

xerophthalmia Ulceration of the cornea occurring in vitamin A deficiency.

xeroradiography Technique for soft tissue radiography using special equipment giving a positive print.

xerosis Abnormal dryness, *e.g.* of the conjunctiva or the skin.

xerostomia Dryness of the mouth.

xiphoid process Small cartilage at the lower end of the sternum.

x-rays Photons with a frequency distribution higher than the ultraviolet range of the electromagnetic spectrum. *See* RADIATION.

Y

yaws Framboesia. Tropical disease which resembles syphilis, caused by Treponema pertenue.

Y chromosome Sex chromosome found only in the heterogametic sex (male). It is shorter than the X chromosome and usually carries few major genes.

yeast Unicellular fungi (Ascomycetes) which possess enzymes capable of converting sugars into ethanol with the release of carbon dioxide. Yeasts are also used as sources of protein and vitamins.

yellow fever Virus-mediated disease, transmitted by mosquitoes, characterized by fever, prostration, jaundice and gastrointestinal haemorrhage.

Z

zero Nought, nothing.

Ziehl–Neelsen's stain Staining technique used to identify tubercle bacilli by their ability to retain the stain when treated with acid; hence acid-fast bacilli.

zinc Important dietary trace element. Deficiency in pregnancy is associated with fetal malformation and possibly growth retardation. In adults it is associated with poor wound healing. Zinc compounds have many therapeutic uses particularly as antiseptics and astringents.

Zollinger–Ellison syndrome
Increased production of acid gastric juice in response to gastrin secreted by pancreatic neoplasm, resulting in peptic ulceration and inactivation of enzymes of the small intestine which operate only in the alkaline range.

zona   Literally a girdle and applied to mean shingles. *See* HERPES. *Z. pellucida*: membrane surrounding the ovum.

zonula ciliaris   Suspensory ligament of lens in the eye.

zoogloea layer   Colonies of bacteria in a jelly-like layer. Found on the top of a sand filter bed. This layer contains algae and protozoa and helps in water purification.

zoology   That part of biology which deals with the study of animal life.

zoonosis   A disease occurring in man and animals and transmissible between them.

zoosperm   Spermatozoa.

zoster   Shingles. *See* HERPES.

zygoma   The cheekbone.

zygote   The cell formed by combination of ovum with spermatozoon.

Appendixes

Appendix 1

BLOOD

The figures given below represent the approximate ranges of normal values for the constituents of the peripheral blood.

Red cells

Haemoglobin	12–18 g/dl
Red cells	3.9–6.5 × 10^{12}/litre
Reticulocytes (newly formed red cells)	less than 1 per cent of total red cells
Mean cell volume (MCV)	75–95 fl
Packed cell volume (PCV or Haematocrit)	0.41
Mean cell haemoglobin content (MCH)	27–32 pg
Mean cell haemoglobin concentration (MCHC)	30–35 g/dl

White cells

Total white cells	4.0–10.0 × 10^9/litre
Neutrophilis	60–70 per cent
Lymphocytes	25–35 per cent
Basophilis	1 per cent
Esosinophils	1–4 per cent
Monocytes	4–8 per cent
Platelets (thrombocytes)	150–400 × 10^9/litre

Blood chemistry

Urea	2.5–6.6 mmol/litre
Uric acid (men)	0.15–0.4 mmol/litre
Uric acid (women)	0.1–0.35 mmol/litre
Cholesterol	3.6–7.8 mmol/litre
Bilirubin	less than 17 μmol/litre
Calcium	2.25–2.6 mmol/litre
Phosphate	0.8–1.45 mmol/litre
Bicarbonate (CO_2)	
adults	23–31 mmol/litre
children	18–23 mmol/litre
Fasting blood sugar (glucose)	
adults	3.6–5.6 mmol/litre (65–100 mg/100 ml)
children	2.2–5.6 mmol/litre (40–100 mg/100 ml)
Potassium	3.5–5.5 mmol/litre
Sodium	133–144 mmol/litre
Chloride	96–106 mmol/litre
Total plasma proteins	62–82 g/litre
albumin	36–52 g/litre
globulin	24–37 g/litre
fibrinogen	1.5–4.0 g/litre

Appendix 2

DESIRABLE WEIGHTS OF ADULTS ACCORDING TO HEIGHT AND FRAME

MEN

cm	height without shoes ft	in	small frame kg	lb
155.0	5	1	50.8–54.4	112–120
157.5	5	2	52.2–55.8	115–123
160.0	5	3	53.5–57.2	118–126
162.5	5	4	54.9–58.5	121–129
165.0	5	5	56.2–60.3	124–133
167.5	5	6	58.1–62.1	128–137
170.0	5	7	59.9–64.0	132–141
172.5	5	8	61.7–65.8	136–145
175.0	5	9	63.5–68.0	140–150
177.5	5	10	65.3–69.9	144–154
180.0	5	11	67.1–71.7	148–158
182.5	6	0	68.9–73.5	152–162
185.0	6	1	70.8–75.7	156–167
187.5	6	2	72.6–77.6	160–171
190.0	6	3	74.4–79.4	164–175

MEN

| medium frame | | large frame | |
kg	lb	kg	lb
53.5–58.5	118–119	57.2–64.0	126–141
54.9–60.3	121–133	58.5–65.3	129–144
56.2–61.7	124–136	59.9–67.1	132–148
57.6–63.0	127–139	61.2–68.9	135–152
59.0–64.9	130–143	62.6–70.8	138–156
60.8–66.7	134–147	64.4–73.0	142–161
62.6–68.9	138–152	66.7–75.3	147–166
64.4–70.8	142–156	68.5–77.1	151–170
66.2–72.6	146–160	70.3–78.9	155–174
68.0–74.8	150–165	72.1–81.2	159–179
69.9–77.1	154–170	74.4–83.5	164–184
71.7–79.4	158–175	76.2–85.7	169–189
73.5–81.6	162–180	78.5–88.0	173–194
75.7–83.9	167–185	80.7–90.3	178–199
78.0–86.2	172–190	82.6–92.5	182–204

Desirable weights of adults according to height and frame

WOMEN

| | height without shoes | | small frame | |
cm	ft	in	kg	lb
142.5	4	8	41.8–44.5	92–98
145.0	4	9	42.7–45.9	94–101
147.5	4	10	43.6–47.2	96–104
150.0	4	11	44.9–48.5	99–107
152.5	5	0	46.3–49.9	102–110
155.0	5	1	47.6–51.3	105–113
157.5	5	2	49.0–52.6	108–116
160.0	5	3	50.3–54.0	111–119
162.5	5	4	51.7–55.8	114–123
165.0	5	5	53.5–57.6	118–127
167.5	5	6	55.3–59.4	122–131
170.0	5	7	57.2–61.2	126–135
172.5	5	8	59.0–63.5	130–140
175.0	5	9	60.8–65.3	134–144
177.5	5	10	62.6–67.1	138–148

WOMEN

| medium frame | | large frame | |
kg	lb	kg	lb
43.5–48.5	96–107	47.2–54.0	104–119
44.5–49.9	98–110	48.1–55.3	106–122
45.8–51.3	101–113	49.4–56.7	109–125
47.2–52.6	104–116	50.8–58.1	112–128
48.5–54.0	107–119	52.2–59.4	115–131
49.9–55.3	110–122	53.5–60.8	118–134
51.3–57.2	113–126	54.9–62.6	121–138
52.6–59.0	116–130	56.7–64.4	125–142
54.4–61.2	120–135	58.5–66.2	129–146
56.2–63.0	124–139	60.3–68.0	133–150
58.1–64.9	128–143	62.1–69.9	137–154
59.9–66.7	132–147	64.0–71.7	141–158
61.6–68.5	136–151	65.8–73.9	145–163
63.5–70.3	140–155	67.6–76.2	149–168
65.3–72.1	144–159	69.4–78.5	153–173

Appendix 3

ABBREVIATIONS

ABPN	Association of British Paediatric Nurses
ADMS	Assistant Director of Medical Services
ADNS	Assistant Director of Nursing Services
ADS	Alzheimer's Disease Society
AEMT	Association of Emergency Medical Technicians
AHA	Area Health Authority
AIDNS	Association of Integrated and Degree Courses in Nursing
AIMS	Association for Improvements in the Maternity Service
AIMSW	Associate of the Institute of Medical Social Workers
AMS	Army Medical Service
ARMS	Action for Research into Multiple Sclerosis
ASNA	Amalgamated School Nurses' Association
ASTMS	Association of Scientific, Technical and Managerial Staffs
BA	Bachelor of Arts
BACUP	British Association of Cancer United Patients and their Families and Friends
BASc	Bachelor of Applied Science
BASE	British Association for Service to the Elderly
BASW	British Association of Social Workers

BCh, BChir	Bachelor of Surgery
BChD	Bachelor of Dental Surgery
BHMA	British Holistic Medical Association
BDA	British Dental Association
BDS	Bachelor of Dental Surgery
BDSc	Bachelor of Dental Science
BHyg	Bachelor of Hygiene
BM	Bachelor of Medicine
BMA	British Medical Association
BMJ	British Medical Journal
BMedSc	Bachelor of Medical Science
BN	Bachelor of Nursing
BNF	British National Formulary
BPharm	Bachelor of Pharmacy
BRCS	British Red Cross Society
BS	Bachelor of Surgery
BSc	Bachelor of Science
BUPA	British United Provident Association
BVMS	Bachelor of Veterinary Medicine and Surgery
CCD	Central Council for the Disabled
CIH	Certificate in Industrial Health
ChB	Bachelor of Surgery
ChM	Master of Surgery
CGC	Committee on Gynaecological Cytology
CHSM	Centre for Health Service Management
CMB	Central Midwives' Board
CNN	Certificated Nursery Nurse
CNO	Chief Nursing Officer
COHSE	Confederation of Health Service Employees
COMA	Committee on Medical Aspects of Food Policy

COTS	Childlessness Overcome Through Surrogacy
CPH	Certificate in Public Health
CSP	Chartered Society of Physiotherapists
CSS	Council for Science and Society
DA	Diploma in Anaesthetics
DBO	Diploma of the British Orthoptic Council
DAP&E	Diploma in Applied Parasitology and Entomology
DAv Med	Diploma in Aviation Medicine
DCh	Doctor of Surgery
DCH	Diploma in Child Health
DChD	Doctor of Dental Surgery
DCM	Diploma in Community Medicine
DCMT	Diploma in Clinical Medicine of the Tropics
DCP	Diploma in Clinical Pathology
DCPath	Diploma of the College of Pathologists
DCR	Diploma of the College of Radiographers
DDM	Diploma in Dermatological Medicine
DDR	Diploma in Diagnostic Radiology
DDS	Doctor of Dental Surgery
DFHom	Diploma of the Faculty of Homoeopathy
DHSS	Department of Health and Social Security
DHyg	Doctor of Hygiene
DIH	Diploma in Industrial Health
DipCD	Diploma in Child Development
DipCOT	Diploma of the College of Occupational Therapists
DipEd	Diploma in Education
DipPharmMed	Diploma in Pharmaceutical Medicine
DipRG	Diploma in Remedial Gymnastics
DipTP	Diploma for Teachers of Physiotherapy
DLO	Diploma in Laryngology and Otology

DM	Doctor of Medicine
DMD	Doctor of Dental Medicine
DMedRehab	Diploma in Medical Rehabilitation
DMJ	Diploma in Medical Jurisprudence
DMR	Diploma in Medical Radiology
DMRD	Diploma in Medical Radiodiagnosis
DMRE	Diploma in Medical Radiology and Electrology
DMRT	Diploma in Medical Radiotherapy
DMSA	Diploma in Medical Services Administration
DMV	Doctor of Veterinary Medicine
DN	Diploma in Nursing
	District Nurse
DNE	Diploma in Nursing Education/ Director of Nurse Education
DNS	Director of Nursing Services
DO	Diploma in Ophthalmology
DObstRCOG	Diploma of the Royal College of Obstetricians and Gynaecologists
DOrth	Diploma in Orthodontics
DOMS	Diploma in Ophthalmic Medicine and Surgery
DPA	Diploma in Public Administration
DPD	Diploma in Public Dentistry
DPH	Diploma in Public Health
DPhil	Doctor of Philosophy
DPM	Diploma in Psychological Medicine
DPhysMed	Diploma in Physical Medicine
DR	Diploma in Radiology
DRO	Disablement Resettlement Officer
DRCOG	Diploma of the Royal College of Obstetricians and Gynaecologists
DRCPath	Diploma of the Royal College of Pathologists

DRM	Diploma in Radiation Medicine
DS	Doctor of Surgery
DSc	Doctor of Science
DSM	Diploma in Social Medicine
DTCH	Diploma in Tropical Child Health
DTH	Diploma in Tropical Hygiene
DTM	Diploma in Tropical Medicine
DTMH	Diploma in Tropical Medicine and Hygiene
DTPH	Diploma in Tropical Public Health
DV&D	Diploma in Venereology and Dermatology
ECFMG	Education Council for Foreign Medical Graduates
EDTNA	European Dialysis and Transplant Nurses' Association
EMAS	Employment Medical Advisory Services
EMS	Emergency Medical Service
EXTEND	Exercise Training for the Elderly and/or Disabled
FACT	Fertility Action Campaign for Treatment
FCOT	Fellow of the College of Occupational Therapists
FCPath	Fellow of the College of Pathologists
FCP	Fellow of the College of Clinical Pharmacology
FCPS	Fellow of the College of Physicians and Surgeons
FCS	Fellow of the Chemical Society
FCSP	Fellow of the Chartered Society of Physiotherapists
FDS	Fellow in Dental Surgery
FFARCS	Fellow of the Faculty of Anaesthetists of the Royal College of Surgeons

FFCM	Fellow of the Faculty of Community Medicine
FFD	Fellow of the Faculty of Dental Surgeons
FFHom	Fellow of the Faculty of Homoeopathy
FFR	Fellow of the Faculty of Radiologists
FHA	Fellow of the Institute of Hospital Administrators
FIBiol	Fellow of the Institute of Biology
FLCO	Fellow of the London College of Osteopathy
FLCOM	Fellow of the London College of Osteopathic Medicine
FPA	Family Planning Association
FPC	Family Practitioner Committee
FPC	Family Planning Clinic
FPS	Fellow of the Pharmaceutical Society
FRCD	Fellow of the Royal College of Dentists
FRCGP	Fellow of the Royal College of General Practitioners
FRCN	Fellow of the Royal College of Nursing
FRCOG	Fellow of the Royal College of Obstetricians and Gynaecologists
FRCP	Fellow of the Royal College of Physicians
FRCPath	Fellow of the Royal College of Pathologists
FRCPE	Fellow of the Royal College of Physicians, Edinburgh
FRCPI	Fellow of the Royal College of Physicians, Ireland
FRCPsych	Fellow of the Royal College of Psychiatrists
FRCR	Fellow of the Royal College of Radiologists
FRCS	Fellow of the Royal College of Surgeons
FRCSE	Fellow of the Royal College of Surgeons, Edinburgh
FRCSI	Fellow of the Royal College of Surgeons, Ireland

FRS	Fellow of the Royal Society
FSR(R)	Fellow of the Society of Radiographers (Radiography)
FSR(T)	Fellow of the Society of Radiographers (Radiotherapy)
FSS	Fellow of the Statistical Society
GMC	General Medical Council
GP	General Practitioner
HDD	Higher Dental Diploma
HVCert	Health Visitor's Certificate
ICN	International Council of Nurses
	Infection Control Nurse
ICNA	Infection Control Nurses' Association
IHF	International Hospitals Federation
IOTT	Institute of Operating Theatre Technicians
IPPF	International Planned Parenthood Federation
IPPNW	International Physicians for the Prevention of Nuclear War
JCC	Joint Committee on Contraception
	Joint Consultative Committee
JNCC	Joint Negotiating and Consultative Committee
LDS	Licentiate in Dental Surgery
LDSc	Licentiate in Dental Science
LEA	Local Education Authority
LLB	Bachelor of Laws
LLCO	Licentiate London College Osteopathy
LMS	Licentiate in Medicine and Surgery

LMSSA	Licentiate in Medicine and Surgery of the Society of Apothecaries, London
LRCP	Licentiate of the Royal College of Physicians
LRCPE	Licentiate of the Royal College of Physicians, Edinburgh
LRCSI	Licentiate of the Royal College of Physicians, Ireland
LRCS	Licentiate of the Royal College of Surgeons
LRCSE	Licentiate of the Royal College of Surgeons, Edinburgh
LRCSI	Licentiate of the Royal College of Surgeons, Ireland
LSA	Licentiate of the Society of Apothecaries, London
LSM	Licentiate of the School of Medicine
MAO	Master of the Art of Obstetrics
MAOT	Member of the Association of Occupational Therapists
MB	Bachelor of Medicine
MBBS	Bachelor of Medicine, Bachelor of Surgery
MBChB	Bachelor of Medicine, Bachelor of Surgery
MC, MCh, MChir	Master of Surgery
MCB	Master of Clinical Biochemistry
MChD	Master of Dental Surgery
MChS	Member of the Society of Chiropidists
MD	Doctor of Medicine
MDD	Doctor of Dental Medicine
MENCAP	Royal Society for Mentally Handicapped Children and Adults
MFCM	Member of the Faculty of Community Medicine

MFHom	Member of the Faculty of Homoeopathy
MHyg	Master of Hygiene
MIH	Master of Industrial Health
MIND	National Association for Mental Health
MLCO	Member of the London College of Osteopathy
MLCOM	Member of the London College of Osteopathic Medicine
MO	Medical Officer
MPS	Member of the Pharmaceutical Society
MRC	Medical Research Council
MRCGP	Member of the Royal College of General Practitioners
MRCOG	Member of the Royal College of Obstetricians and Gynaecologists
MRCP	Member of the Royal College of Physicians
MRCPath	Member of the Royal College of Pathologists
MRCPsych	Member of the Royal College of Psychiatrists
MRCS	Member of the Royal College of Surgeons
MRCVS	Member of the Royal College of Veterinary Surgeons
MRO	Member of the Register of Osteopaths
MS	Master of Surgery
MSA	Member of the Society of Apothecaries
MSc	Master of Science
MSRG	Member of the Society of Remedial Gymnasts
MSR(R)	Member of the Society of Radiographers (Radiography)
MSR(T)	Member of the Society of Radiographers (Radiotherapy)

NAC	National Association for the Childless
NALGO	National Association of Local Government Officers
NDCS	National Deaf Children's Society
NHI	National Health Insurance
NHS	National Health Service
NUPE	National Union of Public Employees
OPCS	Office of Population and Census Surveys
OT	Occupational Therapist
PhD	Doctor of Philosophy
PHLS	Public Health Laboratory Service
PMO	Principal Medical Officer
PNA	Psychiatric Nurses' Association
RADAR	Royal Association for Disability and Rehabilitation
RADC	Royal Army Dental Corps
RAMC	Royal Army Medical Corps
RCM	Royal College of Midwives
RCN	Royal College of Nursing
RGN	Registered General Nurse
RHA	Regional Health Authority
RHV	Registered Health Visitor
RMN	Registered Mental Nurse
SANDS	Stillbirth and Neonatal Death Society
SCM	State Certified Midwife
SEN	State Enrolled Nurse
SHO	Senior House Officer
SMO	Senior Medical Officer
SPOD	Sexual and Personal Relationships of the Disabled